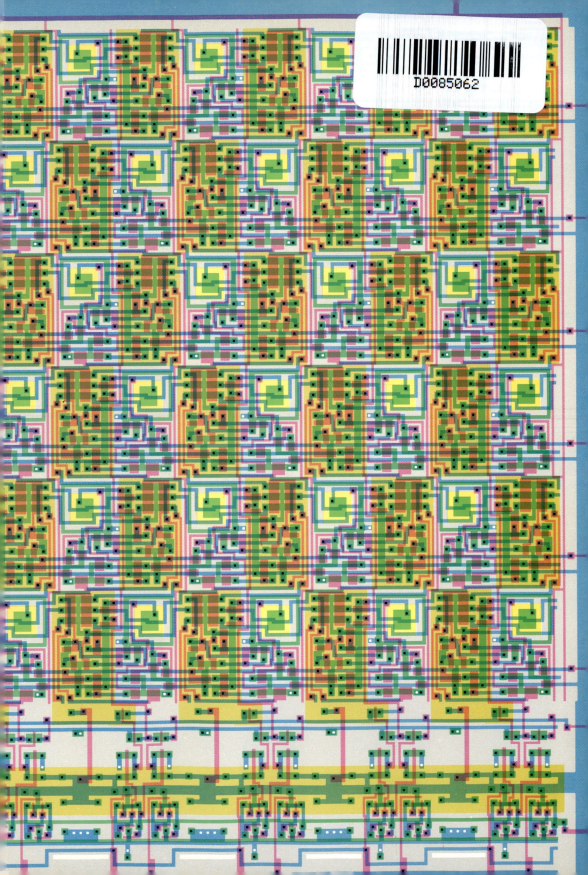

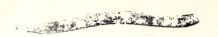

ANALOG VLSI AND
NEURAL SYSTEMS

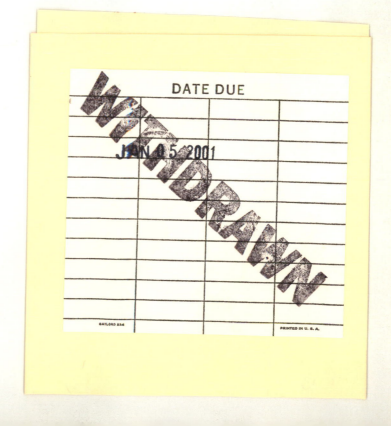

ANALOG VLSI AND NEURAL SYSTEMS

Carver Mead

California Institute of Technology

ADDISON-WESLEY PUBLISHING COMPANY

Reading, Massachusetts • Menlo Park, California • New York
Don Mills, Ontario • Wokingham, England • Amsterdam • Bonn
Sydney • Singapore • Tokyo • Madrid • San Juan

This book is in the **Addison-Wesley VLSI System Series**
Lynn Conway and Charles Seitz, **Consulting Editors**

This book is in the **Addison-Wesley Computation and Neural Systems Series**
Christof Koch, **Consulting Editor**

Peter S. Gordon, **Sponsoring Editor**
Bette J. Aaronson, **Production Supervisor**
Lyn Dupré, **Development Editor and Copy Editor**
Vanessa Piñeiro, **Text Designer**
Alan Anders and Edward K. Shurla, **Illustrators**
Calvin W. Jackson, Jr., **Compositor**
Marshall Henrichs, **Cover Designer**
Hugh Crawford, **Manufacturing Supervisor**

Library of Congress Cataloging-in-Publication Data

Mead, Carver.   Analog VLSI and neural systems / Carver A. Mead.
        p.   cm.
    Bibliography: p.
    Includes index.
    ISBN 0-201-05992-4
    1. Neural computers. 2. Integrated circuits—Very large scale integration. I. Title.
QA76.5.M39 1989
621.395—dc19   88-14635
                                                                    CIP

In memory of my parents

Grace Martha Mead
1908–1978
James Arnold Mead
1904–1980

The VLSI System Series

Lynn Conway and Charles Seitz, *Consulting Editors*

Analog VLSI and Neural Systems	Carver Mead, 1989
Circuits, Interconnections, and Packaging for VLSI	H. Brian Bakoglu, 1989
The CMOS3 Cell Library	Edited by Dennis V. Heinbuch, 1988
Computer Aids for VLSI Design	Steven M. Rubin, 1987
VLSI Signal Processing: A Bit-Serial Approach	Peter Denyer and David Renshaw, 1985
The Design and Analysis of VLSI Circuits	Lance A. Glasser and Daniel W. Dobberpuhl, 1985
Principles of CMOS VLSI Design: A Systems Perspective	Neil Weste and Kamran Eshraghian, 1985
The VLSI Designer's Library	John Newkirk and Robert Mathews, 1983
Introduction to VLSI Systems	Carver Mead and Lynn Conway, 1980

The Computation and Neural System Series

Christof Koch, *Consulting Editor*

Analog VLSI and Neural Systems	Carver Mead, 1989

FOREWORD

Carver Mead's new book, *Analog VLSI and Neural Systems,* not only carries the seeds of still another technical revolution, but also reveals much of the way in which one of our generation's most creative researchers develops, validates, and teaches a revolutionary idea. We are delighted to add this remarkable book to the VLSI Systems Series, and to offer it as the first book in the Computation and Neural Systems Series. The biologically inspired analog VLSI systems that Mead and his students and colleagues have designed and tested over the past several years will be of great interest to the VLSI design and engineering community, as well as to the rapidly growing community of researchers studying neural networks, connectionist models, and the structure and function of the nervous system.

VLSI system ideas are derived from many sources. In the past, they came nearly exclusively from computational functions involving the storage, communication, and processing of digital information. There is nothing in the technology itself, however, that restricts microelectronic devices to digital signals. The development of systems that are inspired by the analog computations performed by living neurons requires different "building-block" circuits and compositional paradigms. The circuits and systems presented in this book are truly ingenious. The subthreshold region of operation of field-effect transistors—unfamiliar territory to most designers of digital VLSI circuits—is used to make elegantly simple analog circuits that operate at extremely low power levels. The strategies for achieving collective behavior, such as the "winner-take-all" network, are quite different from their possible digital counterparts. Nonetheless, the experienced VLSI designer will recognize in the system examples an adherence to structuring by repetition and hierarchy that is characteristic of the Mead–Conway style of digital VLSI designs.

Mead's experiments have a motivation and significance that go beyond VLSI design to the desire to understand neurobiological circuits. Most models and theories concerned with various aspects of neuronal information processing are simulated on serial or parallel digital computers. However, by building working systems such as the "silicon retina," in which the image brightness can vary over five orders of magnitude, the hardware designer must cope with all aspects of noisy, real-life physical environments. Furthermore, the physical restrictions on the density of wires, and the cost of communications imposed by the spatial layout of electronic circuits are related to the constraints under which biological organisms evolved. Thus, the silicon medium provides both the computational neuroscientist and the engineering community with tools to test theories under realistic and real-time conditions. In a nutshell, understanding any system means engineering it. Mead's approach ultimately may lead to a synthetic neurobiology.

In addition to acknowledging the signficance of this book's contents, we admire the way that *Analog VLSI and Neural Systems* teaches its subject; it starts from fundamental principles, and works up to system examples.

The VLSI Systems Series—The subject of VLSI systems spans a broad range of disciplines, including semiconductor devices and processing; integrated electronic circuits; digital logic; design disciplines and tools for creating complex systems; and the architecture, algorithms, and applications of complete VLSI systems. The Addison-Wesley VLSI Systems Series comprises a set of textbooks and research references that present the best current work across this exciting and diverse field, with each book providing a perspective that ties its subject to related disciplines.

The Computation and Neural Systems Series—Over the past 600 million years, biology has solved the problem of processing massive amounts of noisy and highly redundant information in a constantly changing environment by evolving networks of billions of highly interconnected nerve cells. It is the task of scientists—be they mathematicians, physicists, biologists, psychologists, or computer scientists—to understand the principles underlying information processing in these complex structures. At the same time, researchers in machine vision, pattern recognition, speech understanding, robotics, and other areas of artificial intelligence can profit from understanding features of existing nervous systems. Thus, a new field is emerging: the study of how computations can be carried out in extensive networks of heavily interconnected processing elements, whether these networks are carbon- or silicon-based. Addison-Wesley's new Computation and Neural Systems Series will reflect the diversity of this field with textbooks, course materials, and monographs on topics ranging from the biophysical modeling of dendrites and neurons, to computational theories of vision and motor control, to the implementation of neural networks using VLSI or optics technology, to the study of highly parallel computational architectures.

For the VLSI Systems Series: Lynn Conway
                                                                  Ann Arbor, Michigan

                                                                  Charles Seitz
                                                                  Pasadena, California

For the Computation and Neural Systems Series: Christof Koch
                                                                  Pasadena, California

PREFACE

The viewpoint described in this book is the result of my conviction that the nervous system of even a very simple animal contains computing paradigms that are orders of magnitude more effective than are those found in systems made by humans. After many years of study, I have become confident that the powerful organizing principles found in the nervous system can be realized in our most commonly available technology—silicon integrated circuits. Integrated-circuit fabrication has evolved to the point where systems of the scale of small, but identifiable, parts of the nervous system can be emulated on a single piece of silicon. Continuing evolution of the technology should further extend the available complexity level by another two orders of magnitude within the next decade. It is clear to me that we will develop silicon neural systems, and that learning how to design them is one of the great intellectual quests of all time. We are not limited by the constraints inherent in our fabrication technology; we are limited by the paucity of our understanding.

The challenge in understanding these systems arises because they are analog and highly nonlinear, and because they compute functions of many input variables. In addition, the efficient mapping of a system onto its implementation medium—be it neuron or silicon—is the essence of the design problem. Once we are able to design systems of this kind, we will have extended our notion of computation into application areas that are intractable for even the largest digital computers.

In addition, this technology provides an ideal synthetic medium in which neurobiologists can model organizational principles found in various biological systems.

We are witnessing the birth of a new discipline. This book is designed to serve as the text for a course on this topic. It begins by introducing the most elementary concepts, and finishes by describing design examples of considerable complexity. The course should be appropriate for advanced undergraduates and beginning graduate students from several disciplines—biology, physics, electrical engineering, and computer science. Due to that diversity of educational background, the book is self-contained, assuming only a knowledge of mathematics at the level of differential equations, a familiarity with basic physics (including electrical concepts), and a general knowledge of biology. I have taught such a course for four years, using preliminary versions of the material presented in this text. After they had taken that course, students were able to design complete systems of the general scale described in Part IV, and to test those systems successfully in the laboratory.

In Part I, I present background material in basic electronics, transistor physics, and neurobiology, emphasizing the similarity in fundamental principles across these disciplines. Detailed treatments of integrated-circuit fabrication and MOS transistor physics have been included as Appendixes A and B.

In Part II, I discuss computations that are not explicit functions of time, and introduce the use of the two independent electrical variables—voltage and current—to represent different signals at the same point in space. I then apply this important principle to the design of circuits that aggregate many input signals into a single useful computation. Appendixes C and D are extensions of this material.

In Part III, I examine a number of circuits that compute explicit functions of time. First, for students not already familiar with linear system theory, I introduce the complex plane as a representation of the temporal behavior of linear systems. The essential role of nonlinearity in each of the circuit examples is a central theme throughout the book. Nonlinearities have particularly important effects on the time behavior of circuits; these effects are addressed in detail as each circuit is presented.

The four chapters in Part IV describe system-level chips built using the circuits and methodology developed in Parts I, II, and III. The first two examples are presented from an engineering point of view, whereas the last two describe direct attempts to model certain biological structures. From these examples, it is clear that we can now build nontrivial systems that are radically different from those hitherto available. Furthermore, systems of this type scale gracefully to extremely large complexity.

The book is intended primarily as a text for courses in the new discipline, and as a reference for people working in the field. I hope that it will bring to engineers a fresh view of the term *computation*, and will give neurobiologists an effective medium in which to model the objects of their study.

Pasadena, California   Carver Mead

ACKNOWLEDGMENTS

The train of events that led to this book began in 1967, when Max Delbrück introduced me to neurobiology. In 1982, Richard Feynman, John Hopfield, and I jointly taught a course on "The Physics of Computation." As a direct result of that course, I began to see how to undertake the creation of something resembling neural computation in the VLSI medium. That same year, the System Development Foundation initiated a grant that was to be the sole financial support of the work for 5 years. More recently, the Office of Naval Research has provided the principal financial support for the project. Over the entire period, Hewlett-Packard has provided the computing hardware on which all of the work was (and is) done. Every example shown in this book is accompanied by data obtained from a working chip; the fabrication of these circuits (and of countless others that were cast aside as we found better solutions) was accomplished through the MOSIS fabrication service, provided by the good graces of DARPA and NSF.

The first chip-design and data-acquisition tools were pathetic programs that I myself wrote to run on the HP "chipmunk" workstations. Soon after these early forays, software help began to appear. Today, our work is being accomplished within an environment superbly tailored to our needs, made possible by contributions from graduate and undergraduate students associated with the project. VLSI design tools were contributed by David Gillespie, Glenn Gribble, John Lazzaro, Mary Ann

Maher, Martin Sirkin, Massimo Sivilotti, John Tanner, Telle Whitney, and John Wawrzynek. Data are acquired automatically, and are displayed with theoretical curves using programs developed by David Gillespie, Mary Ann Maher, James Campbell, and Jin Luo. We set the type using TEX, and merged with figures using ArborText software, which they kindly made available before the official release. For typesetting of this edition, Blue Sky Research allowed us to use their experimental version of Donald Knuth's Computer Modern fonts rendered by geometric descriptions in the PostScript language. Calvin Jackson and Glenn Gribble developed our document preparation capability to the point where we were able to deliver this entire manuscript to our publisher as a PostScript file.

Data shown in the book were collected by numerous members of the project, foremost among whom is James Campbell, who also contributed in countless other ways. The manuscript has been through numerous iterations; two preliminary versions were used as texts for courses on the subject at California Institute of Technology, Columbia University, Imperial College (London), Lund Technical University (Sweden), Massachusetts Institute of Technology, and the Oregon Graduate Center. The book has benefited immeasurably from careful reviews by John Wyatt, Gordon Shepherd, Eric Vittoz, Michael Godfrey, David Johannsen, Yannis Tsividis, David Feinstein, Mary Ann Maher, Richard Lyon, and Peter Denyer. These individuals have saved future readers many hours of frustration. Lyn Dupré has acted as developmental editor of the material since the earliest version of the manuscript, and has contributed well beyond my most optimistic hopes. Vicki Hester prepared computer-based transcriptions from audio tapes of my first course on this subject. Allison Jackson translated my markings on the final manuscript into text that was used to prepare the index. Angela Blackwell handled all references and permissions. Misha Mahowald provided the quotations for the part openings. Calvin Jackson oversaw the entire development of the book, from original audio recording of class lectures to the final PostScript files: Without his monumental contributions there would be nothing for which to thank anyone else.

This book has been in the making for 3 years. Book writing is known to make an author impatient, moody, and generally unsociable. In trying times, one finds out who one's friends are, and in that regard I have been fortunate indeed. Technical discussions with John Allman, Masakazu Konishi, Paul Müller, Gordon Shepherd, and David Van Essen were of enormous help from the neurobiology side. Yaser Abu-Mostafa, Federico Faggin, John Hopfield, Terrence Sejnowski, and many other friends gave me insights from alternate points of view. These individuals provided encouragement as well as vision. My students have been far more understanding and supportive of their even-more-absent-minded-than-usual professor than I could have hoped for, as has my Person Friday (and Thursday, and Wednesday, and ...), Helen Derevan. Many other friends helped and cared in many ways. I thank all of you.

CONTENTS

P A R T   I   **BASICS**

1

INTRODUCTION   3
A New Approach   7
References   8

2

ECLECTRONICS   11
Electrical Quantities   12
    Energy   13   Fluid Model   14   Capacitance   15   Resistance and
    Conductance   16   Equipotential Regions   17
Schematic Diagrams   17
Linear Superposition   19
Active Devices   19
Thermal Motion   20
    Drift   21   Diffusion   22   Boltzmann Distribution   24

3

TRANSISTOR PHYSICS   27
Boltzian Hydraulics   27
Semiconductors   31
   Atoms and All That   31   Crystals   32   Conduction   32
MOS Transistors   33
Circuit Properties of Transistors   36
Current Mirrors   39
Summary   40
References   41

4

NEURONS   43
Nerve Membrane   45
Electrical Operation   48
   Power Supply   48   Equivalent Circuit   49
The Action Potential   50
   Initiation of the Action Potential   51   Voltage Dependence of the
   Conductances   53
Ionic Channels   54
   Channel Conductance   54   Voltage-Dependent Conductance   57
Computation   58
Synapses   59
References   62

P A R T   II   STATIC FUNCTIONS

5

TRANSCONDUCTANCE AMPLIFIER   67
Differential Pair   67
Simple Transconductance Amplifier   70
Circuit Limitations   71
   Transistor Mismatch   72   Output-Voltage Limitation   72
Voltage Output   75
   Voltage Gain   76
Wide-Range Amplifiers   79
Abstraction   80
Summary   81
References   82

6

ELEMENTARY ARITHMETIC FUNCTIONS   83

Identity Functions   83
    Currents   84   Voltages   84
Addition and Subtraction   85
    Voltages   85   Currents   87
Absolute Value   88
Multiplication   90
    Four-Quadrant Multiplier   90   Limits of Operation   93   Wide-Range
    Multiplier   94
Nonlinear Functions   97
    Exponentials and Logarithms   97   Square Root   98
Summary   99
References   99

7

AGGREGATING SIGNALS   101

Statistical Computation   104
Follower Aggregation   105
    Robustness   106
Resistive Networks   107
    Electrotonic Spread   108   Multiple Inputs   110
Dendritic Trees   111
    Synaptic Inputs   111   Shunting Inhibition   112
Two-Dimensional Networks   112
    Solution for the Hexagonal Network   114   Wiring Complexity   116
The Horizontal Resistor (HRes) Circuit   116
    The Resistive Connection   116   Bias Circuit   118   Networks in
    CMOS   120
Smooth Areas   121
Segmentation   122
Summary   123
References   123

P A R T   III   DYNAMIC FUNCTIONS

8

TIME-VARYING SIGNALS   127

Linear Systems   128

The Resistor–Capacitor (RC) Circuit   129
Higher-Order Equations   130
Complex Numbers   131
    Polar Form   132   Complex Conjugate   133
Complex Exponentials   134
The Heaviside Story   136
Driven Systems   137
Sine-Wave Response   138
    Transfer Function   138   RC-Circuit Example   139
Response to Arbitrary Inputs   140
    Relationship of $H(s)$ to the Impulse Response   144   Impulse
    Response   144
Summary   146
References   146

9

FOLLOWER–INTEGRATOR CIRCUIT   147
Small-Signal Behavior   148
Composition   149
Implementation   151
Delay Lines   152
    Follower–Integrator Delay Line   152   RC Delay Line   155
Large-Signal Behavior   158
    Transient Response   158   Frequency Response   160
Staying Linear   161
Summary   162
References   162

10

DIFFERENTIATORS   163
Differentiation   163
Realizable Differentiator   164
Transient Response   166
Follower-Based Differentiation   167
The Diff1 Circuit   167
    Input Offset   168
The Diff2 Circuit   169
    Effect of Input Offset   169   Transfer Function   170   Frequency
    Response   170   Transient Response   171   Large-Signal
    Response   172

Hysteretic Differentiator   173
   Small-Signal Behavior   174   Large-Signal Behavior   175
   Logarithmic Compression   177   Noise Immunity   177
Summary   178

11

SECOND-ORDER SECTION   179
Small-Signal Analysis   180
   Complex Roots   181   Transient Response   183   Frequency
   Response   184
Large-Signal Behavior   186
   Stability Limit   187   Small-Signal Behavior at Stability Limit   189
   Recovery from Large Transients   190
Summary   191
References   192

12

AXONS   193
The Axon-Hillock Circuit   194
   Capacitive Voltage Divider   196   Feedback Sequence   197
Self-Resetting Neuron   198
   Depolarization   199   Repolarization   200   Saturation   201
Silicon Axon   201
Summary   203

P A R T   I V   SYSTEM EXAMPLES

13

SEEHEAR   207
Biological Basis of the SeeHear System   208
   Biological Visual Systems   209   Auditory Psychophysiology   210
   Main Principles   213
The SeeHear Design   213
   Vision   213   Sound Synthesis   214
The SeeHear Chip   216
   Implementation   218
Performance   221
Summary   226
References   227

14

OPTICAL MOTION SENSOR   229

A Two-Dimensional Analog Motion Detector   230
   Solution of Simultaneous Constraints   233   Constraint-Solving
   Circuits   233
Performance   242
   Characterization of the Motion Output   242   Verification of Constraint-
   Line Behavior   247   Velocity-Space Maps   248
Least-Squares Methods and Gradient-Descent Solutions   251
   Notation   251   The Static Least-Squares Problem   252   The
   Dynamic Least-Squares Problem   253
Summary   254
References   254

15

SILICON RETINA   257

Retinal Structure   258
   Photoreceptor Circuit   260   Horizontal Resistive Layer   261   Triad
   Synapse Computation   262
Implementation   263
Performance   267
   Sensitivity Curves   268   Time Response   269   Edge
   Response   270   Space Constant of the Resistive Network   272
   Mach Bands   275
Summary   276
References   277

16

ELECTRONIC COCHLEA   279

Basic Mechanisms of Hearing   280
   Traveling Waves   281   Sine-Wave Response   282   Neural
   Machinery   282   Outer Hair Cells   283
Wave Propagation   284
   Fluid Mechanics of the Cochlea   285   Scaling   287   Approximate
   Wavenumber Behavior   288
Silicon Cochlea   289
   Basilar-Membrane Delay Line   289   Second-Order Sections in
   Cascade   291   Transistor Parameter Variation   294   Frequency
   Response   295   Transient Response   297

Gain Control 298
Summary 301
References 302

A P P E N D I X E S

CMOS FABRICATION   305

Patterning 306
The Silicon-Gate CMOS Process 308
Yield Statistics 311
Geometric Constraints 312
    Geometric Design Rules 313   Generic Rules 316
References 317

B

FINE POINTS OF TRANSISTOR PHYSICS   319

Subthreshold Operation 320
    Electrostatics 320   Current Flow 322   Drain Conductance 323
Body Effect 325
The General MOS Model 327
    Electrostatics 328   Source Boundary Condition 329   Channel
    Current 330   Long-Channel Limit 332   Short-Channel Transistor
    in Saturation 333   Short-Channel Transistor Below Saturation 334
    Drain Conductance 336
Summary 337
References 337

C

RESISTIVE NETWORKS   339

One-Dimensional Continuous Networks 339
Discrete Networks 340
    Discontinuities in Dendritic Processes 345   Shunting Inhibition 347
    Branches 348
Two-Dimensional Continuous Networks 349
References 351

D

COMPLEXITY IN NEURAL SYSTEMS   353
Analog Factor   354
Entropy Factor   356
References   358

CREDITS   359

INDEX   361

BASICS

The abstract form idea imposed from above, unrelated to the properties of structural elements, has given way to the form-concept in which forms evolve from the roots up, emerging from the properties of the basic units.

—C.F.A. Pantin   *The New Landscape* (1951)

CHAPTER

1

INTRODUCTION

Even the most naive observer can see that the nervous system is vastly different from a computer. Living systems are made from three-dimensional, squishy cells; computers are constructed of rigid inorganic matter in flat, two-dimensional sheets. Living systems are powered by metabolic biochemistry; computers are powered by transformers and rectifiers from the power mains. Living systems have approximately 100-millivolt nerve impulses lasting nearly a millisecond: computers have 5-volt signal levels switching at nanosecond intervals. The destruction of a few percent of the cells in a brain will cause no discernible degradation in performance; the loss of even a single transistor in a computer (save for in its memory) may cause complete loss of functionality. The average nerve cell dissipates power in the 10^{-12}-watt range; the average logic gate in a computer dissipates 10 million times as much.

Nonetheless, a more careful look reveals some underlying similarities between the two kinds of systems. Both process information. Signals are represented as differences in electrical potential, and are conveyed on "wires" formed by surrounding a conducting path with an excellent electrical insulator. Active devices cause electrical current to flow in a second "output" conductor due to the potential in a first "input" conductor. The "output" of an active device has more energy than was present in the "input" to that device; hence, the systems possess "gain"—the essential ingredient for unbounded information processing—

which is accompanied by an unavoidable dissipation of energy. A "power supply" maintains a near-constant average difference in electrochemical potential across the active devices. The active devices are formed of extremely thin *energy barriers* that prevent the flow of current between two electrical nodes. The passage of current is mediated by the potential on a third "control" electrical node. That current varies exponentially with the potential on the control node.

Heartened by these less obvious but deeper similarities between the two systems, we may be tempted to conclude that the brain is, indeed, a digital computer. Its nerve pulses encode information in much the same way as do pulses in a telephone exchange. Neurons perform Boolean AND and OR operations on the way to firing off a nerve pulse to the next stage of computation. Small neural memory elements store information in much the same way as computer memories do. Perhaps we are, after all, on the verge of discerning one of nature's most profound and best-kept secrets: the working of thought itself.

Speculations of this sort were rampant in the late 1940s. A film depicting the operation of the Whirlwind, an early vacuum-tube computer with magnetic-core memory, was called *Faster than Thought* [Bowden, 1953]. The field of artificial intelligence was born. Soon, however, signs of distress could be seen. By 1977, Marvin Minsky, one of the artificial-intelligence pioneers, opened a seminar at Caltech with the following observation:

> *Our first foray into Artificial Intelligence was a program that did a cred-ible job of solving problems in college calculus. Armed with that success, we tackled high school algebra; we found, to our surprise, that it was much harder. Attempts at grade school arithmetic, involving the concept of num-ber, etc., provide problems of current research interest. An exploration of the child's world of blocks proved insurmountable, except under the most rigidly constrained circumstances. It finally dawned on us that the over-whelming majority of what we call intelligence is developed by the end of the first year of life.* [Minsky, 1977]

The visual system of a single human being does more image processing than do the entire world's supply of supercomputers. The digital computer is extremely effective at producing precise answers to well-defined questions. The nervous system accepts fuzzy, poorly conditioned input, performs a computation that is ill-defined, and produces approximate output. The systems are thus different in essential and fundamentally irreconcilable ways. Our struggles with digital computers have taught us much about how neural computation is *not* done; unfortunately, they have taught us relatively little about how it *is* done. Part of the reason for this failure is that a large proportion of neural computation is done in an *analog* rather than in a digital manner.

Perhaps the most rewarding aspect of analog computation is the extent to which elementary computational primitives are a direct consequence of funda-mental laws of physics. In Chapter 3, we will see that a single transistor can take at its gate a voltage-type signal and produces at its drain a current-type signal that is exponential in the input voltage. This exponential function is a direct result of the Boltzmann distribution. We will see that addition and subtraction of currents follows directly from the conservation of charge. In subsequent chapters, we will encounter many examples of computations that follow directly from physical laws.

It is essential to recognize that neural systems evolved without the slightest notion of mathematics or engineering analysis. Nature knew nothing of bits, Boolean algebra, or linear system theory. But evolution had access to a vast array of physical phenomena that implemented important functions. It is evident that the resulting computational metaphor has a range of capabilities that exceeds by many orders of magnitude the capabilities of the most powerful digital computers.

It is the explicit mission of this book to explore the view of computation that emerges when we use this evolutionary approach in developing an integrated semiconductor technology to implement large-scale collective analog computation.

The biological questions asked about neural computation were for many years, and to a large extent still are, basically reductionist. It is tacitly assumed that, if we understand in detail the operation of each molecule in a nerve membrane, we will understand the operation of the brain. It is to this view that our knowledge of computers can bring some insight. A computer is built up of a completely known arrangement of devices; the operation of these devices is understood in minute detail. Yet it is often impossible to derive even a simple proof that a program that we ourselves write will compute the desired result or, for that matter, that the computation will even terminate!

The complexity of a computational system derives not from the complexity of its component parts, but rather from the multitude of ways in which a large collection of these components can interact. Even if we understand in elaborate detail the operation of every nerve channel and every synapse, we will not by so doing have understood the neural computation as a *system*. It is not the neural devices themselves that contain the secret of thought. It is, rather, the organizing principles by which vast numbers of these elementary devices work in concert. Neural computation is an emergent property of the system, which is only vaguely evident in any single component element.

Although study of the elements is an essential step in understanding the system organization, in and of themselves, the elements tell us very little. Furthermore, we have learned enough in recent years concerning the operation of nerves and synapses to know there is no mystery in them. In not a single instance is there a function done by a neural element that cannot, from the point of view of a system designer, be duplicated by electronic devices.

What then is to prevent us from creating a nervous system in silicon? Two barriers have historically blocked the way:

1. Neural systems have far greater connectivity than has been possible in standard computer hardware. Many early attempts to create neural systems failed simply because no workable technology existed for realizing systems of the requisite complexity.

2. Sufficient knowledge of the organizing principles involved in neural systems was not available.

The rapidly developing technology of very large scale integrated (VLSI) circuits has given us a medium in which it is presently possible to fabricate tens of millions of devices (transistors) interconnected on a single silicon wafer. This number will increase by two orders of magnitude before fundamental limitations are encountered [Hoeneisen et al., 1972a]. The densest and most widely available technology uses metal-oxide-silicon (MOS) transistors; it has been primarily conceived as a digital technology, and has been highly evolved for the production of microprocessors, memories, and other digital products. It might therefore be supposed that the most highly evolved fabrication process would not be suitable for the functions required in neural processing. The noise level of a typical device is higher, or the precision with which any two devices can be matched is lower, for example, than are those of technologies historically used for implementing analog functions. We observe, however, that the precision, reliability, and noise properties available in neural wetware fall short of those used in even the most rudimentary electronic systems. This lack of precision and reproducibility at the component level is more than offset by the redundancy introduced at the system level. Whether this property is the primary reason for the large connectivity in neural systems, or whether it is a byproduct of an organizing principle dictated by other system needs, is not a question open to us at the present time. We do know, however, that robustness under failure or imprecision of individual components is one important emergent property of neural systems. If we base our designs on the same organizing principles, we should not be concerned that individual devices will cause system malfunction. To the contrary, we can expect that systems with extraordinary reliability and robustness will result; so much so that useful integration at the scale of a complete wafer is feasible. In the chapters that follow, we will explore many ways in which an ordinary digital technology (complementary MOS, or CMOS) can be used to implement extraordinary systems based on neural paradigms.

In terms of discovering neural organizing principles, we are less well off. Although a great deal of progress has been made in recent years, there is still no global view of the principles and representations on which the nervous system is organized. There has been, however, a striking increase in knowledge of particular systems, due in large part to experimental techniques developed over the past decade. Detailed physiological studies have given us a picture of the mapping from the visual field onto the visual cortex [Schwartz, 1977], and similar information is available for many important auditory areas [Merzenich et al., 1977]. Several authors have put together a more unified view of these findings. Readable accounts of the gross connectivity among major areas of the brain have been given for the visual system [Van Essen, 1984; De Yoe et al., 1988] and the auditory system [Pickles, 1982; Kim, 1984]. A most notable account of the detailed synaptic circuits of each of several areas of the brain is given in *The Synaptic Organization of the Brain* by Gordon Shepherd of Yale University [Shepherd, 1979].

Many people have proposed hypotheses about the way computation is performed in these systems. To date, it has proved difficult if not impossible either to verify or to disprove any given hypothesis concerning the operating principles of even the simplest neural system. Major areas are so richly interconnected, and computation within a given area is so intertwined, that there exists no good way of separating one function from another. Our traditional scientific approach of studying the elements separately in order to understand the whole fails us completely. Simple neural systems based on clear, obvious principles may once have existed, but they are buried by the sands of time. Billions of years of evolution have presented us with highly efficient, highly integrated, and impossibly opaque systems.

A NEW APPROACH

Let us, then, undertake the following program. We have already noted that elementary operations found in the nervous system can be realized in silicon. We also note that many neural areas are thin sheets, and carry two-dimensional representations of their computational space. The retina is the most obvious example of this organization, which also occurs in the visual cortex and in several auditory areas. In both neural and silicon technologies, the active devices (synapses and transistors) occupy no more than 1 or 2 percent of the space—"wire" fills the entire remaining space. We can be confident, therefore, that the limitation of connectivity will force the solution into a very particular form. If the required functions could have been be implemented with less wire, nature would have evolved superior creatures with more computation per unit brain area, and they would have eaten the ones with less well-organized nervous systems.

We will therefore embark on a second evolutionary path—that of a silicon nervous system. As in any evolutionary endeavor, we must start at the beginning. Our first systems will be simple and stupid. But they, no doubt, will be smarter than the first animals were. We are, after all, endowed with the product of a few billion years of evolution with which to study these systems!

The constraints on our analog silicon systems are similar to those on neural systems: wire is limited, power is precious, robustness and reliability are essential. We therefore can expect that the results of our second evolution will bear fruits of biological relevance. The effectiveness of our approach will be in direct proportion to the attention we pay to the guiding biological metaphor. We use the term "metaphor" in a deliberate and well-defined way. We are in no better position to "copy" biological nervous systems than we are to create a flying machine with feathers and flapping wings. But we can use the organizing principles as a basis for our silicon systems in the same way that a glider is an excellent model of a soaring bird.

It is in that spirit, then, that we will proceed. First we will describe the relevant aspects of neural wetware at the level of abstraction where we will be working. We will then develop the operations that are natural to silicon, and examine how they can be used to implement certain known neural functions. Finally, we will show several examples of complete subsystems that have metaphors drawn, in one way or another, from biology.

It is the author's conviction that our ability to realize simple neural functions is strictly limited by our understanding of their organizing principles, and not by difficulties in implementation. If we *really* understand a system, we will be able to build it. Conversely, we can be sure that we do not fully understand a system until we have synthesized and demonstrated a working model.

The silicon medium can thus be seen to serve two complementary but inseparable roles:

1. To give computational neuroscience a synthetic element, allowing hypotheses concerning neural organization to be tested
2. To develop an engineering discipline by which collective systems can be designed for specific computations

The success of this venture will create a bridge between neurobiology and the information sciences, and will bring us a much deeper view of computation as a physical process. It also will bring us an entirely new view of information processing, and of the awesome power of collective systems to solve problems that are totally intractable by traditional computer techniques.

REFERENCES

Bowden, B.V. *Faster than Thought*. London: Sir Isaac Putnam & Sons Ltd., 1953.

De Yoe, E.A. and Van Essen, D.C. Concurrent processing streams in monkey visual cortex. *Trends in NeuroSciences*. 11:219, 1988.

Hoeneisen, B. and Mead, C.A. Fundamental limitations in microelectronics— I. MOS technology. *Solid-State Electronics*, 15:819, 1972a.

Kim, D.O. Functional roles of the inner– and outer–hair-cell subsystems in the cochlea and brainstem. In Berlin, C.I. (ed), *Hearing Science: Recent Advances*. San Diego, CA: College-Hill Press, 1984, p. 241.

Merzenich, M.M., Roth, G.L., Andersen, R.A., Knight, P.L., and Colwell, S.A. Some basic features of organization of the central auditory nervous system. In Evans, E.F. and Wilson, J. (eds), *Psychophysics and Physiology of Hearing*. New York: Academic Press, 1977, p. 485.

Minsky, M. Personal communication.

Pickles, J.O. *An Introduction to the Physiology of Hearing*. Orlando, FL: Academic Press, 1982.

Schwartz, E. Spatial mapping in the primate sensory projection: Analytic structure and relevance to perception. *Biological Cybernetics*, 3:181, 1977.

Shepherd, G.M. *The Synaptic Organization of the Brain*. 2nd ed., New York: Oxford University Press, 1979.

Van Essen, D.C. Functional organization of primate visual cortex. In Peters, A. and Jones, E.G. (eds), *Cerebral Cortex,* vol 3. New York: Plenum Press, 1984, p. 259.

ECLECTRONICS

This chapter introduces a relation between the study of biological neural systems and that of electronic neural systems. The chapter title, **eclectronics**, is derived in the following manner:

ec·lec·tic **1.** selecting what is thought best in various doctrines, methods, or styles. **2.** consisting of components from diverse sources.

e·lec·tron·ic of, based on, or operated by the controlled flow of charge carriers, especially electrons.

e·lec·tron·ics the science and technology of electronic phenomena and devices.

ec·lec·tron·ics the common framework of electrical properties used for information processing in both brain and silicon.

As we have mentioned, both neural and electronic systems represent information as electrical signals. Neurobiologists deal with neural systems, and have evolved a viewpoint, notation, jargon, and set of preconceptions that they use in any discussion of neural networks. Likewise, electrical engineers have developed an elaborate language and symbolism that they use to describe and analyze transistor circuits. In both cases, the language, viewpoint, and cultural bias derive partly from the properties inherent in the technology, and partly from the perspectives and ideas of early influential workers in the field. By now, it is extremely difficult to separate the conceptual framework and vernacular of either field from the properties of the devices and systems being studied.

Because it is the express purpose of this book to explore the area of potential synergy of these two fields, we must develop a common conceptual framework within which both can be discussed. Such an undertaking will, of necessity, require a reevaluation of the underlying assumptions of the existing lore. In particular, it will be possible neither to preserve all the detailed distinctions prevalent in the current literature in either field, nor to pay lip service to the many schools of thought that intersect in a plethora of combinations. Rather, we will present a simple, unifying perspective within which the function of either technology can be visualized, described, and analyzed. Such a viewpoint is possible for two reasons:

1. The operation of elementary devices in both technologies can be described by the aggregate behavior of *electrically charged entities* interacting with *energy barriers*. In both cases, the rate at which dynamic processes take place is determined by the energy due to random thermal motion of the charged entities, which is accurately described by the Boltzmann distribution. The steady-state value of any quantity of interest is, in both cases, the result of equalization of the rate of processes tending to increase, and those tending to decrease, that quantity's value.

2. The properties of devices in both technologies are not well controlled. The operation of any robust system formed from the devices of either technology, therefore, must not be dependent on the detailed characteristics of any particular device. For system purposes, a device can be adequately described by an abstraction that captures its essential behavior and omits the finer detail.

In the process of any simplification, it is, by definition, necessary to omit detail. By "essential behavior," we mean those relationships that are necessary to reason about the correct operation of the system. We will attempt to develop a simplification that does not lose these relationships. In other words, as far as they go, the explanations in this book are intended to provide a conceptually correct foundation in the following sense: Gaining a deeper understanding of any given point should not require unlearning any conceptualization or formulation. History alone will determine the extent to which we approach this ideal.

ELECTRICAL QUANTITIES

WARNING: If you are already familiar with electric circuits, Boltzmann statistics, energy diagrams, and neural and transistor physics, you will be bored to tears with the following material—we urge you to skip the remainder of this chapter. If you have a background in solid-state physics, you should read the introduction to the elements of neuroscience in Chapter 4. If you are an expert in neuroscience, you should read the introduction to transistor operation in Chapter 3. Read the following discussion if you lack a firm preparation in either discipline.

Energy

All electrical mechanisms are concerned with the interaction of electrical **charges**. The concept of an elementary charge is so ingrained in our curricula that we seldom question its origin. The electrical force f_e that attracts two electrical charges q_1 and q_2 of opposite type (one positive and the other negative) is

$$f_e = \frac{1}{4\pi\epsilon} \frac{q_1 q_2}{r^2} \tag{2.1}$$

where ϵ is called the **permittivity** of the medium in which the charges are embedded. When ϵ is given in terms of ϵ_0, the permittivity of free space (vacuum), it is called the **dielectric constant** of the medium. In the units we will use, $\epsilon_0 = 8.85 \times 10^{-12}$ farads per meter.

To aid us in visualizing the interaction of electrical charges, we will first examine the analogous behavior of masses interacting through the force of gravity. The gravitational force f_g between two masses m_1 and m_2 due to their mutual gravitational attraction is

$$f_g = G \frac{m_1 m_2}{r^2} \tag{2.2}$$

where G is the gravitational constant. Note that Equation 2.2 is of exactly the same form as Equation 2.1.

Gravitational force plays a key role in our everyday experience. We could not get up in the morning, throw a baseball, drive a car, or water a lawn without an intuitive understanding of its operation. Yet no one but the astronauts has experienced gravitation in the form shown in Equation 2.2. Being earthbound mortals, we walk on the surface of a planet of mass M and of radius r. We must be content to manipulate a mass m that is infinitesimal compared with M over distances that are much smaller than r. Under those conditions, the gravitational law we encounter in daily life is a simplified form of Equation 2.2, in which M, r, and G can all be lumped into a new constant g, defined by

$$f_g = m \frac{MG}{r^2}$$

$$= mg \tag{2.3}$$

The quantity f_g in Equation 2.3 is called the **weight** of the object. The quantity

$$g = \frac{MG}{r^2}$$

is the force per unit mass, and is called the **gravitational field** due to the mass M.

We also know from common experience that an expenditure of energy is required to raise a mass to a higher elevation; that energy can be recovered by allowing the mass to fall in the gravitational field. The amount of **potential energy** (PE) stored in a mass at height h above the surface of the earth is just

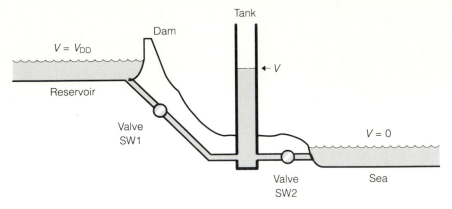

FIGURE 2.1 Hydraulic analogy of electronic or neural circuit. The power supply is a reservoir of water at potential V_{DD}. The reference potential is sea level, corresponding to ground in an electrical circuit. The water level in the tank corresponds to the output voltage. The tank can be filled by opening valve SW1, or emptied by opening valve SW2.

the integral of the force over the distance h. For values of h much smaller than r, the gravitational force is nearly constant and

$$\text{PE} = mgh$$

The quantity gh is called the **gravitational potential**. It is the energy per unit mass of matter at height h above the earth's surface. We will use the symbol V for potential in both gravitational and electrical paradigms, to emphasize the similarity of the underlying physics. In both cases, the field is the gradient of the potential.

Fluid Model

In all system-level abstractions of device behavior, be those devices neural or electronic, electrical charges are present in sufficient number that they cannot be accounted for individually. In both disciplines, they are treated as an *electrical fluid,* the flow of which is called the **electrical current**. We can extend the gravitational-energy concepts of the preceding section to give us an intuitively simple yet conceptually correct picture of the operation of electrical systems. In this analog, shown in Figure 2.1, water represents the electrical fluid. The gravitational potential V, which is directly proportional to the height of the water, represents the **electrical potential**.

The electrical potential V also is called the **voltage;** the two terms are synonymous and are used interchangeably. The quantity of water represents the quantity of electrical charge Q. There is an underlying granularity to these quantities: Water is made up of water molecules; charge in a neuron is made up of ions; charge in a transistor is made up of electrons. In all cases, we can discuss the quantity in terms of either the number of elementary particles or a more convenient macroscopic unit. For water, we use liters; for electrical charge we use **coulombs**. (Throughout this book, we will use the meter-kilogram-second-ampere [MKSA] system of units.) The magnitude q of the charge on an electron or monovalent ion is 1.6×10^{-19} coulombs. Similarly, we can measure the flow—or current—in terms of elementary particles per second or in macroscopic units. For water, we use liters per second; for the electrical current I, we use coulombs per second. Electrical current is such an important and universally used quantity that it has a unit of its own: 1 coulomb per second is called an **ampere**, or **amp.**

In all cases, it requires 1 unit of energy to raise a quantity of 1 unit to a potential of 1 unit. In the MKSA system, the unit of energy is the **joule**. To raise 1 kilogram 1 meter above the surface of the earth requires 1 joule of energy. To raise the potential of 1 coulomb of charge by 1 volt requires 1 joule of energy. It is often convenient to discuss microscopic processes in terms of the *energy per particle*. The energy required to raise the potential of one electronic charge by 1 volt is 1 **electron volt**. An electron volt is, of course, 1.6×10^{-19} joule.

Let us reexamine Figure 2.1. We see a reservoir filled with water, the surface level of which is called V_{DD} (dermis of the dam water). The reservoir is used to fill a tank, under the control of valve SW1. To empty the tank, we can open valve SW2, allowing water to discharge into the sea. Note that, with this system, the height of water in the tank cannot exceed V_{DD}, and cannot be reduced below sea level. We can measure the height of water from any reference point we choose. There is an advantage, however, to one particular choice. If we choose sea level as the **reference potential** $(V = 0)$, the height always will be positive or zero. In an electric circuit, it is useful to have such a reference potential, from which all voltages are measured. The reference corresponding to sea level is called **ground**.

The electrical equivalent of the reservoir in Figure 2.1 is called a **power supply**. The reservoir can be kept full only if the water is replenished after it is depleted. In many cases, a pump is used for this purpose. So we need a mechanism to run the pump when the reservoir level is low, and to shut off the pump when the surface is above the desired level.

In neurons, voltage-sensitive pumps run by metabolic processes in the cell actively pump potassium ions into and sodium ions out of the cell's cytoplasm. Potassium ions exist as a minority ionic species in the extracellular fluid. This ionic gradient acts as the power supply for electrical activity in the neuron.

In an electronic circuit, a reservoir of charge is provided either by an electrochemical process (as in a battery), or by an active circuit that monitors the potential of the reservoir and adds charge as required. Such a circuit is called a **regulated power supply**.

Capacitance

For the moment, we will consider the role of the apparatus of Figure 2.1 to be the manipulation of the water level in the tank to the desired level. By closing valve SW1 and opening SW2, we can reduce the level to zero. The amount of water required to increase the level in the tank by a certain amount—say, 1 meter—is obviously dependent on the cross-sectional area of the tank. That area can be expressed in acres, square feet, or some other arbitrary unit. For consistency, however, it is convenient to express it as the quantity of water required to raise the water level by 1 unit of potential. In an electrical circuit, such a storage tank is called a **capacitor**, and the electrical charge required to raise the potential level by 1 volt is its **capacitance**. The unit of capacitance—coulombs per volt—is called the **farad**. The total charge Q on a capacitor, like the total water in the tank, is related to C, the capacitance, and to V, the voltage, by the expression

$$Q = CV \tag{2.4}$$

Current I is, by definition, the rate at which charge is flowing:

$$I = \frac{dQ}{dt}$$

In the particular case where the capacitance C is constant, independent of the voltage V, the current flowing into the capacitor results in a rate of change of the potential

$$I = C\frac{dV}{dt}$$

In our water analogy, constant capacitance corresponds to a tank with constant cross-sectional area, independent of elevation.

Resistance and Conductance

If both valves in Figure 2.1 are opened, water will flow from the reservoir into the sea at a finite rate, restricted by the diameter of the pipe through which it must pass. If the water level in the reservoir is increased, water will flow more quickly. If the diameter of the pipe is decreased, water will flow more slowly. The property of the pipe that restricts the flow of water is called **resistance**. The electrical element possessing this quality is called a **resistor**. A current I through a resistor of resistance R is related to the voltage difference V between the two ends of the resistor by

$$V = IR \tag{2.5}$$

A voltage of 1 volt across a unit resistance will cause a current flow of 1 amp. The unit of resistance, the volt per amp, is called an **ohm**.

It often is convenient to view an electrical circuit element in terms of its *willingness* to carry current rather than of its reluctance to do so. When a nerve membrane is excited, it passes more current than it does when it is at rest. When a transistor has a voltage on its gate, it carries more current than it does when its gate is grounded. For this reason, both biological and electronic elements are described by a **conductance** G. The conductance is defined as the current per unit voltage:

$$G = \frac{1}{R} = \frac{I}{V}$$

The unit of conductance, the amp per volt, is called a **mho**. In the neurobiology literature, the mho is called the **siemens**.

Equipotential Regions

We are all familiar with bodies of water that have flat surfaces (lakes, oceans), and with others that have sloping surfaces (rivers, streams). In Figure 2.1, we can identify regions in which the water level is flat (independent of position on the surface). The reservoir, the sea, and the inside of the tank are examples. To a first approximation, the water level in such **equipotential regions** will stay flat whether or not water is flowing in the pipes. In an electrical circuit, equipotential regions are called **electrical nodes**. By definition, a node is a region characterized by a single potential. As we proceed, we often will describe the dependence of one potential on that of other nodes, and will talk about that potential's evolution with respect to time. For these discussions, we will refer to names or labels attached to the nodes. Because there is a one-to-one relationship between nodes and voltages, we often will use the voltage label as the name of the node—as "I_1 and I_2 join at the V_1 node." This convention also will be applied to resistors and capacitors: The same label will be used for both their *name* and their *value*. This abuse of notation will be indulged only where there is a one-to-one correspondence, and thus no confusion can result.

SCHEMATIC DIAGRAMS

Once we have identified the nodes, we can construct an abstraction of the physical situation by lumping all the charge storage into capacitive elements, and all the resistance to current flow into resistors. The abstraction can be expressed either as a coupled set of differential equations or as a diagram called a **schematic**. Most people find it convenient to develop a schematic from the physical system, and then to write equations for the schematic. A schematic for Figure 2.1 is shown in Figure 2.2.

In any abstraction, certain details of the physical situation are omitted. The idealizations in Figure 2.2 are as follows:

1. We have treated the two valves as *switches*; they can be either on or off, but they cannot assume intermediate values

2. We have neglected the volume of water stored in the pipes

3. We have treated the reservoir and the mechanism by which it is kept full as a lumped constant *voltage source*, shown as a battery

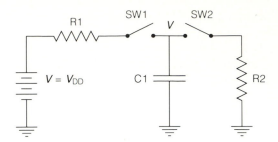

FIGURE 2.2   Schematic diagram representing the essential behavior of the physical system shown in Figure 2.1. The resistor R1 corresponds to the friction in the upper pipe, and R2 to that in the lower pipe. The capacitor represents the water-storage capacity of the tank. The two switches are analogous to the two valves. The battery is an abstraction of the reservoir, and must include a mechanism that keeps it full.

4. We have neglected any voltage drop (difference in water level) in the upper reservoir caused by water flowing out of the pipe through SW1

5. We have assumed all dependencies to be *linear*, as defined by Equations 2.5 and 2.4

The assumption of linearity in item 5 is a property, not of the schematic representation, but rather of the individual components. Many elements in both biological and electronic systems are highly nonlinear. The nonlinearities produced by most physical devices are smooth, however, and can be treated as linear for small excursions from any given operating point. We will encounter many examples in which the locally linear approximation gives us valuable information about an inherently nonlinear system.

These five idealizations have allowed us to construct a precise mathematical **model**, embodied in Figure 2.2. We will need such a model to analyze any physical system, because the myriad details in any real system are intractable to analysis. We intend the model to capture all effects that are relevant at the level of detail we are considering, and to omit the potentially infinite detail that would not affect the outcome in any substantial way. It is clear that no analysis can be any better than the model on which it is based. Constructing a good model requires consummate skill, judgment, experience, and taste. Once we have constructed an elegant model, analysis may present mathematical difficulties but does not require conceptual advances.

Models required for biological systems often are inherently *nonlinear*, in the sense that no linear system will behave even qualitatively as the observed system does. Analysis techniques for nonlinear systems have not evolved to nearly the level of generality as have those for linear systems. For this reason, when we wish to model a biological system, we have to pay more attention to the qualitative aspects of its behavior. Our models generally will evolve as we increase our understanding of the system. In fact, we can argue that the best models in a complex discipline *are* the embodiment of the understanding of that discipline.

The remainder of this book is devoted to a modeling technique quite different from any previously attempted. Not only are the resulting models directly related to the system under study, but the models themselves are real-time working physical systems. They can be used directly in engineering applications.

LINEAR SUPERPOSITION

Idealization 5 in the previous section has put us in a position to state the single most important principle in the analysis of electrical circuits: the **principle of linear superposition**. For any arbitrary network containing resistors and voltage sources, we can find the solution for the network (the voltage at every node and the current through every resistor) by the following procedure. We find the solution for the network in response to each voltage source individually, with all other voltage sources reduced to zero. The full solution, including the effects of all voltage sources, is just the sum of the solutions for the individual voltage sources. In addition to linearity of the component characteristics, there must be a well-defined reference value for voltages (ground), to which all node potentials revert when *all* sources are reduced to zero.

This principle applies to circuits containing current sources as well as to those containing voltage sources. It applies even if the sources are functions of time, as we will discuss in Chapter 8. It also applies to circuits containing capacitors, provided that any initial charge on a capacitor is treated as though it were a voltage source in series with the capacitor. Finally, the principle is applicable to networks containing transistors, or other elements with smooth nonlinearities, if the signal amplitudes are small enough that the circuit acts linearly within the range of signal excursions.

The analytical advantage we derive from this principle lies in the ability it gives us to treat the contribution of each individual input in isolation, knowing that the effect of each input is independent of the values of the other inputs. Thus, we need not worry that several inputs will combine in strange and combinatorially complex ways.

ACTIVE DEVICES

Although there are many details of any technology that can be changed without compromising our ability to create useful systems, there is one essential ingredient without which it simply is not possible to process information. That key ingredient is *gain*.

The nervous system is constantly bombarded by an enormous variety of sensory inputs. Perhaps the most important contribution of early sensory information-processing centers is to inhibit the vast majority of unimportant and therefore unwanted inputs, in order to concentrate on the immediately important stimuli. Of course, all inputs must be available at all times, lest an unseen predator leap suddenly from an inhibited region. Therefore, any real-time system of this sort will, at any time, develop its outputs from a small subset of its inputs. Because every input is the output of some other element, it follows that every element must be able to drive many more outputs than it receives as active inputs at any given time. An elementary device therefore must have **gain**—it must be able to supply more energy to its outputs than it receives from its input signals. Devices with this capability are called **active devices**.

In Figure 2.2, the active devices are shown as switches, but we have not specified what is required to open or close them. In both biology and electronics, valves are controlled not by some outside agent, as tacitly assumed in Figure 2.2, but rather by the *potential at some other point in the system*. Furthermore, valves cannot be treated as switches that are purely on or off; they assume intermediate values. Active devices play a central role in information processing; we will take a much closer look at how they work. In fact, this task will occupy us for the next two chapters.

THERMAL MOTION

The systems of particles that we will discuss—molecules in a gas, ions in a solution, or electrons in a semiconductor crystal—seem superficially so different that mentioning them in the same sentence may appear to be ridiculous. For many phenomena, we must exercise great care when drawing parallels between the behavior of these systems. For the phenomena of importance in computation, however, there is a deep similarity in the underlying physics of the three systems: in all cases, the trajectory of an individual particle is completely dominated by thermal motion. Collisions with the environment cause the particle to traverse a *random walk*, a familiar example of which is Brownian motion. We have no hope of following the detailed path of any given particle, let alone all the paths of a collection of particles. The quantities we care about—electrical charge, for example—are in any case sums over large numbers of particles. It suffices, then, to treat the average motion of a particle in a statistical sense.

By making three simplifications, we can derive the important properties of a collection of particles subject to random thermal motion by an intuitive line of reasoning:

1. We treat the inherently three-dimensional process as a one-dimensional model in the direction of current flow

2. We replace the distributions of velocities and free times by their mean values

3. We assume that electric fields are sufficiently small that they do not appreciably alter the thermal distribution

Although the resulting treatment is mathematically rough-and-ready, it is both mercifully brief and conceptually correct.

Drift

In any given environment, a particle will experience collisions at random intervals, either with others of its own kind (as in a gas), or with other thermally agitated entities (as in a semiconductor crystal lattice). In any case, there will be some **mean free time** (t_f) between collisions. We will make the simplest assumption about a collision: that all memory of the situation prior to the collision is lost, and the particle is sent off in a random direction with a random velocity. The magnitude of this velocity is, on average, v_T.

If the particle is subject to some external force f, from gravity or from an electric field, it will accelerate during the time it is free in accordance with Newton's law:

$$f = ma$$

Over the course of the time the particle is free, the particle will move with increasing velocity in the direction of the acceleration. Although the initial velocity is random after a collision, the small incremental change in velocity is always in the direction of the force. Over many collisions, the random initial velocity will average to zero, and we can therefore treat the particle as though it accelerated from rest after every collision. The distance s traveled in time t by a particle starting from rest with acceleration a is

$$s = \frac{1}{2}at^2$$

In the case of our model, over the time t_f between collisions, the acceleration $a = f/m$ will cause a net change δh in the position h of the particle:

$$\delta h = \frac{1}{2}at_f^2 = \frac{f}{2m}t_f^2$$

The average **drift velocity** (v_{drift}) of a large collection of particles subject to the force f per particle is just the net change in position δh per average time t_f between collisions:

$$v_{\text{drift}} = \frac{\delta h}{t_f} = \frac{ft_f}{2m} \tag{2.6}$$

Equation 2.6 describes the behavior of a uniform distribution of electrons or ions with charge q in the presence of an electric field E. The force on each particle is

$$f = qE$$

and therefore the drift velocity is linear in the electric field:

$$v_{\text{drift}} = \frac{qt_f}{2m}E = \mu E \tag{2.7}$$

The constant $\mu = qt_f/2m$ is called the **mobility** of the particle.

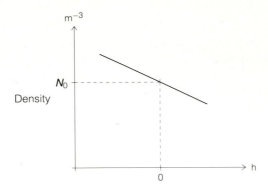

FIGURE 2.3 Density of particles as a function of some spatial dimension h. At $h = 0$, the particle density is N_0 per cubic meter. Particles will diffuse from regions of higher density (low h) to regions of lower density (high h).

Diffusion

In all structures that are interesting from an information-processing point of view, such as transistors and nerve membranes, there are large spatial gradients in the concentration of particles. Under such circumstances, there is a **diffusion** of particles from regions of higher density to those of lower density. Consider the situation shown in Figure 2.3. Particles diffusing from left to right cross the origin at some rate proportional to the gradient of the density N (number of particles per unit volume). That flow rate (J), given in particles per unit area per second, can be viewed as a movement of all particles to the right with some effective **diffusion velocity** (v_{diff}):

$$J = N v_{\text{diff}} \tag{2.8}$$

For electrically charged particles, J usually is given in terms of charge per second per unit area (current per unit area), and is called the **current density**. This electrical current density is equal to the particle density given by Equation 2.8, multiplied by q.

A simple model of the diffusion process is shown in Figure 2.4. We have divided the spatial-dimension axis (h) into compartments small enough that a particle can, on the average, move from one to the other in one mean free time (t_f). Due to the local density gradient, there are $N_0 + \Delta N$ particles in the left compartment, but only N_0 particles in the right compartment. One t_f later, half of the particles in each compartment will have moved to the right, and half will have moved to the left. There is, therefore, a net movement of $\Delta N/2$ particles to the right. This flow is purely the result of the random movement of particles; the particles' individual velocities have no preferred direction. So $\Delta N/2$ particles move a distance $v_T t_f$ every t_f. Because there are N_0 total particles, the average velocity v_{diff} per particle in the $+h$ direction is $v_T \Delta N/(2N_0)$. The width of each

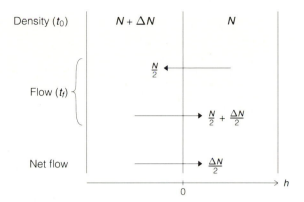

FIGURE 2.4 Flow of particles due to random thermal motion. The higher density to the left of the origin results in more particles crossing the axis to the right than to the left. The net flow to the right is the difference between these two rates.

compartment is $v_T t_f$, so

$$\Delta N \approx \frac{dN}{dh} v_T t_f$$

The diffusion velocity can thus be written in terms of the gradient of the particle distribution,

$$v_{\text{diff}} = -\frac{1}{2N} \frac{dN}{dh} t_f v_T^2 \tag{2.9}$$

The negative sign arises because the net flow of particles is from higher density to lower density.

In a one-dimensional model, a particle in thermal equilibrium has a mean kinetic energy that defines its **temperature** (T):

$$\frac{1}{2} m v_T^2 = \frac{1}{2} kT$$

Here k is Boltzmann's constant, m is the mass of the particle, and v_T is called the **thermal velocity**. At room temperature, kT is equal to 0.025 electron volt. Substituting v_T^2 into Equation 2.9, we obtain

$$v_{\text{diff}} = -\frac{1}{2N} \frac{dN}{dh} kT \frac{t_f}{m}$$

$$= -D \frac{1}{N} \frac{dN}{dh} \tag{2.10}$$

The quantity $D = kT t_f / 2m$ is called the **diffusion constant** of the particle. Comparing Equation 2.7 with Equation 2.10, we can see that the mobility and diffusion constants are related:

$$D = \frac{kT}{q}\mu \qquad (2.11)$$

Although the preceding derivation was approximate, Equation 2.11 is an exact result called the **Einstein relation**; it was discovered by Einstein during his study of Brownian motion. It reminds us that drift and diffusion are not separate processes, but rather are two aspects of the behavior of an ensemble of particles dominated by random thermal motion.

The processes of drift and diffusion are the stuff of which all information-processing devices—both neural and semiconductor—are made. To understand the physics of active devices, we need one more conceptual tool—the energy diagram. Like a schematic, the energy diagram is a pictorial representation of a model. With the Boltzmann distribution, it forms a complete basis for the device physics that follows. We will discuss the Boltzmann distribution next, and will return to the energy diagram in Chapter 3.

Boltzmann Distribution

We all know that the earth's atmosphere is held to the earth's surface by gravitational attraction. Gas molecules have weight, and thus are subject to a force toward the center of the earth. If the temperature were reduced to absolute zero, the entire atmosphere would condense into a solid sheet about 5 meters thick. The distribution of matter in the atmosphere is the result of a delicate balance: Thermal agitation, through random collisions between molecules, tends to spread matter uniformly throughout space. Gravitational attraction tends to concentrate matter on the surface of the planet. In quantitative terms, the gravitational force produces a *drift velocity* toward the surface given by Equation 2.6, where the force f is just the weight w of each molecule, which we will assume to be independent of the height h over a small range of elevation. As molecules drift toward the surface, the density increases at lower elevations and decreases at higher elevations, thus forming a density gradient. This density gradient causes an upward *diffusion* of molecules, in accordance with Equation 2.10. Equilibrium is reached when the rate of diffusion upward due to the density gradient is equal to the rate of drift downward. Setting the two velocities equal, we obtain

$$v_{\text{drift}} = \frac{wt_f}{2m} = v_{\text{diff}} = -\frac{1}{2N}\frac{dN}{dh}kT\frac{t_f}{m}$$

We cancel out t_f and m, leaving a relationship between density and height:

$$\frac{1}{N}\frac{dN}{dh}kT = -w \qquad (2.12)$$

Integration of Equation 2.12 with respect to h yields

$$kT \ln \frac{N}{N_0} = -wh \qquad (2.13)$$

where N_0 is the density at the reference height $h = 0$. Exponentiation of both sides of Equation 2.13 gives

$$N = N_0 e^{-\frac{wh}{kT}} \qquad (2.14)$$

The density of molecules per unit volume in the atmosphere decreases exponentially with altitude above the earth's surface.[1] The quantity wh is, of course, just the potential energy of the molecule.

Equation 2.13 can be generalized to any situation involving thermally agitated particles working against a gradient of potential energy. For charged particles, the potential energy is qV, and Equation 2.13 takes the form

$$V = -\frac{kT}{q} \ln \frac{N}{N_0} \qquad (2.15)$$

The voltage V developed in response to a gradient in the concentration of a charged species, and exhibiting the logarithmic dependence on concentration shown in Equation 2.15, is called the **Nernst potential**. In the electrochemistry and biology literature, kT/q is written RT/F. Exponentiation of Equation 2.15 leads to

$$N = N_0 e^{-\frac{q}{kT}V} \qquad (2.16)$$

Equation 2.16 is called the **Boltzmann distribution**. It describes the exponential decrease in density of particles in thermal equilibrium with a potential gradient. It is the basis for all exponential functions in the neural and electronic systems we will study.

---

[1] This treatment ignores all the complications present in a real atmosphere: convection, multiple gases, and so on.

CHAPTER

3

TRANSISTOR PHYSICS

The active devices in electronic systems are called **transistors**. Their function is to control the flow of current from one node based on the potential at another node. In terms of our analog of Figure 2.1 (p. 14), we construct a valve that is operated by the level in another tank. Although it is easy to imagine mechanical linkages that could cause a valve to operate, we will not succumb to the temptation to use that model. Rather, we will describe a somewhat less familiar but still intuitive model that accurately embodies all the necessary physics of the transistor.

BOLTZIAN HYDRAULICS

We saw in Chapter 2 that the density of gas molecules in the atmosphere decreases exponentially with height. For the planet Earth, the gravitational attraction, temperature, and molecular weight are such that the atmospheric density decreases by a factor of e for each approximately 20-kilometer increase in elevation. It is easy to imagine a planet with much higher gravitational attraction, lower temperature, and heavier molecules, such that the change in elevation required to decrease the density by a factor of e would be about 1 meter. Because such a planet would not be a hospitable place to live, we will travel to it only to illustrate the principles on which transistors operate. We will call this imaginary planet Boltzo.

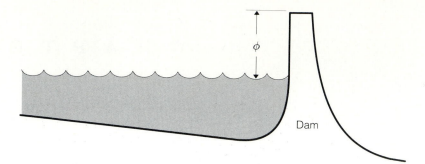

FIGURE 3.1   Cross-section of reservoir showing water level a distance ϕ below the top of the dam. Any water vapor must rise to this height to spill over the dam.

We will use a hydraulic power system similar to that shown in Figure 2.1 (p. 14). If we locate our Boltzian reservoir about 200 meters above sea level, the potential energy of a water molecule in the reservoir (measured in units of kT) will be about equal to that of an electron in the 5-volt power supply of an electronic circuit. (Had we located our reservoir at an altitude of 25 meters, we would have approximated the operation of a neural system, but that story is a bit more complicated. We will content ourselves for the moment with creating a hydraulic transistor.)

Early Boltzian engineers constructed a dam in the bottom of a deep canyon, as shown in Figure 3.1. The purpose of the dam was to create a reservoir to store water. When the rains were heavy and the reservoir nearly full, however, the Boltzians noticed that the water level did not stay constant, even if no water was withdrawn from the reservoir. They made an exhaustive search, but found no sign of leakage. Finally, they sought the advice of a wise and venerable Boltzian philosopher. After surveying the situation, he gave his reply: "Contemplate atop the dam in the quiet of the night."

This pronouncement instantly became the subject of much discussion in learned circles—what could he possibly mean by such a reply? One young engineering student named Lily Field grew tired of the endless arguments. Against prevailing sentiment, she undertook the long journey to the dam site. Sitting atop the massive structure as the noises of the day faded into darkness, she contemplated the meaning of the philosopher's words. All wind had ceased; not a blade of grass or a leaf stirred. Still she had the strong sense of a cold and heavy force against her back. Holding out her silk scarf like a sail, she noticed that it billowed out, as if pressed by some invisible force. When she raised it to eye level, the billowing was considerably weaker. She found a long stick, attached the scarf to its tip, and held it aloft; the billowing effect was scarcely detectable.

The mystery was solved. The water was not escaping in liquid form at all— it was *evaporating*, and the vapor was pouring over the dam in enormous quantities. There was a source of water behind the dam, and no source on the opposite side of the dam. There was thus a difference in density of water vapor on the two

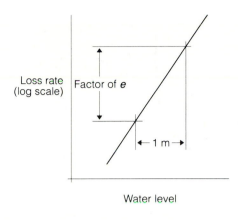

FIGURE 3.2 Loss rate of water vapor over the dam of Figure 3.1 as a function of water level in the reservoir. The distance ϕ decreases as the water level rises. Because the vapor density decreases exponentially with height above the water level, the loss rate increases exponentially with the water level.

sides of the dam. Water vapor was *diffusing* from the region of high vapor density to the region of low density. The density gradient, and hence the diffusion rate, was proportional to the density at the top of the dam. Because the density of the vapor decreased exponentially with height above the water level, the effect was noticeable only when the reservoir was very nearly full.

When Field returned to the city, she looked up data on the water loss rate and level over the several years that the dam had been operating. She plotted the log of the loss rate as a function of the height of the water level in the reservoir. The result was a straight line, as shown in Figure 3.2. For each meter that the water level rose, the loss rate increased by a factor of e.

Field presented her findings in a poster session at the next International Hydraulics Conference (IHC); her study soon became the talk of the entire meeting. A special evening discussion session was organized. Field showed the data, and pointed out that the engineers could greatly reduce the vapor loss by extending the height of the dam only a few meters. The additional structure would be required to support not the weight of liquid water, but only the density gradient of water *vapor*, so it could be constructed of light material such as wood or plastic, rather than of massive reinforced concrete.

In an invited paper at the IHC the following year, Dr. Field presented a mechanism for controlling the flow of vapor over the dam, shown in Figure 3.3. A barrier of light material is allowed to slide vertically in a slot in the middle of the dam. The barrier is supported on a series of floats. The floats are buoyed up by water from another reservoir or tank. If the level in the second tank is high, the barrier will be high and the flow of vapor over the dam will be low. If the level in the second tank is low, the barrier will be low, and the flow of vapor over the dam will be large. The flow rate I across the barrier will be directly proportional to the density gradient in the horizontal direction. That gradient will, in turn, be proportional to the density of water vapor at height ϕ above the liquid surface, given in Equation 2.14 (p. 25):

$$I = I_0 e^{-\frac{w\phi}{kT}} \tag{3.1}$$

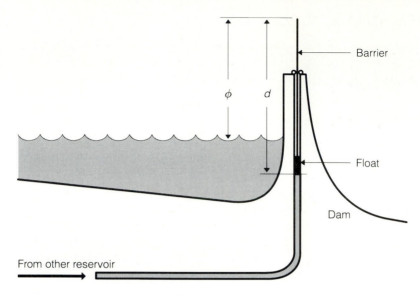

FIGURE 3.3 Hydraulic transistor. The barrier floats on water in a chamber filled from another reservoir. The water-vapor flow rate is an exponentially decreasing function of the water level in the second reservoir.

From the basic dimensions of the structure, Equation 3.1 can be expressed as

$$I = I_0 e^{-\frac{w}{kT}(h_2 - h_1 + d)} \tag{3.2}$$

where h_1 is the elevation of the main reservoir and h_2 is the elevation in the control reservoir. The physical height d of the barrier can be factored into a new preexponential constant,

$$I_1 = I_0 e^{-\frac{wd}{kT}}$$

The product wh of the molecular weight w and the reservoir level h is just the potential energy per molecule P. Equation 3.2 can thus be expressed as

$$I = I_1 e^{\frac{P_1 - P_2}{kT}} \tag{3.3}$$

The current decreases exponentially with the energy difference between the control reservoir and source reservoir. Equation 3.3 is the basic governing equation for the operation of a transistor. The only difference between Boltzo and silicon is that, in the latter, gravitational forces have been replaced by electrostatic ones. The Boltzian landscape is the energy profile of our electronic structures. Cross-sections of the energy terrain are called **energy diagrams**, and appear in all discussions of electron device physics. We will see the energy diagram for an MOS transistor later in this chapter.

SEMICONDUCTORS

All physical structures—neural, electronic, or mechanical—are built out of atoms. Before proceeding, we will briefly review the properties of these basic building blocks out of which transistors and neurons are made.

Atoms and All That

Atoms can be viewed as a swarm of electrons circulating around a nucleus containing protons and neutrons. The negatively charged electrons are, of course, attracted to the positively charged nucleus, and will orbit as close to it as the laws of quantum mechanics allow. An **element** is a type of atom; each atom of a given element will have the same number of electrons. The total number of electrons in orbit around an atom of a particular element is called the **atomic number** of that element. The electrons are arranged in quantum-mechanical orbits or shells. There is a maximum number of electrons each shell can hold. We can thus classify elements according to the number of electrons in the outermost shell. Such a classification is called a **periodic table** of the elements. A simplified periodic table showing the elements with which we will be concerned is given in Table 3.1.

Hydrogen, the element with atomic number 1, has one lone proton for a nucleus, and one electron in the innermost shell. It is a Group I element; the group number refers to the number of electrons in the outermost shell. The first shell can contain at most two electrons. Helium, a Group Zero element, has two electrons in its inner shell, which is therefore full. After one shell is full, additional electrons are forced to populate the next larger shell. The element lithium, atomic number 3, has the first shell full with two electrons, and one electron in the second

TABLE 3.1 Simplified periodic table of the elements, showing the valence and position of elements that form semiconductor crystals. The Group IV elements shown form a diamond lattice. Silicon is by far the most commonly used semiconductor. Boron, aluminum, and gallium are acceptor impurities in silicon; phosphorus and arsenic are donors. In addition, Group III elements can combine with Group V elements to form diamondlike crystals in which alternate lattice sites are occupied by atoms of each element. The best known of these Group III–V semiconductors is gallium arsenide, which is used for microwave transistors and light-emitting diodes. Group II–VI crystals also are semiconductors. Zinc sulfide is a common phosphor in television display tubes, and cadmium sulfide was the earliest widely used photosensitive material.

I	II	III	IV	V	VI	VII	Zero
H							He
Li	Be	B	C	N	O	F	Ne
Na	Mg	Al	Si	P	S	Cl	Ar
K	Zn	Ga	Ge	As	Se	Br	Kr
Rb	Cd	In	Sn	Sb	Te	I	Xe

shell. It is therefore a Group I element. The second, third, and fourth shells can each hold eight electrons. Neon, with atomic number 10, has both its first and second shells full.

In the world of atoms, having a full outer shell is a happy circumstance. So happy, in fact, that atoms fortunate enough to attain this condition have absolutely no desire to interact with other atoms. Such elements as helium, neon, and argon are **inert gases**, the ultimate snobs of the atomic pecking order. Other, less fortunate atoms strive mightily to emulate their austere brethren by forming alliances with similar atoms. These alliances, called **covalent bonds**, are based on sharing electrons such that all parties to the charade can make believe they have a full shell, even though some of the electrons that fill the outer shell are shared with neighbors. Small communal aggregates of this sort are called **molecules**. An example is methane, CH_4. Carbon, being a Group IV atom, has four electrons with which to play, but is desperately seeking four more to fill its outer shell. Each hydrogen has only one electron with which to play, but needs only one more to fill its outer shell. The ultimately blissful arrangement results when each of the four hydrogens shares its electron with the carbon, and the carbon shares one electron with each hydrogen. Not quite neon, but not too bad!

Crystals

Molecules can satisfy a social need for a few atoms, but for regimentation on a massive scale there is no substitute for a **crystal**. In the simplest crystal, every atom is an equivalent member of a vast army, arrayed in three dimensions as far as the eye can see. Three elements in Group IV of the periodic table crystallize naturally into a remarkable structure called the **diamond lattice**: carbon, silicon, and germanium. Each atom is covalently bonded to four neighbors arranged at the corners of a regular tetrahedron. Group IV is unique in chemistry. Eight electrons are required to complete an atomic shell. Atoms with four electrons can team up with four neighbors, sharing one electron with each. Such an arrangement fills the shell for everyone; no electrons are left over, and no bond is missing an electron. A pure crystal formed this way is called an **intrinsic** semiconductor; it is an electrical insulator, because there are no charged particles free to move around and to carry current.

Conduction

If we alter the crystal by replacing a small fraction of its atoms with impurity atoms of Group V, the crystal becomes conductive. The addition of impurities is called **doping**. Group V elements have one *more* electron than the four needed for the covalent bonds. This extra electron is only weakly bound to the impurity site in the lattice; at room temperature, it is free to move about and to carry current. Such atoms are called **donors**, because they donate a free electron to the crystal. The free electrons are negative, and a semiconductor crystal doped with donors is said to be **n-type**. The entire crystal is charge neutral, because it is made of atoms that have as many positively charged protons in their nuclei as they have electrons in their shells. When an electron leaves its donor, the donor is said to be **ionized**. An ionized donor has a positive charge because it has lost one electron.

It also is possible to dope a Group IV semiconductor with atoms of Group III. These impurities have one *less* electron than is required for the four covalent bonds. Group III dopants are therefore called **acceptors**. The absence of one electron in a bond is called a **hole**. We can think of the hole as mobile at room temperature, moving about the crystal. (It is actually electrons that move, and the "motion" of the hole is in the opposite direction. We think of the hole as a "bubble" in the electronic fluid.) The hole, being the absence of an electron, carries a *positive* charge. Once the hole has been filled, the acceptor acquires a negative charge, and is said to be **ionized**. Doping a semiconductor with acceptors renders it conductive, the current being carried by positive holes. Such a crystal is called **p-type**.

It is thus possible to provide either positive or negative charge carriers by doping the crystal appropriately. The concentration of dopants can be controlled precisely over many orders of magnitude, from lightly doped (approximately 10^{15} atoms per cubic centimeter) to heavily doped (approximately 10^{19} atoms per cubic centimeter). Heavily doped n-type material is called $n+$, and heavily doped p-type material is called $p+$. The density of impurity atoms is always small compared to the approximately 5×10^{22} atoms per cubic centimeter in the crystal itself.

Because electrons and holes are both charged, and are both used to carry current, we refer to them generically as **charge carriers**.

MOS TRANSISTORS

A cross-section of the simplest transistor structure is illustrated in Figure 3.4. It shows an intrinsic substrate into which two highly doped regions have been fabricated. Consistent with our hydraulic analogy, one of the highly doped regions is called the **source**, and the other is called the **drain**. The entire surface is covered with a very thin layer of SiO_2 (quartz), which is an excellent electrical insulator. On top of the insulator is a metallic control electrode, called the **gate**, that spans the intrinsic region between source and drain. Current flows from source to drain in the region just under the gate oxide called the **channel**. This structure was first described by a freelance inventor named Lilienfeld in a patent issued in 1933 [Lilienfeld, 1928]. It is called an MOS transistor because the active region consists of a metallic gate, an oxide insulator, and a semiconductor channel. In today's technology, the metallic gate often is made of heavily doped polycrystalline silicon, called **polysilicon** or **poly** for short. The details of how transistors are fabricated are the subject of Appendix A. At this point, we will consider the electrical operation of such a transistor.

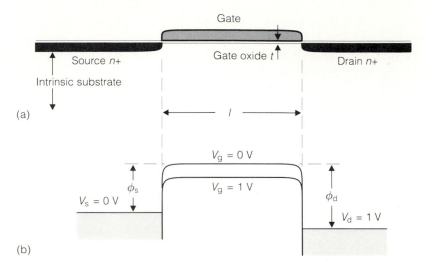

FIGURE 3.4   Cross-section (a) and energy diagram (b) of an *n*-channel transistor. In a typical 1988 process, the gate-oxide thickness is approximately 400 angstroms (0.04 micron), and the minimum channel length *l* is approximately 1.5 microns. When the circuit is in operation, the drain is biased positively; hence, the barrier for electrons is greater at the drain than at the source. Applying a positive voltage at the gate lowers the electron barrier at both source and drain, allowing electrons to diffuse from source to drain.

In Figure 3.4, an energy diagram of the cross-section of part (a) is shown in part (b). The energy of the charge carrier is plotted upward. The surface of the electronic "fluid" is called the **Fermi level**. The drain Fermi level is lower than that of the source by qV_{ds}, where V_{ds} is the drain voltage relative to the source, and q is the electronic charge.

The gate oxide is very thin compared to the source–drain spacing. In a typical 1988 process, the source–drain spacing l is 1.5 microns and the oxide thickness t is 400 angstroms (100 angstroms is equal to 0.01 micron). For this reason, the potential in the channel at the surface of the silicon, just under the gate, is dominated by the gate voltage. There are fringe effects of the source and drain voltages, which will be discussed in Appendix B. For the moment, we will ignore those effects. As a first approximation, then, we assume that any change in the potential on the gate will be reflected in an equal change in potential in the channel. As the gate potential is lowered, the lowest potential will be at the silicon surface. As this barrier between source and drain is lowered, more charges can flow along the surface from source to drain. The barrier for two gate voltages is shown in Figure 3.4(b). The device is exactly analogous to Dr. Field's hydraulic transistor, described at the beginning of the chapter.

The barrier ϕ_s from source to channel is lower than ϕ_d from drain to channel, so more charges will be able to surmount ϕ_s than can climb over ϕ_d. The charge-

carrier density at the source end of the channel thus will be larger than that at
the drain end of the channel. Current flows through the channel by diffusion,
from the region of high density at the source to that of low density at the drain.
We will now compute the channel current.

The carrier density N_s at the source end of the channel is given by Equation 2.16 (p. 25):

$$N_s = N_0 e^{-\frac{\phi_s}{kT}} \tag{3.4}$$

where N_0 is the carrier density at the Fermi level. A similar relation holds for N_d,
the carrier density at the drain end of the channel:

$$N_d = N_0 e^{-\frac{\phi_d}{kT}} \tag{3.5}$$

When the transistor was fabricated, there was a built-in barrier ϕ_0 between
source and channel. The control of this barrier is the most crucial element of a
high-quality processing line. As the gate potential is lowered, the barrier will be
lowered accordingly:

$$\phi_s = \phi_0 + q(V_g - V_s) \tag{3.6}$$

$$\phi_d = \phi_0 + q(V_g - V_d) \tag{3.7}$$

We can now write the barrier energies in Equations 3.4 and 3.5 in terms of the
source, gate, and drain voltages:

$$N_s = N_0 e^{-\frac{\phi_0 + q(V_g - V_s)}{kT}} \tag{3.8}$$

$$N_d = N_0 e^{-\frac{\phi_0 + q(V_g - V_d)}{kT}} \tag{3.9}$$

From Equations 3.8 and 3.9, we can compute the gradient of carrier density
with respect to the distance z along the channel (z is equal to zero at the source).
Because no carriers are lost as they travel from source to drain, the current is
the same at any z, and the gradient will not depend on z. The density thus will
be a linear function of z:

$$\frac{dN}{dz} = \frac{N_d - N_s}{l} = \frac{N_1}{l} e^{-\frac{qV_g}{kT}} \left(e^{\frac{qV_d}{kT}} - e^{\frac{qV_s}{kT}} \right) \tag{3.10}$$

where $N_1 = N_0 e^{-\phi_0/(kT)}$.

The electrical current is just the total number of charges times the average
diffusion velocity given in Equation 2.10 (p. 23). The current per unit channel
width w is thus

$$\frac{I}{w} = qN v_{\text{diff}} = -qD\frac{dN}{dz} \tag{3.11}$$

where D is the diffusion constant of carriers in the channel. Substituting Equation 3.10 into Equation 3.11, we obtain the general form of the MOS transistor current:

$$I = I_0 e^{-\frac{qV_g}{kT}} \left(e^{\frac{qV_s}{kT}} - e^{\frac{qV_d}{kT}} \right) \tag{3.12}$$

The accumulated preexponential constants have been absorbed into one giant constant I_0.

For a transistor with its source connected to the power supply rail, V_s is equal to zero, and Equation 3.12 becomes:

$$I = I_0 e^{-\frac{qV_{gs}}{kT}} \left(1 - e^{\frac{qV_{ds}}{kT}} \right) \tag{3.13}$$

where V_{gs} and V_{ds} are the gate-to-source and drain-to-source voltages, respectively.

Because there are charge carriers with positive as well as negative charge, there are two kinds of MOS transistor: Those using electrons as their charge carriers are called **n-channel**, whereas those using holes are called **p-channel**; the technology is thus called **complementary MOS**, or CMOS. For positive q (*p*-channel device), the current increases as the gate voltage is made negative with respect to the source; for negative q (*n*-channel device), the opposite occurs. kT is the thermal energy per charge carrier, so the quantity kT/q has the units of potential; it is called the **thermal voltage**, and its magnitude is equal to 0.025 volt at room temperature. A carrier must slide down a potential barrier of kT/q to raise its energy by kT. As we noted in Chapter 2, electrochemists and biologists write RT/F in place of kT/q. The way it is written does not change its value.

We have made a number of simplifying assumptions, which will be addressed in Appendix B. Equation 3.12, however, captures all the essential quantitative principles of transistor operation. Notice that, in Equation 3.10, the roles of the source and of the drain are completely symmetrical; therefore, if we interchange them, the magnitude of the current given by Equation 3.12 is identical, with the current flowing in the opposite direction.

The energy diagrams for both types of transistors are identical to that shown in Figure 3.4, but the energy axis has a different meaning. For a *p*-channel device, upward means higher energy for positive charges, or positive voltage. For an *n*-channel device, upward means higher energy for negative charges, or negative voltage. Opposite charges attract. An *n*-channel device requires positive gate voltages to attract negative electrons out of its source into its channel; a *p*-channel device requires negative gate voltages to attract positive holes out of its source into its channel.

CIRCUIT PROPERTIES OF TRANSISTORS

The symbols used in schematic diagrams for both *n*- and *p*-channel transistors are given in Figure 3.5, which shows the source, gate, and drain terminals. We put a bubble on the gate of the *p*-channel symbol to remind us that the

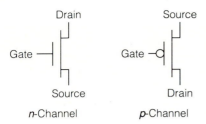

FIGURE 3.5 Circuit symbols for *n*- and *p*-channel transistors. These abstractions are used in schematic diagrams of transistor circuits. Note that the assignment of source and drain depends on the voltages to which these terminals are connected, because the physical device structure is symmetrical.

transistor turns on as we make the gate more negative relative to the source. We normally will draw the positive supply at the top of the diagram, and the most negative supply at the bottom. For this reason, the *sources* of *p*-channel devices usually are located at the *top*, whereas those of *n*-channel devices normally are at the *bottom*. Implicit in the schematic is a shadow of the Boltzian landscape, with upward meaning positive voltage, as in the energy diagram for *p*-channel transistors. Positive current (the flow of positive charges) is from high to low. Ground, the reference level, is the most negative supply, or sea level, for positive charges.

The measured current–voltage characteristics of a typical transistor are shown in Figure 3.6. The drain current is zero for $V_{ds} = 0$, as expected. For a given gate voltage, the drain current increases with V_{ds} and then saturates after a few kT/q, as predicted by Equation 3.13. The current in the flat part of the curves is nearly independent of V_{ds} and is called the **saturation current**, I_{sat}. A plot of the saturation current as a function of gate voltage V_{gs} is shown in Figure 3.7. I_{sat} increases exponentially with V_{gs} as predicted by Equation 3.13,

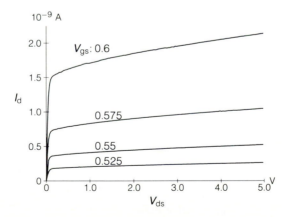

FIGURE 3.6 Drain current as a function of drain–source voltage for several values of gate–source voltage. The channel length of this transistor is 6 microns. The drain current increases rapidly with drain voltage, and saturates within a few kT/q to a gently sloping region of nearly constant current. The slope in the saturation region is due to the change in channel length with drain voltage. The slope in this region is proportional to drain current.

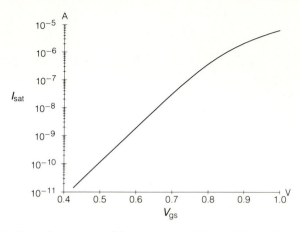

FIGURE 3.7   Saturation current of the transistor of Figure 3.6 as a function of gate voltage. The drain voltage was fixed at 2 volts. The current is an exponential function of gate voltage over many orders of magnitude. In this region, the current increases by a factor of e every 37 millivolts, corresponding to κ = 0.676. Above approximately 0.8 volt, the limiting effects of mobile charge on the current are evident. The nominal "threshold" of the device is approximately 0.9 volt.

but the voltage required for a factor of e increase in I_{sat} is 37 millivolts, rather than the 25 millivolts we expected.

In our simplified derivation, we assumed that the gate voltage was 100-percent effective in reducing the barrier potential. This assumption is valid for a structure built on an intrinsic substrate, as shown in Figure 3.4. Real transistors, such as those from which the data of Figure 3.7 were taken, are not built on intrinsic substrates. The n-channel transistors are fabricated on p-type substrates, and vice versa. Charges from the ionized donors or acceptors in the substrate under the channel reduce the effectiveness of the gate at controlling the barrier energy (see Appendix B). For our purposes, the effect can be taken into account by replacing kT/q by $kT/(q\kappa)$ in the gate term in Equation 3.12, and rescaling I_0. Equation 3.12 can thus be written

$$ I = I_0 e^{-\frac{q\kappa V_{\text{g}}}{kT}} \left(e^{\frac{qV_{\text{s}}}{kT}} - e^{\frac{qV_{\text{d}}}{kT}} \right) \tag{3.14} $$

The transistor shown has a value of κ approximately equal to 0.7. The values of κ can vary considerably among processes, but are reasonably constant among transistors in a single fabrication batch. Throughout this book, we will treat kT/q as the unit of voltage. Because this quantity appears in nearly every expression, we have developed a shorthand notation for it. If the magnitude of kT/q is used to scale all voltages in an expression—as, for example, when a voltage appears as the argument of an exponential—we often will write the voltage as though it were dimensionless. Using this notation, we can write Equation 3.14 for an

n-channel transistor as follows:

$$I = I_0 e^{\kappa V_g}\left(e^{-V_s} - e^{-V_d}\right) = I_{sat}\left(1 - e^{-V_{ds}}\right) \quad (3.15)$$

Where V_{ds} is the drain–source voltage. For a p-channel device, the signs of all voltages are reversed.

At the upper end of the current range of Figure 3.7, the current increases less rapidly than does the exponential predicted by Equation 3.15. This deviation from the exponential behavior occurs when the charge on the mobile carriers becomes comparable to the total charge on the gate. The gate voltage at which the mobile charge begins to limit the flow of current is called the **threshold voltage**. For gate voltages higher than threshold, the saturation current increases as the square of the gate voltage. Most circuits described in this book operate in **subthreshold**—their gate voltages are well below the threshold voltage. Typical digital circuits operate well above threshold. The detailed model described in Appendix B describes transistor characteristics over the entire range of operation.

Subthreshold operation has many advantages, three of which we are now in a position to appreciate:

1. Power dissipation is extremely low—from 10^{-12} to 10^{-6} watt for a typical circuit

2. The drain current saturates in a few kT/q, allowing the transistor to operate as a current source over most of the voltage range from near ground to V_{DD}

3. The exponential nonlinearity is an ideal computation primitive for many applications

We will encounter many more beneficial properties, and some limitations, of subthreshold operation as we proceed.

CURRENT MIRRORS

An often-used circuit configuration is shown in Figure 3.8. Here, each transistor is **diode-connected**; that is, its gate is connected to its drain. For a typical process, values of I_0 are such that even the smallest drain current used (10^{-12} amp) requires V_{gs} approximately equal to 0.4 volt. Higher drain currents

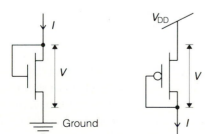

FIGURE 3.8 Diode connected n- and p-channel transistors. Because the drain–source voltage is always a few hundred millivolts, a device in this configuration is guaranteed to be saturated. The current–voltage characteristic is thus exponential, like that of Figure 3.7.

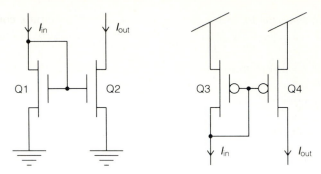

FIGURE 3.9 Current mirror connected *n*- and *p*-channel transistors. This configuration turns a source of current (the input) into an equal *sink* of current (the output). Reflecting currents in this manner is the most common operation in analog circuit design.

require higher values. Thus, the drain curves of Figure 3.6 are well into saturation for any useful V_{gs}. For this reason, the current through these diode-connected transistors has the same exponential dependence on voltage as that shown for the saturation current in Figure 3.7.

It is common to have a current of a certain sign—for example, a source of positive charges—and an input that requires an equal but opposite current— for example, a source of negative charges. A simple circuit that performs this inversion of current polarity is shown in Figure 3.9. The input current I_{in} biases a diode-connected transistor Q1. The resulting V_{gs} is just sufficient to bias the second transistor Q2 to a saturation current I_{out} equal to I_{in}. The value of I_{out} will be nearly independent of the drain voltage of Q2 as long as Q2 stays in saturation. A similar arrangement is shown for currents of the opposite sign using *p*-channel transistors Q3 and Q4. The *p*-channel circuit *reflects* a current to ground into a current from V_{DD}, so it is called a **current mirror**. The *n*-channel current mirror reflects a current from V_{DD} into a current to ground. We will use these circuit configurations in nearly every example in this book.

SUMMARY

We have seen how we can construct a physical structure that allows a voltage on one terminal to control the flow of current into another terminal. Although the first proposal for a device of this type was made in the 1930s [Lilienfeld, 1926], it took 3 decades to reduce the ideas to a production process. By the 1960s, MOS technology came into its own—today, it is the major technology on which the computer revolution has been built. For our purposes, MOS transistors are controlled sources of both positive and negative current. Their control terminals do not draw current from the nodes to which they are connected. MOS transistors are, in that sense, the most ideal active devices extant. The exponential dependence of drain current on gate voltage allows us to control current levels over many orders of magnitude. We will develop increasingly complex configurations of these simple elements, culminating in complete neural subsystems for vision and hearing.

REFERENCES

Lilienfeld, J.E. Method and apparatus for controlling electric currents. Patent (1,745,175: January 28, 1930): October 8, 1926.

Lilienfeld, J.E. Device for controlling electric current. Patent (1,900,018: March 7, 1933): March 28, 1928.

4

NEURONS

The basic *anatomical* unit in the nervous system is a specialized cell called the **neuron**. An artist's view of a typical neuron is shown in Figure 4.1. Many extensions of the single cell are long and filamentary; these structures are called **processes**. Every neuron plays several functional roles in a neural system:

1. Metabolic machinery within the cell provides a power source for information-processing functions. In addition, the cell enforces a certain unity for biochemical mechanisms throughout its extent.

2. A tree of processes called **dendrites** is covered with special structures called **synapses**, where junctions are formed with other neurons. These synaptic contacts are the primary information-processing elements in neural systems.

3. Processes act as wires, conveying information over a finite spatial extent. The resistance of fine dendrites allows the potential at their tips to be computed with only partial coupling to other computations in the tree.

4. Temporal integration of signals occurs over the short term through charge storage on the capacitance of the cell membrane, and over the longer term by means of internal second messengers and complex biochemical mechanisms.

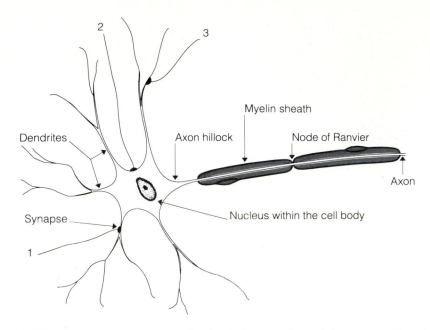

FIGURE 4.1　Conceptual structure of a classical neuron. Synaptic inputs are collected by the dendritic tree and are integrated on the capacitance of the cell body. When the potential at the axon hillock exceeds threshold, a nerve pulse is generated and is propagated down the axon. The capacitance of the axon to the extracellular fluid is reduced by the myelin sheath. Breaks in the sheath (nodes of Ranvier) allow periodic restoration of the pulse.

Axons (numbered 1, 2, and 3) from other neurons synapse onto their target neuron in different ways. Axon 1 synapses onto the trunk of a particular dendritic structure; axon 2 synapses onto the cell body; axon 3 synapses onto a more distal dendrite. (*Source:* Adapted from [Katz, 1966].)

5. Certain neurons are equipped with a long, specialized process called an **axon**. The axon is used for "digitizing" data for local transmission, and for transmitting data over long distances.

We shall first review the classical doctrine of how a neuron operates. We then shall be in a position to integrate several more recent findings, out of which a considerably richer and more complex picture emerges. The classical neuron is equipped with a tree of filamentary dendrites that aggregate synaptic *inputs* from other neurons. The input currents are integrated by the capacitance of the cell until a critical **threshold** potential is reached, at which point an *output* is generated in the form of a nerve pulse—the **action potential**. This output pulse propagates down the axon, which ends in a tree of synaptic contacts to the dendrites of other neurons.

The resistance of a nerve's cytoplasm is sufficiently high that signals cannot be transmitted more than about 1 millimeter before they are hopelessly spread out in time, and their information largely lost. For this reason, axons are equipped with an active amplification mechanism that restores the nerve pulse as it propagates. In lower animals, such as the squid, this restoration is done continuously along the length of the axon. In higher animals, many axons are wrapped with a special insulating material called **myelin**, which reduces the capacitance between the cytoplasm and the extracellular fluid, and thereby increases the velocity at which signals propagate. The sheaths of these myelinated axons have gaps called **nodes of Ranvier** every few millimeters. These nodes act as repeater sites, where the signal is periodically restored. A single myelinated fiber can carry signals over a distance of 1 meter or more.

Even the most casual exploration of nervous tissue with an electrode reveals a host of signals encoded as trains of action potentials. For this reason, the mechanism of initiation of the nerve pulse, and of its restoration as it propagates down the axon, became the center of early physiological investigations. The first quantitative work was carried out by Hodgkin, Huxley, and Katz [Hodgkin et al., 1952a; Hodgkin et al., 1952b; Hodgkin et al., 1952c; Hodgkin et al., 1952d] on the giant axon of the squid—an unmyelinated structure nearly 1 millimeter in diameter. This classic investigation revealed the following fascinating story:

1. The cytoplasm in the cell's interior is normally **polarized**—charged to a potential of approximately −80 millivolts with respect to the extracellular fluid

2. This potential difference is supported across a **cell membrane** so thin that it can be resolved only by an electron microscope

3. If sufficient current is injected into the cytoplasm in the direction to depolarize the membrane to a threshold potential of approximately −40 millivolts, a nerve pulse is initiated

4. The pulse travels in both directions from the initiation point, and its shape rapidly becomes independent of the mechanism through which the initiation took place

What are the mechanisms by which the axon initiates and propagates the action potential? That question motivated a sustained investigation by many workers over more than 5 decades. In any great scientific detective story, the resolution of a mystery at one level sharpens the focus of the researchers, and creates pressing questions at the next level. In the following sections, we will trace the story of the axon clue by clue. In the process, we will see how the nerve membrane is constructed, and how the electrical mechanism embedded in that membrane is responsible for the active transmission of nerve pulses. Only after we understand the axon will we be in a position to investigate how information processing is done in the dendritic tree of the neuron. That story is still unfolding.

NERVE MEMBRANE

All electrical activity in a neuron takes place in the thin membrane that electrically separates the neuron's interior from the extracellular fluid. The nerve membrane is formed from phospholipid molecules arranged in a **bilayer** about

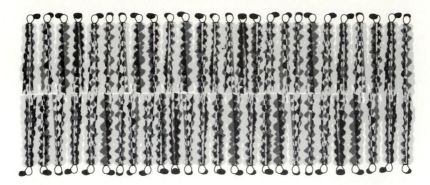

FIGURE 4.2 Cross-section of the bilayer structure that forms the nerve membrane. Individual lipid molecules have polar head-groups containing positive (white) and negative (black) charges. The hydrocarbon tails of the lipid molecules turn inward to avoid confronting the water (not shown). The energy of the electric dipole head-groups is much lower in the water surrounding the entire configuration than in hydrocarbon, which stabilizes the entire structure. The energy of an ion is much higher in the hydrocarbon membrane core, where the polarizability is low, than it is in the water, where the polarizability is high. The membrane thus forms an energy barrier to the passage of ions.

50 angstroms (5×10^{-9} meter) thick. The approximately 100-millivolt potential across the membrane creates an electric field of approximately 2×10^7 volts per meter—only 10 times less than the maximum field that can be supported reliably by the silicon dioxide insulator of a MOS transistor. How can so thin a structure be formed, and how can it be stable enough to support such large electrical gradients?

The structure of the bilayer is shown in Figure 4.2. The polar head-groups at one end of the lipid molecules bind to the aqueous solution, whereas the hydrocarbon chains on the other end of the molecules are hydrophobic. A highly stable structure is formed by two layers, oriented with hydrocarbon chains facing one another in the membrane's interior. The binding forces responsible for the great stability of the bilayer structure result from the interaction of water with charges in the polar head-group of each lipid molecule. The greedy oxygen atom in a water molecule forcibly removes an electron from each of its smaller hydrogen sidekicks. The oxygen end of the molecule thus becomes *negative,* and the hydrogen end is left *positive.* When another polar object is immersed in water, water molecules in its vicinity **polarize**—they orient such that the positive parts of the object are surrounded by negative ends of water molecules, and negative parts snuggle up to positive ends of other water molecules.[1] In such an arrangement, everyone is warm and happy—in technical terms, the energy of the system has been reduced.

In the bilayer, the hydrophilic polar head-groups of the lipid molecules face

---

[1] This use of the term *polarize* (from physics) should not be confused with the neurobiological usage, where the word means to charge the interior of a neuron to a negative potential. The only similarity between the two uses is that they both involve electrostatic potentials.

outward into the aqueous solution on either side, to which they are attracted by these electrostatic forces. Each head-group is an **electric dipole**, a positive and a negative charge separated by some distance. The energy of these charges in water is much lower than in the hydrocarbon phase, and results in the stability of the bilayer structure. The entire structure is a wonderful example of *self-assembly*. A tiny drop of lipid on the surface of a dish filled with water will spread out into a monolayer—the molecules immediately bury their head-groups in the water, leaving their hydrocarbon tails sticking straight up into the air. If we place a fine wire parallel to the surface and immerse it slowly through the monolayer into the water, the wire will carry the two halves of the monolayer with it. The exposed nonpolar hydrocarbon surfaces of the two halves join quickly to avoid confronting the hostile water molecules. We now have two monolayers back to back, forming the membrane structure shown in Figure 4.2. This monolayer technique is routinely used to create artificial bilayers in the laboratory.

Nature has evolved a great trick—the use of the electrical polarizability of water to attract charged sites on molecules. This technique is the ultimate basis of the three-dimensional conformation of most biologically important entities. It is the primary reason that the plan for building a three-dimensional organism can be embedded in a one-dimensional genetic code. Biological molecules fold into their stable conformations in reaction to the same hydrophobic and hydrophilic forces that organize the lipid bilayer. If there were to be a secret of life as we know it, this would be it.

In quantitative terms, we can estimate the energy of a single charge in water or hydrocarbon in the following way. The **permittivity** ϵ is a measure of the polarizability of a medium. The permittivity of free space is

$$\epsilon_0 = 8.85 \times 10^{-12} \frac{\text{coulombs per meter}^2}{\text{volts per meter}} \qquad \text{(farads per meter)}$$

The permittivity of water is about 80 times that of free space, whereas that of the hydrocarbon phase in the interior of the membrane is only about two times that of free space. The energy of a charged ion in either phase can be calculated by integrating the energy required to assemble the charge q in this position from a large number of infinitesimal charges at infinity. The potential for a given accumulated charge can be calculated by integration of Equation 2.1 (p. 13) with respect to r, from infinity to the **ionic radius** r_i. The result of this integration is

$$V = \frac{q}{r_i} \frac{1}{4\pi\epsilon}$$

The potential computed in this way also is the energy per unit charge required to add an infinitesimal charge dq to the total charge. The total energy W is given by

$$W = \frac{1}{4\pi\epsilon} \int_0^q \frac{q'}{r_i} dq' = \frac{q^2}{r_i} \frac{1}{8\pi\epsilon} \tag{4.1}$$

The energy of an ion such as sodium, which has a 1-angstrom radius in water, is approximately 0.1 electron volts. In the interior of the bilayer, the energy is approximately 2.4 electron volts, which is approximately 100 kT. The difference between the two energies is an **energy barrier** that prevents ions in the aqueous phase from entering the membrane. The energy barrier is strictly the result of the difference between the polarizability of water and that of the hydrocarbon phase.

ELECTRICAL OPERATION

The energy barrier formed by the nerve membrane is so high that, at room temperature, vanishingly few ions are able to surmount it. For this reason, it is possible to treat the membrane as a perfect insulator. Any current flow through it will have to be mediated by some agent other than the bare ions in the aqueous solution on either side. It is by the manipulation of these agents that living systems achieve the gain in signal energy required for information processing. What kind of agents operate in the nerve membrane, and what operations do they perform?

Power Supply

Before there is gain, there must be a power supply. The most basic charge-transfer agents in all nerve membranes are the metabolically driven **pumps** that actively expel sodium ions from the cytoplasm and concomitantly import potassium ions from the extracellular fluid. As a result of this pumping process, the cytoplasm is enriched in potassium and depleted of sodium, whereas the converse is true of the seawater outside the cell. The concentrations of relevant ions inside and outside a nerve cell are shown in Table 4.1 [Katz, 1966 (p. 43)].

A concentration gradient of any charged particles can be used to power electrical activity. Suppose, for the moment, that the membrane is permeable to only one type of ion—potassium, for example. Due to the gradient in density, ions will diffuse out of the cell, causing a net negative charge to accumulate inside the cell. This negative charge will accumulate on the capacitance of the cell membrane, causing a negative potential in the cytoplasm relative to the

TABLE 4.1 Typical concentrations of ions inside neural processes and in the extra-cellular fluid. (*Source:* Adapted from [Katz, 1966].)

Ion*	Concentration (mM/l)		Reversal potential (mV)
	Inside	Outside	
K^+	400	10	−92
Na^+	50	460	55
Cl^-	40	540	−65

* K^+: potassium; Na^+: sodium; Cl^-: chlorine.

extracellular fluid. This situation is an exact analog to the one that created the exponential density gradient in the atmosphere in Chapter 2. The diffusion of ions outward will be exactly counterbalanced by the drift inward when the voltage across the membrane reaches the value V_r such that the relation of Equation 2.15 (p. 25) is satisfied:

$$V_r = -\frac{kT}{q} \ln \frac{N_{\text{in}}}{N_{\text{ex}}} \qquad (4.2)$$

Here N_{ex} is the ion density in the extracellular fluid, and N_{in} is the density in the cytoplasm. All voltages are referred to the extracellular fluid. If we artificially raise the potential inside the cell above (more positive than) V_r, we will cause a positive current to flow outward. If we reduce the potential inside the cell below (more negative than) V_r, we will cause a positive current to flow inward. For this reason, V_r is called the **reversal potential** for the ion at the ionic concentration ratio given in Equation 4.2. The reversal potentials for the three ionic species also are given in Table 4.1. In operational terms, we can think of the sodium reversal potential as the positive power-supply rail for the nerve, and the potassium reversal potential as the negative rail.

We should note that the concentrations shown in Table 4.1 are for the giant axon of the squid; they vary considerably among species, and even among cell types in a given organism. There is recent evidence that different regions of the same neuron may have different ionic concentrations to achieve different synaptic behavior at different but electrically related points.

Equivalent Circuit

A schematic diagram that summarizes the contribution of the three ionic

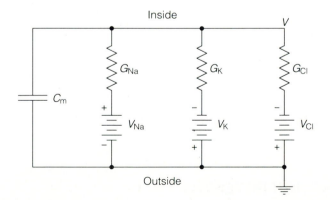

FIGURE 4.3 Equivalent circuit of a patch of nerve membrane. The batteries represent the reversal potentials for particular ions; the conductances represent the membrane permeability for the same ion. The membrane capacitance is shown as a lumped capacitor.

gradients to the membrane current is shown in Figure 4.3. From it, we can visualize the operation of the membrane over a wide range of conditions. In this diagram, the Vs are the reversal potentials of the ions, and the Gs are the conductances of the membrane for the flow of these ions. Using Figure 4.3, we can compute the membrane current I for any given cytoplasmic potential V, and for any values of ionic conductances:

$$I = (V_K - V)G_K + (V_{Na} - V)G_{Na} + (V_{Cl} - V)G_{Cl} \qquad (4.3)$$

Any net current will charge or discharge the capacitance of the membrane until the current is reduced to zero. Hodgkin et al. [Hodgkin et al., 1952b] found that, under normal conditions, the chloride current can be neglected. Making this assumption, we can solve Equation 4.3 for the voltage V_0 at which the current is zero:

$$V_0 = \frac{V_K G_K + V_{Na} G_{Na}}{G_K + G_{Na}}$$

V_0 is called the **resting potential** of the cytoplasm, because it is the potential at which the cell will come to rest if left electrically undisturbed. In a typical neuron, G_K is approximately 20 times G_{Na}. Using that value, and the concentrations given in Table 4.1, V_0 is −85 millivolts. The resting potential can vary considerably from one set of experimental conditions to another.

We have come to a solution of the first riddle in the axon story: A neuron at rest is **polarized** to a negative potential because its membrane is selectively permeable to potassium. A nerve pulse is a transient excursion of the cytoplasmic potential in a positive direction; it is an example of an **excitatory** signal because it **depolarizes** the membrane. If the membrane is charged more negatively than its resting voltage, it is said to be **hyperpolarized**, in which case the signal is **inhibitory**.

We achieve electrical activity in a patch of nerve membrane by making one or more of the ionic conductances dependent on some **control quantity**. That quantity can be the voltage (as in the axon), the concentration of a chemical substance (as in chemical synapses), the intensity of light (as in photoreceptors), or the degree of mechanical deflection (as in the hair cells in the ear). We will first see how these conductances are responsible for the generation and propagation of the action potential in an axon. In later sections, we will consider other ways that the potential inside the neuron is manipulated by the nervous system to accomplish information-processing tasks.

THE ACTION POTENTIAL

We have seen that the membrane potential can be manipulated by any agent that selectively increases the permeability of the membrane to one ionic species. How can agents of this kind be employed to initiate and propagate an action potential?

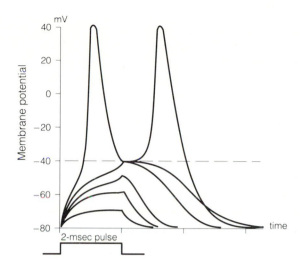

FIGURE 4.4 Response of the axon to stimulation by 2-millisecond current pulses of increasing magnitude. When the pulse drives the potential of the cytoplasm higher than −40 millivolts relative to the extracellular fluid, an action potential is generated. Once this action potential is triggered, it acquires a constant shape, independent of the circumstances under which it originated. Marginal cases result in either a delayed action potential or a delayed falling transient, as shown by the rightmost two curves. (*Source:* Adapted from [Katz, 1966].)

Initiation of the Action Potential

If we inject small pulses of current into the cytoplasm, the potential will respond as shown in Figure 4.4. For current levels that depolarize the membrane less than approximately 20 millivolts from its resting state, the potential shows a somewhat sluggish response that saturates after a few milliseconds. This type of response is characteristic of any circuit consisting of a capacitance in parallel with a conductance, as we will discuss in Chapter 8. In the case of the axon, the capacitance is that of the membrane, and the conductance is due to the potassium permeability. At higher current levels, we observe an exponential increase in the cell potential, culminating in the explosive generation of an action potential. If we terminate the current pulse before the potential has reached approximately −40 millivolts, the membrane recovers, and no pulse is generated. Once the potential is more positive than approximately −40 millivolts, however, a pulse is generated even if the driving current is terminated. That potential is therefore a **threshold**, beyond which a self-reinforcing reaction is underway, and no recovery is possible.

All the information we have presented so far was known by 1950. The key question was, *what mechanism was responsible for the self-reinforcing reaction?* That question was unraveled by the detective work for which Hodgkin and Huxley received the Nobel Prize in 1963. The giant axon of the squid is large enough

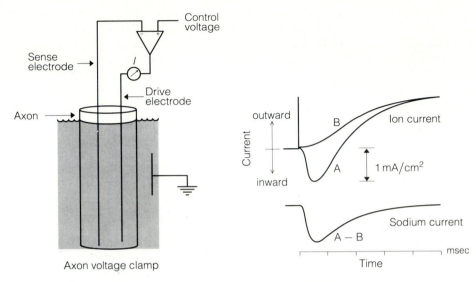

FIGURE 4.5   Schematic of the arrangement used by Hodgkin, Huxley, and Katz to measure the current through the membrane of a squid axon under conditions where the membrane potential was controlled precisely. The sense electrode assumes the potential of the cytoplasm. The amplifier generates a current *I* proportional to the difference between the actual potential and the desired potential. This current is in the direction to move the actual potential toward the desired value. The current is sensed by an oscilloscope, shown as a meter on the diagram; the extracellular fluid is ground for the entire arrangement. (*Source:* [Hodgkin et al., 1952a].)

   The waveforms shown are a simplification of records taken, using this apparatus, for a step increase in membrane potential. The initial transient is the current required to charge the membrane capacitance. Curve A is the total current as a function of time. Curve B is the potassium current alone. The difference, A − B, is thus attributed to the sodium current, which rises to a maximum and then decays.

that an insulating rod carrying two independent electrodes can be placed inside it. Hodgkin and Huxley used the voltage-clamp arrangement shown in Figure 4.5.

   When a voltage step from approximately −60 millivolts to near 0 millivolts was applied to the membrane, the current waveform labeled A in Figure 4.5 was observed. A transient *inward* current was followed by a sustained *outward* current. From Figure 4.3, we can see that there is only one source of inward-directed current—the sodium gradient. To check this conjecture, Hodgkin and Huxley replaced most of the sodium ions in the extracellular fluid with choline—large organic ions that cannot pass through the membrane. In this way, the researchers could approximately equalize the sodium concentration on the two sides of the membrane, thereby reducing the sodium reversal potential to zero and eliminating the sodium current at this voltage. Hodgkin and Huxley attributed the resulting current waveform (labeled B in Figure 4.5) to potassium. The difference between the two waveforms had to be the sodium current under normal conditions, as shown in the bottom trace in Figure 4.5.

In response to a depolarization of the membrane, there is a transient increase in the sodium conductance, followed by a delayed but prolonged increase in the potassium conductance. The currents through these conductances, acting on the capacitance of the membrane, create the action potential. Although this picture explains the qualitative shape of the action potential once the pulse is triggered, it tells us nothing about the mechanism that leads to the threshold, and to the all-or-nothing response. To understand that behavior, we must know how the conductances depend on the membrane potential.

Voltage Dependence of the Conductances

By carrying out similar experiments at several depolarizing potentials, Hodgkin and Huxley gathered data on the time course of the two currents as a function of the membrane potential. From these data, they reconstructed the time dependence of the sodium and potassium *conductances* for different membrane potentials. Plots of the peak sodium conductance and the sustained potassium conductance as functions of the membrane potential are plotted in Figure 4.6. At low current levels, both conductances are exponential functions of the membrane potential, increasing by a factor of e for every approximately 4-millivolt increase in voltage. At higher current levels, both curves saturate—altogether reminiscent of the dependence of transistor current on gate voltage shown in Figure 3.7 (p. 38). The quantitative difference between the transistor current and the nerve current is that the latter has an exponential characteristic that is six

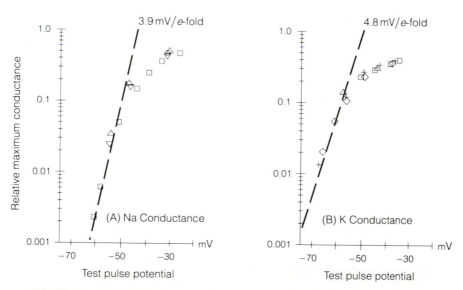

FIGURE 4.6   Exponential current–voltage characteristic of voltage-dependent channels. At high voltages, the fraction of channels that are open approaches unity, causing a saturation of the curves. (*Source:* [Hodgkin et al., 1952b, p. 464].)

times steeper than that of the former! It is this exponentially increasing current that gives the axon membrane the gain required to produce the self-reinforcing reaction leading to the all-or-nothing response.

Although Hodgkin and Huxley did not address the mechanism by which this remarkable exponential dependence comes about, their findings did allow them to reconstruct the initiation and propagation of the action potential. The summary in their 1952 paper is still the best short description of the phenomenon extant:

> *When the membrane potential is suddenly reduced (depolarization), the initial pulse of current through the capacity of the membrane is followed by large currents carried by ions (chiefly sodium and potassium), moving down their own electrochemical gradients. The current carried by sodium ions rises rapidly to a peak and then decays to a low value; that carried by potassium ions rises much more slowly along an S-shaped curve, reaching a plateau which is maintained with little change until the membrane potential is restored to its resting value.*
>
> *These two components of the membrane current are enough to account qualitatively for the propagation of an action potential, the sequence of events at each point on the nerve fibre being as follows: (1) Current from a neighbouring active region depolarizes the membrane by spread along the cable structure of the fibre ('local circuits'). (2) As a result of this depolarization, sodium current is allowed to flow. Since the external sodium concentration is several times greater than the internal, this current is directed inwards and depolarizes the membrane still further, until the membrane potential reverses its sign and approaches the value at which sodium ions are in equilibrium. (3) As a delayed result of the depolarization, the potassium current increases and the ability of the membrane to pass sodium current decreases. Since the internal potassium concentration is greater than the external, the potassium current is directed outwards. When it exceeds the sodium current, it repolarizes the membrane, raising the membrane potential to the neighbourhood of the resting potential, at which potassium ions inside and outside the fibre are near to equilibrium.* [Hodgkin et al., 1952b, p. 470]

IONIC CHANNELS

The question of electrical activity in the axon has been sharpened still further—*what is the mechanism by which the membrane conductance achieves its remarkable exponential dependence?* To find the answer, we need to take a close look at the sodium current.

Channel Conductance

A close look at the sodium current, finally captured in 1986 by Keller [Keller et al., 1986] and his coworkers, is shown in Figure 4.7. The ion-specific conductance changes in discrete steps; the height of each step is approximately linear

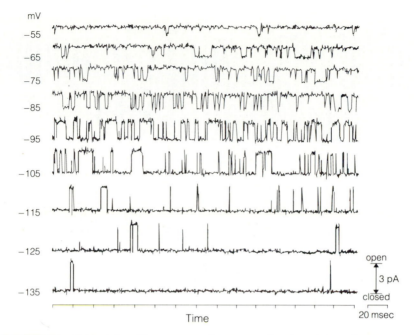

FIGURE 4.7 Current through nerve membrane as a function of time, for several membrane voltages. Upward steps are due to formation of sodium channels; downward steps are due to the channels' disappearance. The height of a single step is the current in a single channel, which increases approximately linearly with applied voltage, measured with respect to the sodium resting potential.

Several charges are pulled through the membrane when a channel is formed; hence, the average number of channels penetrating the membrane decreases exponentially with applied voltage. (*Source:* Adapted from [Keller et al., 1986].)

in the membrane potential relative to the reversal potential of the ion. At low currents, the number of steps and the width of each step are both exponential functions of the membrane potential. At any given voltage, the steps are all the same height. This remarkable finding suggests that each step is the result of an atomic action on the part of a single molecular entity. The molecular entities responsible for selective permeability of nerve membranes to specific ions are aggregates called **channels**. The channels responsible for propagating the nerve pulse in an axon are *voltage-controlled.*

Because the detailed structure has not been worked out for either the sodium or the potassium channels, we will exercise a bit of artistic license to visualize how one of these channels might operate. The result of this creative endeavor is shown in Figure 4.8.

Imagine a molecule about 50 angstroms long, with two positive charges on one end of a long hydrocarbon backbone and two negative charges on the other. The backbone is sprinkled with occasional polar groups along its length. We suppose that, in their normal stable configuration (shown in the highly schematized

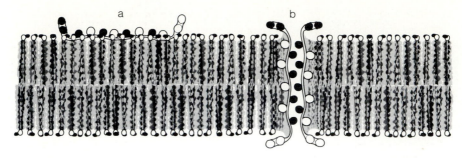

FIGURE 4.8 Cross-section of the bilayer structure of Figure 4.2 showing a conceptual model of how a voltage-controlled channel might operate. A triad of molecules can exist in two stable configurations: (a) lying flat on one surface, or (b) penetrating the membrane. Each molecule of the triad has two positive (white) charges on one end, and two negative (black) charges at the other. Six charges are carried through the membrane when the triad switches from one configuration to the other. The energy of the penetrating configuration is dependent on the voltage across the membrane, whereas that of the flat configuration is not. The fraction of triads that are in the penetrating configuration thus will be exponentially dependent on the membrane voltage. The penetrating configuration provides a tortuous path lined with negative ions—the open channel—through which a small positive ion can pass.

rendition in Figure 4.8a), triads of these molecules are lying on one surface of the membrane in the form of a triangle, the positive end of one next to the negative end of its neighbor. The hydrocarbon backbones of all three are buried in the membrane to get away from the water. A single molecule would be capable of penetrating the membrane, placing the positively charged head-group on the opposite side of the membrane from the negatively charged tail-group.

The energy of such an isolated molecule in this new conformation would be much higher than that of the molecule in the original state, because the polar groups on the hydrocarbon backbone would be directly confronted with the low-permittivity membrane center. The triad of molecules could penetrate the membrane as a group, however, each one lowering the energy that the others must pay to get through the membrane. The symbiosis would allow each molecule to turn its backbone to the membrane's hydrocarbon interior and share polar groups with the other two in the triangular space between them. This configuration of our imaginary triad (shown in Figure 4.8b) would have six elementary positive charges on one side of the membrane, and six negative charges on the other. The transition from the surface configuration to the penetrating configuration would carry six charges from one side of the membrane to the other.

If it were indeed possible to construct a triad capable of this type of behavior, many of such triads would have been tried in the long course of evolution. Some, no doubt, would have a little space running down the center through which some enterprising ion might pass, in constant contact with a polar group from one molecule or another. In other words, the penetrating configuration of the triad might function as a *channel* for ionic flow through the membrane. If the ion were too small, its energy in the center of the membrane would be too high, as per Equation 4.1. If the ion were too large, it could not fit through the space between polar groups. But an ion of just the right size might squeeze through, nicely shielded from the hostile hydrocarbon by the polar groups of the molecules in the triad. In this way, a particular molecule could form channels with a high degree of specificity for one ion.

The foregoing discussion is highly idealized, and in detail it is certainly not correct for any particular channel. It is, however, consistent in broad outline with the known properties of voltage-dependent channels. A detailed discussion of the known properties of channels can be found in Hille [Hille, 1984].

Voltage-Dependent Conductance

We can analyze the voltage dependence of the triads described in the previous section using a **two-state model**. Let us call the penetrating configuration the **open state,** and the surface configuration the **closed state**, of the triad. The two states have different energies; a transition from one state to the other will be associated with a **transition energy** E_t. The transition from the closed to the open state transports charges through the membrane, so the transition energy is voltage-dependent. The energy is lowered by the number of **gating charges** n transported through the membrane by the formation of the channel, times the potential V across the membrane:

$$E_t = E_0 - Vnq$$

where E_0 is the transition energy at zero membrane voltage.

Suppose there are N total triads associated with a particular membrane, and that, at a given time, N_c of them are closed and N_o of them are open. Recall the Boltzmann distribution of Chapter 2, from Equation 2.16 (p. 25) we know that

$$\frac{N_o}{N_c} = e^{-E_t/(kT)} \tag{4.4}$$

Because $N_o + N_c = N$, we can write Equation 4.4 in terms of the fraction $\theta = N_o/N$ of channels in the open state:

$$\frac{\theta}{1 - \theta} = e^{-E_0/(kT)} e^{qnV/(kT)}$$

For θ much less than 1, the θ in the denominator will be negligible and the number of open channels will be an exponential function of the membrane voltage V. The average conductance of the membrane as a whole is the number of open channels multiplied by the conductance of each channel. For high values of V, θ will saturate at 1, all the channels will be open, and the conductance of the membrane will saturate, exactly as shown by the experimental data in Figure 4.6.

By this mechanism, the conductance for a given ion can be made to depend exponentially on the membrane potential. The dependence is very steep, because a number of gating charges is involved in the reaction that opens the channel. For Figure 4.6, taken from the giant axon of the squid, there are approximately six gating charges involved. Recent work on the node of Ranvier of the frog suggests that two molecules form a channel in that system [DuBois et al., 1983]. The voltage dependence of Figure 4.7 gives approximately four gating charges. It thus seems that vertebrates employ a channel formed of two molecules, each carrying two charges through the membrane. If the charges in the reaction do not go all the way through the membrane, the energy they contribute is only a fraction of qV, and hence noninteger quantities often are observed.

The exponential dependence of conductance on membrane potential is a result of the behavior of the *population of channels*, rather than of the conduction property of any given channel. A close look at the current in Figure 4.7 reveals a discrete increase in current as each channel opens, and an equal decrease as each channel closes. The size of an individual step is roughly linear in the difference between the membrane voltage and the reversal potential for the selected ion, indicating that an individual channel is **ohmic** (current proportional to voltage). The rate at which channels open increases, and the rate at which they close decreases, with voltage. Both dependencies are exponential, and can be seen clearly in Figure 4.7. The number of channels open at any time is a result of the balance of these two processes.[2]

The exponential current–voltage relation in the nerve is a result of the same physical laws responsible for the exponential transistor characteristic. There is an energy barrier between a state in which current can flow and one in which current cannot flow. The height of that barrier is dependent on a control voltage. The Boltzmann distribution determines the fraction of the total population that is in the conducting state. In the transistor, the electrons in the channel form the population in question, and these same electrons carry the current. In the nerve membrane, the channels form the population in question, and ions in the channels carry the current. In both cases, the number of individual charges in transit is exponential in the control voltage, and the transport of these charges results in a current that varies exponentially with the control voltage.

COMPUTATION

We have traced the ideas elucidated in one of the great endeavors in intellectual history; in the process, we have learned a great deal about the electrical machinery in the neuron. At one time, people might have supposed that understanding the action potential would be the key that would unlock a full

---

[2] This mechanism by which very steep exponentials can be created by a population of individual ohmic channels was first worked through quantitatively for the antibiotic alamethicin in artificial bilayer membranes [Eisenberg et al., 1973]. The technology for similar quantitative work for real nerve channels in natural membranes has become available only recently. A quantitative model of sodium channels from the node of Ranvier in the frog is given by DuBois and colleagues. [DuBois et al., 1983].

understanding of neural information processing in the brain. It is now clear that, although we have a good understanding of how the nervous system *transmits* information over large distances, this knowledge does not shed much light on how the information is *computed.* We have yet to find a single unifying principle in neural computation that shines with the same clarity as the axon story does; that work is ahead of us. The balance of this book describes one approach (of many) to a deeper understanding of the basic principles underlying neural computation. This quest will require the work of specialists in many fields over many years.

A few comments may serve to render our task a bit less daunting. Computation in neural systems uses the same kind of machinery that we have already encountered in the axon story. Once we can control the ionic conductances, we can manipulate the resting potential of the membrane. An increase in sodium conductance depolarizes the membrane, and is the action responsible for initiation of a nerve pulse. An increase in potassium conductance can hyperpolarize the membrane, and hence acts as an inhibitory influence.

If the chloride reversal potential is near the resting potential, as is often the case, an increase in chloride conductance will not have much effect on the potential of the membrane, but can decrease the effect of either a sodium or a potassium conductance by requiring more current for a given excursion in potential. This reduction in the sensitivity of the membrane by increasing its conductance to the resting potential is called **shunting inhibition**.

These and other methods of manipulating the membrane potential operate in the richly branched tree of dendrites to produce the complex interaction of electrical and chemical signals that is *neural computation.* Interactions in the dendritic tree can all work in a continuous analog fashion, as indicated by Equation 4.3. They neither require nerve pulses for their operation, nor necessarily result in the generation of a nerve pulse. In fact, the vast majority of computation in the nervous system is done with slowly varying analog potentials in the dendritic trees of neurons. These signals come about through the actions of synaptic contacts with other neurons. The result of the computation may or may not ever be converted into an action potential to be transmitted to the far reaches of the brain.

The synapses provide an entirely new class of function in dendritic computations. We can say that the synapse is to computation what the voltage-controlled channel is to communication. The story of the synapse is still being worked out, and the following section gives only the briefest account of this fascinating and rapidly evolving field.

SYNAPSES

We have seen how the *potential across a nerve membrane* can cause an *exponential change in current through the same membrane.* This action is appropriate for the propagation of an action potential, but is not sufficient for general compu-

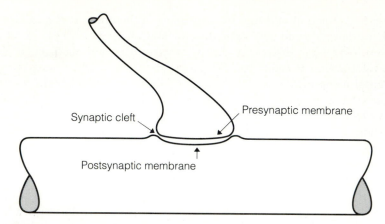

FIGURE 4.9 Simplified sketch of a synapse. Depolarization of the presynaptic membrane results in neurotransmitter release. Neurotransmitter diffuses across the synaptic cleft, resulting in the opening of receptor channels in the postsynaptic membrane. Postsynaptic current flows from the cytoplasm to the extracellular fluid.

tation. What we need is the ability to control the *conductance through a second membrane*. The ability to control the current into or out of one electrical node by the potential on another node is the key ingredient that makes all information processing possible. This capability results in a natural *direction* in the flow of information; in neural systems, it is provided by *synapses*. These specialized structures are the central information-processing devices in neural systems.

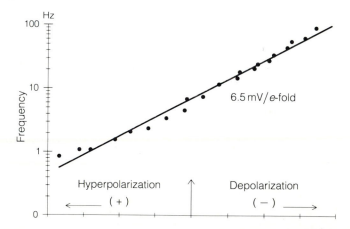

FIGURE 4.10 Exponential dependence of postsynaptic current on presynaptic membrane potential. The frequency of miniature end-plate potentials (plotted vertically) is a measure of current through the postsynaptic membrane. The current is extremely noisy, due to the quantal nature of neurotransmitter release. The solid line is an exponential fit to the experimental data (filled circles). (*Source:* Adapted from [Shepherd, 1979].)

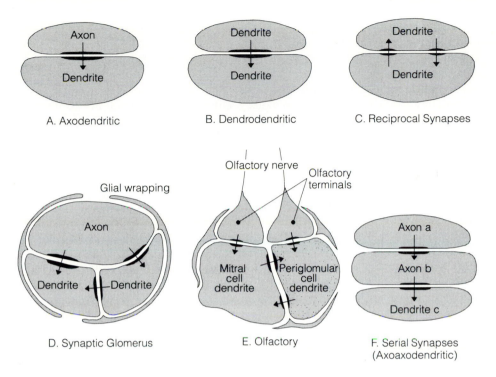

FIGURE 4.11 Examples of synaptic microcircuits by which neural processes interact. Structures of this kind are found in many parts of the nervous system, indicating that much of the neural computation is local in nature. (*Source:* Adapted from [Shepherd, 1979].)

A drawing depicting a typical synaptic arrangement is shown in Figure 4.9. The function of a synapse is to control the conductance of the membrane separating the interior of the postsynaptic cell from the extracellular fluid. That conductance is controlled by the potential across the presynaptic membrane. The detailed mechanism by which synapses operate is extremely interesting, and will no doubt be the subject of study for many years. We will present here only the essential principles of synapse operation. There are several excellent reviews of the subject at various levels of detail [Shepherd, 1979].

Inside the presynaptic membrane is a high concentration of specific **neurotransmitter** molecules. When the presynaptic membrane is depolarized, calcium channels allow calcium ions (Ca^{2+}) to flow into the presynaptic cell from the synaptic cleft. The calcium ions activate the subcellular machinery that causes release of neurotransmitter molecules into the synaptic cleft, where these molecules diffuse to the postsynaptic membrane and initiate a chain of events that results in the opening of ion-specific channels. The quantity of neurotransmitter released, and therefore the change in conductance of the postsynaptic membrane, is an exponential function of the presynaptic potential, as shown in Figure 4.10.

If the channels opened by the neurotransmitter are specific for sodium, for example, a depolarization of the presynaptic membrane will result in a depolarization of the postsynaptic membrane, and the synapse is said to be **excitatory.** If the neurotransmitter leads to the opening of potassium-specific channels, the postsynaptic membrane will be hyperpolarized, and the synapse is said to be **inhibitory**. As we have noted previously, chloride channels can act to increase the conductance of the membrane without appreciable change in potential—synapses leading to this behavior are called **shunting**. Within these broad categories, many variations are possible. In addition, synapses are known that open channels for molecules other than sodium, potassium, or chloride. We shall not discuss any of these complexities here.

A single synapse is the neural counterpart of a transistor. The tip of every neural process ends in a synapse, and there are many synaptic contacts along the branches of the dendritic tree as well. As in electronic computational machinery, synapses occur not in isolation, but rather in *circuit arrangements*. Dendrites form a wide variety of synaptic connections with dendrites and axons of other neurons. The specialization of function of the many areas in the nervous system is largely a result of these synaptic circuit arrangements. Cross-sections through several representative synaptic structures are shown in Figure 4.11. Specific circuits for many parts of the brain are discussed in Gordon Shepherd's excellent book *The Synaptic Organization of the Brain* [Shepherd, 1979]. In addition, a lucid popular account has appeared in *Scientific American* [Shepherd, 1978]. Many of these arrangements have (not altogether by accident) parallels in circuits we will discuss in subsequent chapters.

REFERENCES

DuBois, J.M., Schneider, M.F., and Khodorov, B.I. Voltage dependence of intramembrane charge movement and conductance activation of batrachotoxin-modified sodium channels in frog node of Ranvier. *Journal of General Physiology,* 81:829, 1983.

Eisenberg, M., Hall, J.E., and Mead, C.A. The nature of the voltage-dependent conductance induced by alamethicin in black lipid membranes. *Journal of Membrane Biology,* 14:143, 1973.

Hille, B. *Ionic Channels of Excitable Membranes.* Sunderland, MA: Sinauer Associates, 1984.

Hodgkin, A.L., Huxley, A.F., and Katz, B. Measurement of current–voltage relations in the membrane of the giant axon of Loligo. *Journal of Physiology,* 116:424, 1952a.

Hodgkin, A.L. and Huxley, A.F. Current carried by sodium and potassium ions through the membrane of the giant axon of Loligo. *Journal of Physiology,* 116:449, 1952b.

Hodgkin, A.L. and Huxley, A.F. The components of membrane conductance in the giant axon of Loligo. *Journal of Physiology,* 116:473, 1952c.

Hodgkin, A.L. and Huxley, A.F. The dual effect of membrane potential on sodium conductance in the giant axon of Loligo. *Journal of Physiology,* 116:497, 1952d.

Katz, B. *Nerve, Muscle, and Synapse.* New York: McGraw-Hill, 1966.

Keller, B.U., Hartshorne, R.P., Talvenheimo, J.A., Catterall, W.A., and Montal, M. Sodium channels in planar lipid bilayers. *Journal of General Physiology.* 88:1, 1986.

Shepherd, G.M. Microcircuits in the nervous system. *Scientific American,* 238(2):93, February 1978.

Shepherd, G.M. *The Synaptic Organization of the Brain.* 2nd ed., New York: Oxford University Press, 1979.

STATIC FUNCTIONS

To accumulate characters in stable and coherent aggregates, life has to be very clever indeed. Not only has it to invent the machine but, like an engineer, so design it that it occupies the minimum space and is simple and resilient.

— Teilhard de Chardin   *The Phenomenon of Man* (1955)

5

TRANSCONDUCTANCE AMPLIFIER

In this chapter, we will discuss our first circuit. It is the most important circuit that we will treat, because we will use it for almost everything we do. The circuit is called the transconductance amplifier. We will explain how it works and examine some of its characteristics.

This amplifier is a device that generates as its output a current that is a function of the difference between two input voltages, V_1 and V_2; that difference is called the **differential input** voltage. The circuit is called a **differential transconductance amplifier**. An ordinary *conductance* turns a voltage difference across two terminals into a current through the *same* two terminals. A *transconductance* turns a voltage difference *somewhere* into a current *somewhere else*. In the transconductance amplifier, a voltage difference between two inputs creates a current as the output.

DIFFERENTIAL PAIR

Many circuits take an input signal represented as a *difference between two voltages*. These circuits all use some variant of the **differential pair** shown in Figure 5.1 as an input stage. Because the differential pair is so universally useful, we will analyze its characteristics here; then we will show how it is used in the transconductance amplifier.

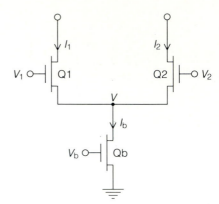

FIGURE 5.1   Schematic of the differential pair. The bias current I_b is set by the bias voltage V_b, and is divided between I_1 and I_2 depending on the difference between V_1 and V_2.

The bottom transistor Qb is used as a current source; under normal circumstances, its drain voltage V is large enough that the drain current I_b is saturated at a value set by the gate voltage V_b. The manner in which I_b is divided between Q1 and Q2 is a sensitive function of the difference between V_1 and V_2, and is the essence of the operation of the stage.

From Equation 3.15 (p. 39), we know that the saturated drain current I_{sat} is exponential in the gate and source voltages

$$I_{\mathrm{sat}} = I_0 e^{\kappa V_g - V_s}$$

Applying this expression to Q1 and Q2, we obtain

$$I_1 = I_0 e^{\kappa V_1 - V} \qquad \text{and} \qquad I_2 = I_0 e^{\kappa V_2 - V} \tag{5.1}$$

The sum of the two drain currents must be equal to I_b:

$$I_b = I_1 + I_2 = I_0 e^{-V} \left(e^{\kappa V_1} + e^{\kappa V_2} \right)$$

We can solve this equation for the voltage V:

$$e^{-V} = \frac{I_b}{I_0} \frac{1}{e^{\kappa V_1} + e^{\kappa V_2}} \tag{5.2}$$

Substituting Equation 5.2 into Equation 5.1, we obtain expressions for the two drain currents:

$$I_1 = I_b \frac{e^{\kappa V_1}}{e^{\kappa V_1} + e^{\kappa V_2}} \qquad \text{and} \qquad I_2 = I_b \frac{e^{\kappa V_2}}{e^{\kappa V_1} + e^{\kappa V_2}} \tag{5.3}$$

If V_1 is more positive than V_2 by many $kT/(q\kappa)$, transistor Q2 gets turned off, so essentially all the current goes through Q1, I_1 is approximately equal to I_b, and I_2 is approximately equal to 0. Conversely, if V_2 is more positive than V_1 by many $kT/(q\kappa)$, Q1 gets turned off, I_2 is approximately equal to I_b, and I_1 is approximately equal to 0. The two currents out of a differential pair are shown as a function of $V_1 - V_2$ in Figure 5.2.

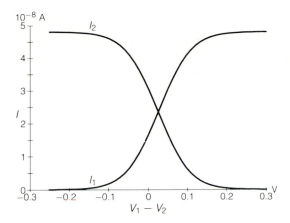

FIGURE 5.2   Output currents of the differential pair as a function of differential input voltage. The sum of the two currents is equal to the bias current I_b. The curves do not cross at zero input-voltage difference due to mismatch between Q1 and Q2.

The differential transconductance amplifier, like many other circuits that we will study, uses various kinds of current mirrors to generate an output current that is proportional to the difference between the two drain currents. This difference is

$$I_1 - I_2 = I_b \frac{e^{\kappa V_1} - e^{\kappa V_2}}{e^{\kappa V_1} + e^{\kappa V_2}} \tag{5.4}$$

Multiplying both the numerator and denominator of Equation 5.4 by $e^{-(V_1+V_2)/2}$, we can express every exponent in terms of voltage differences. The result is

$$I_1 - I_2 = I_b \frac{e^{\kappa(V_1-V_2)/2} - e^{-\kappa(V_1-V_2)/2}}{e^{\kappa(V_1-V_2)/2} + e^{-\kappa(V_1-V_2)/2}}$$

$$= I_b \tanh \frac{\kappa(V_1 - V_2)}{2} \tag{5.5}$$

The tanh is one of the few functions in the world that displays truly civilized behavior. It goes through the origin with unity slope, becomes $+1$ for large positive arguments, and becomes -1 for large negative arguments. How about the factor of two in the denominator of Equation 5.5—where did it come from? Let us examine what happens when only small changes are made in V_1 and V_2. We increase V_1 and decrease V_2 such that V is kept constant. The current through Q2 goes down exponentially and the current through Q1 goes up exponentially. The difference in voltages, however, is twice as large as V_2 relative to V, or as V_1 relative to V. That is why the curves of Figure 5.2 take twice as much voltage to saturate as do the single transistor curves in Chapter 3; this is the origin of the factor of two in Equation 5.5.

SIMPLE TRANSCONDUCTANCE AMPLIFIER

The schematic for the transconductance amplifier is shown in Figure 5.3. The circuit consists of a differential pair and a single current mirror, like the one shown in Figure 3.9 (p. 40), which is used to subtract the drain currents I_1 and I_2. The current I_1 drawn out of Q3 is reflected as an equal current out of Q4; the output current is thus equal to $I_1 - I_2$, and is therefore given by Equation 5.5.

We can measure the current out of the amplifier as a function of the input voltages using the setup shown in Figure 5.4. We are using a current meter with its primary input connected to the amplifier output and its *reference input* connected to a voltage source V_{out}. A perfect current meter has zero resistance; real current meters have sophisticated feedback arrangements to make their input resistances very small. For that reason, the voltage on the output node of the amplifier will be V_{out}. For now, we will simply set V_{out} in the midrange between V_{DD} and ground. In later sections, we will investigate the effect of V_{out} on the performance of the circuit.

The current out of the simple amplifier is plotted as a function of $V_1 - V_2$ in Figure 5.5. The curve is very close to a tanh, as expected. We can determine the effective value of $kT/(q\kappa)$ by extrapolating the slope of the curve at

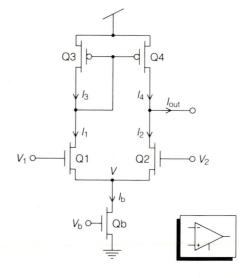

FIGURE 5.3 Schematic diagram of the simple transconductance amplifier. The current mirror formed by Q3 and Q4 is used to form the output current, which is equal to $I_1 - I_2$. The symbol used for the circuit is shown in the inset.

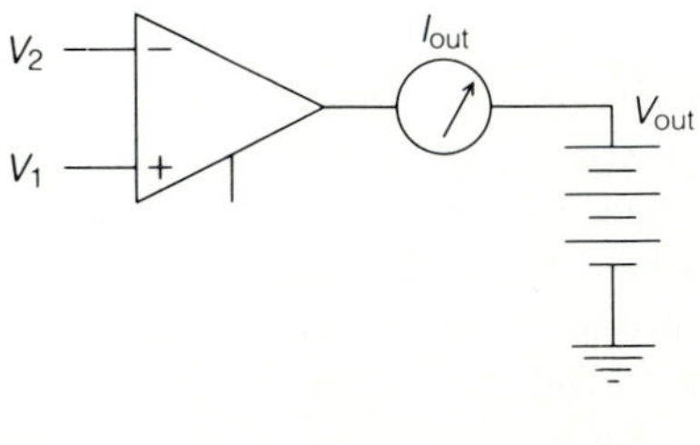

FIGURE 5.4 Arrangement for measuring the output current of the transconductance amplifier. The circuit of Figure 5.3 is represented symbolically.

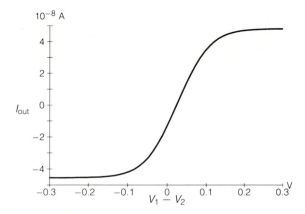

FIGURE 5.5 Output current of the transconductance amplifier as a function of differential input voltage. The mismatch between transistor characteristics can be seen in two ways. For this particular amplifier, the input offset voltage is approximately 25 millivolts, typical for a digital CMOS process. The limiting current for positive inputs is approximately 6 percent larger than that for negative inputs; a more typical variation would be 20 percent.

the origin to the two asymptotes. The difference between the positive and negative intercepts should be $4kT/(q\kappa)$. Using this procedure on Figure 5.5, we obtain the result that $kT/(q\kappa)$ is approximately 43 millivolts, giving κ as approximately 0.58. This value is in good agreement with that obtained from the voltage dependence of the saturation current (Figure 3.7 (p. 38)). The **transconductance** G_m of the amplifier is just the slope of the tanh in Equation 5.5 at the origin. For Figure 5.5, the output current changes 5.6×10^{-8} amp for a 100-millivolt change in $V_\mathrm{in} = V_1 - V_2$. G_m is therefore 5.6×10^{-7} mho. In terms of the circuit variables,

$$G_\mathrm{m} = \frac{\partial I_\mathrm{out}}{\partial V_\mathrm{in}} = \frac{I_\mathrm{b}}{2kT/(q\kappa)} \qquad (5.6)$$

Notice that the transconductance is proportional to the bias current I_b, a fact that will become important when the differential circuit is used to produce a voltage-type output, or as part of a multiplier.

The layout of a typical implementation of the simple amplifier is shown in Plate 7(a).

CIRCUIT LIMITATIONS

Now that we know how an ideal transconductance amplifier works, we can investigate the limitations and imperfect behavior of such circuits in the real world. Deviations from ideal behavior are of two basic sorts:

1. Mismatch between transistors

2. Deviation of a transistor from perfect current–source behavior; this second class of nonideality manifests itself in two ways:

    a. Voltage limitations due to transistors coming out of saturation

    b. Finite slope of the drain curves in saturation

Transistor Mismatch

Unlike people in the United States, not all transistors are created equal. Some are created with higher values of I_0 than are others. The effects of differences of I_0 between transistors can be seen in Figure 5.5. The circuit from which these data were taken is typical: The tanh curve is shifted by about 25 millivolts. In addition, the saturated current coming out of Q4 is not the same as the current coming out of Q2. In other words, the negative asymptote is not the same as the positive asymptote. In Figure 5.5, the difference is about 6 percent.

The Q3–Q4 current mirror does not have 100-percent reflectivity. What we take out of Q3 does not necessarily come out of Q4, because Q4 may have a slightly larger or smaller value of I_0 than does Q3. Differences of a factor of two between I_0 values of nominally identical transistors are observed in circuits such as this. A more typical number for transistors that are physically adjacent is ± 20 percent, corresponding to a difference in gate voltage of ± 10 millivolts.

Note that the difference across a whole chip is not much bigger than a difference between two reasonably closely spaced transistors. The I_0 variation occurs on a small distance scale. For this reason, putting transistors physically close to one another will not eliminate the problem.

One of the things we will emphasize in this book is that we can design circuits in a manner such that these variations *can* be tolerated. The voltage difference matters in some applications; it does not matter in others. It is a good habit not to trust the transistors to be closer than a factor of two in current (approximately ± 30 millivolts in gate voltage). We will try to build circuits that will work in any application given this limitation. The best way to ensure that a circuit will tolerate such variations is to have it **self-compensate** for the voltage offsets.

Self-compensation has another advantage: As circuits age and change and shift with time, the system tunes itself up. More important, in the kinds of applications we will be examining (such as vision and hearing) the systems *must* be self-adjusting. Because we have no idea what the input signals will be, the circuit had better be self-adjusting for whatever operating conditions it encounters.

Output-Voltage Limitation

One small detail we have not mentioned is where the current I_{out} goes. To understand the circuit, we have to be more specific about the I_{out} destination: I_{out} goes into a current meter so that we can measure it. That current meter may be fictitious (invented so that we can reason about the next circuit that we are driving), or it may be a real. In either case, the other end of the meter is at some voltage, which we call V_{out}. This voltage is imposed by the circuit into which this output is fed.

When we construct large integrated systems, it is important that we realize how few *primary inputs* there are compared with the enormous number of interconnections in the computing machinery itself. A 1988 chip may contain approximately 10^6 interconnected transistors in a 40-pin package. The entire auditory system in the brain is stimulated with only two audio input channels. The human visual system, which occupies 40 percent of the brain, is driven by the light impinging on the retina through two small lenses. For this reason, the internal rules of processing, whether of brain or of chip, can (in fact *must*) be made to facilitate the computation process. Interfaces to the outside world will be handled as exceptions.

Thus, from a practical point of view, we should assume that all inputs come from some other circuit, and all outputs go to some other circuit. For the system to work, the preceding circuit had to have an opinion, and the next circuit will certainly have an opinion. The preceding circuit generates the input, and the next circuit receives the output. We have to do something with I_{out}: dump it into a capacitor, for example, or hook it into a current mirror. What we do with it depends on what we are building.

Our first question is: How far we can trust this current I_{out} to be independent of V_{out}? For unlimited variation in V_{out}, the answer is: not at all. Nothing has unlimited range. There is, however, a range of output voltages over which the output current will be nearly constant. For the circuit of Figure 5.3, a plot of the variation of I_{out} as a function of V_{out} for fixed values of V_1 and V_2 is shown in Figure 5.6. There is an upper limit near V_{DD}, where the output current increases rapidly. There also is a lower limit, below which the output current decreases rapidly. In between, the current is not independent of output voltage, but it has a near-constant slope corresponding to a **finite output conductance**. We will discuss the two limits first; then we will examine the effect of the slope in the middle.

Upper limit   We should not expect (or desire) this device to be able to put out a constant current at voltages larger than V_{DD} or smaller than zero. That limitation is important; it means that the circuit cannot generate for the next stage a voltage that is outside those limits. If we raise the output voltage above V_{DD}, the drain of Q4 becomes the source, and we start draining current out of the ammeter down through Q4 to V_{DD}. Q4 will be turned on, because the voltage on its gate is less than V_{DD}—because that voltage is generated by Q3. Even if Q1 is turned off, the worst that can happen is that the voltage on the gate of Q4 will approach V_{DD}. So, if V_{out} gets a few tenths of a volt above V_{DD}, we will start to get an exponential negative increase in I_{out}.

Lower limit   The lower limit to V_{out} is a little more tricky. First, let us consider the case where V_1 is greater than V_2 by several $kT/(q\kappa)$. Under these conditions, V is approximately equal to $\kappa(V_1 - V_{\text{b}})$, I_2 is approximately equal to 0, and I_{out}

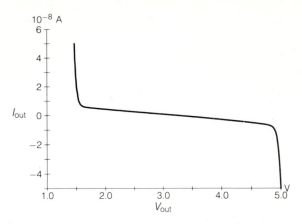

FIGURE 5.6 Dependence of output current of the simple transconductance amplifier on output voltage. The exponential dependencies at the ends are due to the high (V_{DD}) and low (V_{min}) limits discussed in the text. The slope in the midrange, due to the nonzero drain conductance of the output transistors Q2 and Q4, is the output conductance of the amplifier. The curve shown is for V_1 approximately equal to V_2; input-voltage differences cause the entire curve to shift up or down, according to the relationship shown in Figure 5.5.

is positive, approximately equal to I_4. As we lower the output voltage, all is well until V_{out} decreases to less than V, after which the output node becomes the *source* of Q2, and the V node becomes the *drain*. The interchange of source and drain of Q2 results in a reversal of current through Q2—I_2 becomes negative instead of positive. The reversal occurs when V_{out} is equal to $\kappa(V_1 - V_b)$, but is not noticeable in the output current until V_{out} is approximately equal to $\kappa(V_2 - V_b)$, where I_2 becomes comparable with I_1. A further decrease in output voltage results in an exponential increase in I_{out}, because the gate–source voltage of Q2 is increasing. This negative I_2 is supplied by an increase in I_1, which results in an equal increase in output current through Q4. The output current thus increases from two equal contributions of the same sign.

If V_2 is greater than V_1 by several $kT/(q\kappa)$, the same effect can be observed. The output current is negative, and V is equal to $\kappa(V_2 - V_b)$. As we decrease the output voltage, we make the voltage between the source and the drain of Q2 smaller and smaller, Q2 comes out of saturation, and V begins to decrease. As both V_{out} and V decrease, the gate–source voltage of Q2 increases, causing Q2 to conduct more current. The voltage V follows V_{out} more and more closely. There is no noticeable change in output current, however, until V approaches $\kappa(V_1 - V_b)$, at which point the current through Q1 becomes comparable to I_b. As we decrease the voltage at the output node further, I_1 exceeds I_b, and V does not decrease as fast as does V_{out}. Once V is greater than V_{out}, the drain and source of Q2 are interchanged, and the situation is exactly as it was for V_2 greater than V_1. Transistor Q2 starts siphoning charge away from the V node, and the output current increases exponentially.

We call the limitation on the operation of the simple transconductance amplifier imposed by this behavior the "V_{min} problem." We can express the minimum output voltage as

$$V_{min} = \kappa\big(\min(V_1, V_2) - V_b\big) \qquad (5.7)$$

In other words, the amplifier will work with its output voltage up to nearly V_{DD}, and down to V_b below the lowest input signal that we have applied to it, but not lower than that.

We run into two walls, one on the top and one on the bottom. The wall on the top side is not serious; all it does is to prevent us from going right up to V_{DD}. When V_1 is greater than V_2, the current comes out of Q4—so, if we make the output node equal to V_{DD}, we will not get any current out. We cannot quite work up against the rail, but we can get very close. The upper limit on the output voltage is set by the saturation properties of Q4. As long as we stay a few $kT/(q\kappa)$ below V_{DD}, we are fine.

The bottom V_{min} limit is much more serious. It is the biggest problem with this circuit. It forms a *hard limit* below which the circuit does not work, and that limit depends on the input voltage.

VOLTAGE OUTPUT

We call these circuits "transconductance amplifiers" because that is the way in which they are usually used. They also can be used, however, to take a difference in voltage at the input and turn it into a voltage at the output. Instead of measuring I_{out} with an ammeter, we measure V_{out} with a voltmeter. The drain conductances of Q2 and Q4 are used to convert the output current into an output voltage.

The drain current of a transistor is not completely independent of its drain voltage, even in saturation. There is a finite slope of I_d versus V_d given by the **Early effect**, discussed in Appendix B. This effect is responsible for the dependence of output current on output voltage seen between the two limits in Figure 5.6.

The finite output conductance of the circuit can be used to convert the current-type output signal into a voltage-type signal. We take away the V_{out} voltage source completely, and use a voltmeter instead of an ammeter. An ideal voltmeter draws no current from the circuit it is measuring. It is an ideal open-circuit, having zero input conductance (infinite input resistance). The input conductances of real voltmeters vary over many orders of magnitude. A good electrometer has an input resistance greater than 10^{12} ohm; ordinary voltmeters can have resistances many orders of magnitude less. A typical oscilloscope has an input resistance of 10^6 ohm. We must always check that the current drawn by our measuring equipment is small compared with the current flowing in the circuit. Using a good voltmeter, we can observe the voltage at which the output current is equal to zero. That is the **open-circuit output voltage** of the device.

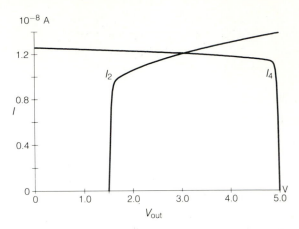

FIGURE 5.7   Current out of the n-channel (Q2) and p-channel (Q4) output transistors of a simple transconductance amplifier, as a function of output voltage, for V_1 approximately equal to V_2. The output current is the difference between the two curves; therefore, the open-circuit output voltage is given by the intersection of these curves.

Consider the combination of Q4 and Q2. In Figure 5.7, we plot the magnitude of I_4 and I_2 versus the output voltage. Current is flowing down from V_{DD} to ground—I_4 is flowing *into* the output node, and I_2 is flowing *out of* the output node. For any given output voltage, the output current is the difference between the two curves. For any particular input voltages, the value of V_{min} will be somewhat below the lowest input—for the operating conditions shown in Figure 5.7, I_2 goes to zero when V_{out} is approximately equal to V_{min}. Because Q4 is a p-channel device, its drain voltage is plotted downward from V_{DD}. The open-circuit voltage is the value at which the two currents are equal; *open-circuit* means *no current*.

We can easily see what the output voltage would do as a function of a difference in the input voltages, if the drain curves for Q2 and Q4 were absolutely flat. When V_1 is a little less than V_2, the output voltage will decrease to nearly V_{min}; when V_1 is a little bigger than V_2, the voltage will increase to almost V_{DD}. The experimental dependence of V_{out} on V_1, for several values of V_2, is shown in Figure 5.8. The output voltage stays at 5 volts until V_1 gets very close to V_2, then it drops rapidly to V_{min}. The sloping line where all curves merge is thus V_{min}.

Instead of an infinite slope in the transition region, which would correspond to infinite gain, which corresponds to output transistors that have zero drain conductance, the actual circuit has a finite slope as a result of its real transistors, which have finite drain conductance.

Voltage Gain

The **voltage gain** A is defined as $\partial V_{out}/\partial V_{in}$, where V_{in} is equal to $V_1 - V_2$. An enlargement of the steep part of the V_2 at 2.5 volt curve in Figure 5.8 is

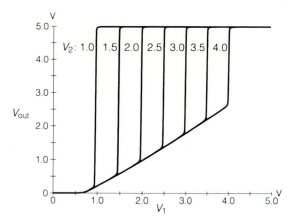

FIGURE 5.8 Open-circuit output voltage of the simple transconductance amplifier as a function of V_1, for several values of V_2. The steep part of the curves occur at V_1 approximately equal to V_2. The sloping lower limit of the output is due to the V_{min} problem.

shown in Figure 5.9. The maximum gain is approximately 143. We can easily compute what the gain of this circuit should be by considering the properties of the output transistors.

An enlargement of the intersection of the Q2 and Q4 drain curves in Figure 5.7 is shown in Figure 5.10. For a certain input-voltage difference, the curves are marked I_2 and I_4. When the input-voltage difference is increased by Δv, both curves change: I_2 decreases to I_2', and I_4 increases to I_4'. Because the bias current I_b is constant, an increase ΔI in I_4 due to a change in input voltage will result in an equal decrease ΔI in I_2, as shown. The total change in output current per unit change in input-voltage difference was defined in Equation 5.6 as the transconductance G_m of the circuit.

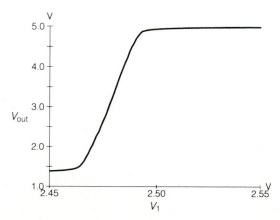

FIGURE 5.9 Expanded view of the center curve (V_2 equal to 2.5 volts) of Figure 5.8.

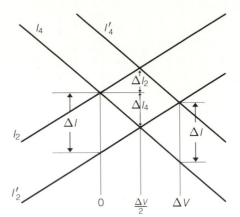

FIGURE 5.10 Expanded view of the intersection of the two curves of Figure 5.7 for two slightly different input voltages. The dependence of output voltage on transistor currents and drain conductances is obtained from the construction shown.

From Figure 5.6, we have seen that the output current *decreases* as the output voltage *increases*. The decrease in the output current per unit change in the output voltage is called the **output conductance** of the circuit.

$$G_{\text{out}} = -\frac{\partial I_{\text{out}}}{\partial V_{\text{out}}} = \frac{\partial I_2}{\partial V_{\text{out}}} - \frac{\partial I_4}{\partial V_{\text{out}}} \tag{5.8}$$

This quantity is the negative of the slope of the central region of Figure 5.6. The output conductance is just the sum of the contributions due to the two output transistors. In Figure 5.6, the output current changes 3.6×10^{-9} amp for a 1 volt change in output voltage. Thus, G_{out} is approximately 3.6×10^{-9} mho.

When the output is open-circuited, the total *increase* $2\Delta I$ in output current due to an increase Δv in input voltage difference is compensated by an equal *decrease* in output current due to the increase ΔV in the output voltage.

$$2\Delta I = \frac{\partial I_{\text{out}}}{\partial V_{\text{in}}} \Delta v = -\frac{\partial I_{\text{out}}}{\partial V_{\text{out}}} \Delta V \tag{5.9}$$

Substituting Equation 5.6 and Equation 5.8 into Equation 5.9, we obtain the open-circuit voltage gain $A = \Delta V / \Delta v$.

$$A = \frac{G_{\text{m}}}{G_{\text{out}}}$$

From the values of G_{m} and G_{out} measured on the simple transconductance circuit, the open-circuit voltage gain should be

$$\frac{5.6 \times 10^{-7}}{3.6 \times 10^{-9}} = 148$$

The result is in good agreement with the measured gain of 143.

In Appendix B, we derive the slope of the transistor drain curve in saturation. The slope of the saturated part of the drain curves of a given transistor has a slope proportional to the current level. In other words, the intercept on the V_{ds}

axis occurs at a voltage V_0 that is approximately independent of the absolute current level:

$$\frac{\partial I_{\text{sat}}}{\partial V_{\text{ds}}} \approx \frac{I_{\text{sat}}}{V_0}$$

V_0 is called the **Early voltage** for the transistor. For open-circuit operation, the steep part of the curves of Figure 5.8 will occur when the current through the two output transistors is equal, and therefore is half of the bias current I_b. Thus, *the output conductance of the amplifier is proportional to the bias current I_b.* The transconductance also is proportional to the bias current (Equation 5.6).

Because both G_m and G_{out} are proportional to the bias current, the explicit dependence on current level cancels out and *the voltage gain is independent of bias current.* We can express the $\partial I / \partial V$ terms in Equation 5.8 in terms of the V_0 values (V_N for Q2 and V_P for Q4):

$$\frac{1}{A} = \left(\frac{1}{V_N} + \frac{1}{V_P} \right) \frac{2}{\kappa} \tag{5.10}$$

where the Vs are expressed in kT/q units.

Equation 5.10 allows us to compute the gain of any output stage composed of complementary p- and n-channel transistors. In Appendix B, we note that the V_0 of a given transistor is proportional to its length. Hence, we can make the gain arbitrarily high by committing a large silicon area to long output transistors. For typical 1988 processes, output transistors 20 microns long will give a voltage gain of approximately 2000.

WIDE-RANGE AMPLIFIERS

A simple transconductance amplifier will not generate output voltages below V_{min}, which, in turn, is dependent on the input voltages. This limitation often is a source of problems at the system level, because it is not always possible to restrict the range of input voltages. We can remove this restriction, however, by a simple addition to the circuit, as shown in Figure 5.11.

Instead of feeding the output directly, the drain of Q2 is connected to the current mirror formed by Q5 and Q6. The currents coming out of Q4 and Q6 now are just the two halves of the current in the differential pair. We then reflect the Q6 current one more time, through Q7 and Q8, and subtract it from I_4 to form the output. As in the simple circuit, the output current is just the difference between I_1 and I_2.

The major advantage of the wide-range amplifier over the simple circuit is that both input and output voltages can run almost up to V_{DD} and almost down to ground, without affecting the operation of the circuit. In other words, we have eliminated the V_{min} problem.

The other nice thing about this circuit is that the current mirrors, such as Q3 and Q5, hold the drain voltages of Q1 and Q2 very nearly constant. In

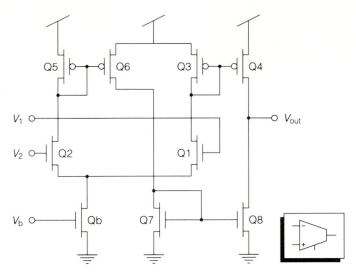

FIGURE 5.11 Schematic of the wide-range transconductance amplifier. This circuit has many advantages over the simple transconductance amplifier of Figure 5.3. The output-voltage range is not affected by the input voltages. The symbol for the circuit is shown in the inset.

diode-connected transistors, the current increases exponentially with the gate voltage, so the drain voltages never get very far below V_{DD}. For that reason, Q2 no longer has a problem associated with its drain conductance; its source–drain voltage is nearly equal to that of Q1. So the drain conductances of Q1 and Q2 are not critical in this circuit. The same thing is true of Q6: Q7 is a diode-connected transistor; it holds the drain voltage of Q6 very nearly constant. The only transistors that work over a large voltage range are Qb, Q4, and Q8, and we can make their channels long to get a low drain conductance (output current that is *nearly independent* of output voltage). Because of their low output conductance, long Q4 and Q8 transistors give the circuit a high voltage gain.

A layout of the improved circuit is shown in Plate 7(b). This new circuit is about twice the size of the simple transconductance amplifier of Plate 7(a). Such wide-range amplifiers have about 10 times the gain of the simple amplifier, and they work all the way down to ground and all the way up to V_{DD}. When we are willing to tolerate an increase of a factor of two in area, we can build a much better amplifier.

ABSTRACTION

The improved wide-range circuit can be used just like our original transconductance amplifier. When we design complex analog systems, we use an amplifier as an elementary component. We will not always distinguish between the simple and wide-range transconductance amplifiers, until we work through a complete implementation. We use the symbol shown in Figure 5.3 as an *abstraction* of the detailed circuit diagram. By convention, the minus input is shown at the top and the plus input at the bottom.

If we wish to distinguish the two circuits, we use a symbol with a wider flattened end to indicate a wide-range amplifier (see Figure 5.11). When we are not sure which circuit to use, we can think about the application and work out its operating range. Most of the time, we need to deal with only the abstraction, in which the output current is a simple function of the difference between the input voltages.

The open-circuit voltage gain of either kind of transconductance amplifier is large. The voltage gain of a simple amplifier like that shown in Plate 7(a) can be 100 to 300; that of a wide-range amplifier like that shown in Plate 7(b) is 1000 to 2000. For this reason, we will often use these amplifiers as "operational amplifiers," as the term is used in classical linear-circuit design. The gain of a classical operational amplifier usually is considerably larger than that we can achieve with the designs described in this chapter. We have chosen to use a symbol for the transconductance amplifier that is similar to that commonly used for an operational amplifier, with the addition of the transconductance control input. This convention is not as confusing as it might appear to be, at first sight, to people familiar with the conventional lore. All amplifiers have a well-defined limit to the current they can supply. Hence, the conventional operational amplifier has all the limitations described for the transconductance amplifier when the former is used in the open-circuit output mode. The classical operational amplifier, however, does not allow its user to control its output-current level. This additional degree of freedom provided by the transconductance amplifier is, as we will see in the following chapters, essential to the full range of techniques necessary for large-scale analog computation. The contrast between common usage and the convention adopted in this book can thus be viewed as follows: The usual treatment of an operational amplifier emphasizes the latter's open-circuit output properties, and treats output-current limitation as a nuisance—as a deviation from ideality. Instead, we choose to view this limitation as a virtue, and to give the designer control over it. The open-circuit behavior then can be viewed as an idealization, achievable only as a limiting case. These issues will become much more clear when we consider the response of systems to time-varying inputs.

SUMMARY

We mentioned that analog circuits can do computations that are difficult or time consuming (or both) when implemented in the conventional digital paradigm. We already have seen that the transconductance amplifier computes a tanh, which is an extremely useful function. It has a very smooth transition from linear behavior for small inputs to behavior that is saturated and does not blow up if we push the input out of limits.

The circuit also is a multiplier, as we can see from Equation 5.5. It multiplies a current by a difference in voltages. Of course, the current I_b is the exponential of the voltage V_b. This circuit can multiply the exponential of one signal by the tanh of some other signal.

We might not, a priori, have chosen this particular function as the most desirable primitive for general analog computation. The same can be said of any synapse in the brain. The point is that we have no reason to expect our preconceptions concerning elementary functions to be particularly reliable. We can be sure, however, that we can learn to build systems out of *any* reasonable set of primitives. We thus follow the time-proven example of evolution, and use primitives that are efficient in the implementation medium. The transconductance amplifier is versatile, and makes efficient use of silicon real estate. Excellent collections of circuits and techniques useful in the design of primitives have been compiled [Gregorian et al., 1986; Vittoz et al., 1977; Vittoz, 1985a; Vittoz, 1985b].

REFERENCES

Gregorian, R. and Temes, G.C. *Analog MOS Integrated Circuits for Signal Processing.* New York: Wiley, 1986.

Vittoz, E.A and Fellrath, J. CMOS analog integrated circuits based on weak inversion operation. *IEEE Journal of Solid-State Circuits*, SC-12:224, 1977.

Vittoz, E.A. Dynamic analog techniques. In Tsividis, Y. and Antognetti, P. (eds), *Design of MOS VLSI Circuits for Telecommunications.* Englewood Cliffs, NJ: Prentice-Hall, 1985a, p. 145.

Vittoz, E.A. Micropower techniques. In Tsividis, Y. and Antognetti, P. (eds), *Design of MOS VLSI Circuits for Telecommunications.* Englewood Cliffs, NJ: Prentice-Hall, 1985b, p. 104.

6

ELEMENTARY ARITHMETIC FUNCTIONS

We have introduced the idea that computation can be done with analog circuits. A computation often is described as a **function** that maps **arguments** into a **result**. In any practical computation system, the arguments have **types**. In digital computers, those types are integer, floating point, Boolean, character, and so on.

In the analog world (physical computation), there are two signal types: *voltages* and *currents*. It would be wonderful if there were elegant ways to do every computation just the way we would like with every signal type, but there are not. The analog art form consists of figuring out how to use particular signal types that lend themselves to certain computations, and thus to end up with the computation that we want.

Introductory computer-science courses often start with the basic algorithms for certain elementary functions that you may want to compute. In this chapter, we present such an introduction for analog circuits.

IDENTITY FUNCTIONS

In any formal system, the first operation anyone discusses is the **identity** operation. In analog systems, we need an identity function to make *copies* of signal values, so they can be used as inputs to several different computations.

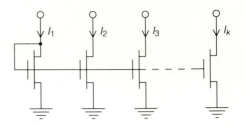

FIGURE 6.1 Current-mirror configuration. A current mirror can be used to make many separate copies of a current-type signal. Here the input current I_1 is replicated in the outputs I_2, I_3, ..., I_k.

Currents

In Chapter 3, we discussed how we can make copies of currents by using a current mirror. For example, if we need to use the value of I in k places, we can use n-channel transistors in the current-mirror configuration to generate current *sinks* of magnitude $I_1, I_2, \ldots, I_k$, as shown in Figure 6.1.

Several nominally identical current *sources* can be made with a p-channel current mirror. The copies are all independent, and how one of them is used does not affect the ways the others can be used. Current mirrors make excellent copies, with certain limitations. As we noted before, transistors cannot be perfectly matched, so one copy can be different from another by up to a factor of two! Hence, this particular identity function really is a multiplication by a random variable. The uncertainty introduced by the random variable may not matter, in which case we can use the current-mirror technique. If we need more precision, we can copy voltages instead of currents.

Voltages

We have a much more precise identity function for voltage-type signals than we have for current-type ones. It is a uniquely useful circuit using an amplifier with open-circuit output that makes good use of its gain; it is called the **unity-gain follower** (Figure 6.2). The term *follower* is used because the output voltage follows (increases or decreases with) the input voltage, without disturbing the circuit that is computing the input. In subsequent chapters, we will describe many unconventional uses of these followers; we will start with the easy, conventional identity function, and will derive the open-circuit input–output relation.

The amplifier multiplies the input voltage difference by its voltage gain A. The difference of the input voltages $(V_{in} - V_{out})$ multiplied by the voltage gain A,

FIGURE 6.2 Schematic of the unity-gain follower. The output current is proportional to the difference between the output voltage and the input voltage. If the follower is connected to a high-resistance load, the output voltage will follow the input voltage.

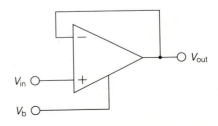

gives us the output voltage V_{out}:

$$V_{out} = A(V_{in} - V_{out})$$

The *transfer function* of the follower V_{out}/V_{in} thus can be written

$$\frac{V_{out}}{V_{in}} = \frac{1}{1 + \frac{1}{A}} \approx 1 - \frac{1}{A}$$

which is the simplest form of the basic equation in feedback-control theory. The follower takes the gain of the amplifier and uses it to make the output as nearly equal to the input as possible; the residual error due to the finite gain is $1/A$. For many applications, the fraction of 1-percent error introduced by a gain of a few hundred is adequately small. In Chapter 9, we will describe a delay line that can have many hundreds of followers connected in cascade, each input being the output of the previous stage. In such applications, we do best using a version of the amplifier that exhibits high voltage gain, as described in Chapter 5.

A particularly attractive property of the follower circuit is that, for static signals, it does not suffer from the V_{min} problem. From Equation 5.7 (p. 75), we know that the simple transconductance amplifier will not work if its output is below

$$V_{min} = \kappa\big(\min(V_1, V_2) - V_b\big) \tag{5.7}$$

In the follower configuration, V_{out} is equal to V_2, and hence V_{out} cannot be below V_{min} as long as the follower is following the input. When the input voltage is decreasing rapidly, and the output voltage cannot keep up, it is possible to have problems due to V_{min}.

ADDITION AND SUBTRACTION

The ability to make copies of signals is important because it allows us to use an intermediate result as input to several subsequent computations. Computation itself, however, is the result of *combining signals* to produce a result that is some function of its inputs. Biological systems have many ways of combining signals, none of which has been well defined in engineering terms. Mathematical notation, although convenient for reasoning about system operation, certainly was not the method used by evolution. Nonetheless, there are many neural operations that can be viewed as sums, differences, multiplications, or divisions. Although we must be careful to avoid an excessively literal interpretation, it is useful to understand how these basic mathematical operations are done in electronic circuits, and to be on the lookout for biological cognates as we proceed.

Voltages

The term **potential difference** is used synonymously with the term *voltage*. Common parlance underscores a fundamental fact about the potential of a single node: in and of itself, it cannot be a *signal*. Any voltage-type signal must have a **reference** at which its value is defined to be zero. The reference usually is the potential on another node. That reference potential can be a constant, such as V_{DD} or ground, or it can be an active signal node. The basic reason that differential amplifiers are effective is that they use a voltage difference directly as their input. If the two inputs are signals that have the same reference, the differential amplifier subtracts the two signals. If, however, the signal itself is the voltage difference between two active nodes, then the amplifier merely amplifies the signal.

The inherently differential nature of signals is the reason voltage sources always are shown with two terminals. Adding or subtracting two voltage differences will eventually require us to make the output of one signal the reference for another. The point can be seen clearly in Figure 6.3. There are two signals, A and B, shown as abstract voltage sources. When the positive terminal of one signal is used as the reference for the other, the sum of the two signals appears across the two remaining terminals. When the two positive terminals are connected to each other, the difference appears between the two reference nodes. With abstract voltage sources, addition operations were trivial because the sources were **floating**: Either terminal could be connected to any potential without disturbing the signal.

What is trivial when we use abstract sources can be a nightmare when we deal with real signals. The problem always can be traced to one question: *Where is the reference?* In biological and electronic systems, signals usually are not floating. If two signals both are referred to ground, we have the situation shown

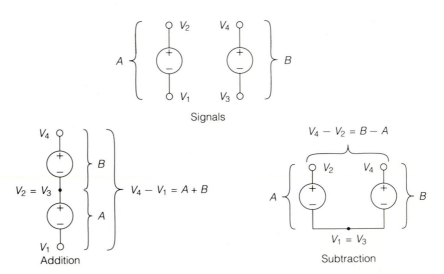

FIGURE 6.3 Addition and subtraction of voltages. These operations require that the output of one voltage source be used as the reference of another. The operations on abstract voltage sources may not be possible in a particular circuit configuration.

in Figure 6.3, and the difference can be taken with a differential amplifier. Under these conditions, however, it is not possible to add the two voltages. In many cases, the situation is not even this nice. Signals often are referred to a potential that is not explicitly available. An example occurs when the offset voltage of an amplifier is much larger than is the signal voltage. The true reference for the signal is the voltage on the negative input of the amplifier plus the offset voltage—a potential that is nowhere available. In biological systems, many signals are referred to the extracellular fluid. Current flowing through the resistance of the fluid can change the local potential in strange and unpredictable ways. Many synaptic arrangements appear to have, as their primary function, the creation of a reference potential. The best-understood example is the horizontal-cell network discussed in Chapter 15. We will have many occasions to revisit these questions in a systems context as we proceed.

Currents

Operations on current-type signals are well defined; they do not suffer from any of the problems mentioned for voltage-type signals. Current is the flow of charge; the zero of current corresponds to no charge moving. The reference for current is thus the coordinate system within which the transistors or neurons are stationary. Unless the circuit is being torn asunder at relativistic velocities (in which case there are more pressing problems), we will have no trouble defining a zero for current.

Addition and subtraction on current-type signals are particularly elegant because they follow from a basic law of physics—Kirchhoff's current law. This law states that the sum of the currents into an electrical node is zero; that is, the sum of the currents out of the node is the same as the sum of the currents into the node.

Kirchhoff's current law is a result of the basic physical concept of *conservation of charge*. Electrical charge is a conserved quantity; it can be neither created nor destroyed. A node cannot, by itself, store any charge. If a node has capacitance with respect to ground, for example, that capacitance is explicitly shown in the schematic as a capacitor with one terminal connected to the node and the other to ground. Any charge flowing into the node will flow out either through the wire to the capacitor, or through some other wire. In physics, this principle is called "conservation of charge"; in electrical engineering, "Kirchhoff's law"; in computer science, "add and subtract."

The basic Kirchhoff adder circuit is shown in Figure 6.4. Positive currents (into the node) are generated by p-channel transistors with their sources at V_{DD}; negative currents (out of the node) are generated by n-channel transistors with their sources at (or near) ground. The transconductance amplifier has the current from one side of a differential pair subtracted from a current from the other side—the simplest possible case of subtraction. Kirchhoff's law generates the difference in the two drain currents.

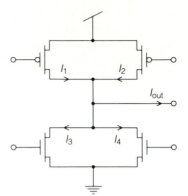

FIGURE 6.4 The Kirchhoff adder. Kirchhoff's law is used to add and subtract current-type signals, shown as the drain currents of two *n*-channel and two *p*-channel transistors. In this example, $I_{out} = I_1 + I_2 - I_3 - I_4$.

The output of the Kirchhoff adder of Figure 6.4 can be used as either a current or a voltage. If it is used in the open-circuit mode, its output voltage will be the output current divided by the output conductance, set by the sum of the drain conductances of all transistors connected to the node. The result is just a generalization of the one we obtained for the transconductance amplifier (Equation 5.8 (p. 78)). Like the transconductance amplifier, the open-circuit Kirchhoff adder has a high gain and a certain offset—its output will therefore be at V_{DD} for most of the range of positive outputs, and at ground for most of the range of negative inputs.

We have just seen how addition and subtraction of currents follows directly from the conservation of charge. This is yet another example of the opportunistic nature of evolution. Neural systems evolved without the slightest notion of mathematics or engineering analysis, but with access to a vast array of physical phenomena that implemented important functions of great strategic value. It is evident that the resulting computational metaphor has a range of capabilities that exceeds by many orders of magnitude that of the most powerful computers. In subsequent chapters, we will encounter many additional examples of computations that follow directly from physical laws.

ABSOLUTE VALUE

In many systems applications, it is not the *signed value* of a signal that is important; rather, it is the *absolute value* of the signal. If the signal is a current, it is extremely easy to take the absolute value with a current mirror. A *p*-channel current mirror can act only as a current source, whereas an *n*-channel current mirror can act only as a current sink. The positive or negative part of any signal represented as a bidirectional current can thus be taken by the appropriate current mirror. The circuit shown in Figure 6.5 creates a current proportional to the absolute value of a voltage difference. Its operation is based on the fact, noted in Chapter 5, that a simple transconductance amplifier can work with its output

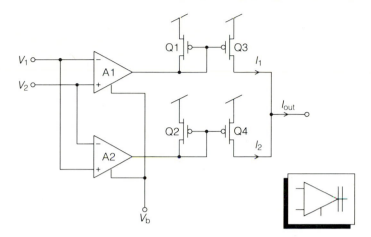

FIGURE 6.5   The absolute-value circuit. The circuit takes a differential voltage as its input and generates a unipolar current as its output. The symbol for the circuit is shown in the inset.

very near to V_{DD}; hence, its output can be worked into a p-channel current mirror. If V_1 is greater than V_2, amplifier A1 creates a current flowing into its output (negative by convention). That current is reflected by the Q1–Q3 current mirror and contributes a positive current to the output. Meanwhile, A2 attempts to put out a positive current. Driving the output voltage toward V_{DD} shuts off the Q2–Q4 current mirror; hence, Q4 contributes no current to the output. When V_2 is greater than V_1, Q4 contributes current to the output, but Q3 is cut off. Therefore, the output current is

$$I_{out} = I_1 + I_2 = I_b \tanh\left(\frac{\kappa|V_1 - V_2|}{2}\right)$$

The I_1 and I_2 currents are the two **half-wave rectified** versions of the input. The sum, I_{out}, is a **full-wave rectified** version of the input. For that reason, we call the absolute-value circuit a **full-wave rectifier**, even though it takes a voltage difference as its input and produces a current as its output.

Because the two halves of the absolute value are generated by separate current mirrors, each half can be copied as many times as necessary. If only one half is needed, one amplifier and one current mirror suffices. Such a **half-wave rectifier** is shown in Figure 6.6.

A great deal of the inhibitory feedback present in biological systems depends on activity in the sensory input channels, but does not depend on the *sign* of the input. For applications such as these, we will find both the full- and half-wave rectifier circuits generally useful. We have created a symbol, or *abstraction*, for these circuits, and for similar circuits with the same function, so that we can represent them conveniently on higher-level circuit diagrams. These abstractions are shown in the lower right-hand corner of Figures 6.5 and 6.6.

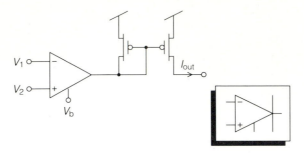

FIGURE 6.6   One half of the absolute-value circuit. This configuration gives an output current that is a half-wave rectified version of the input voltage. The symbol for this circuit is shown in the inset.

MULTIPLICATION

We already mentioned that the transconductance amplifier of Figure 5.3 (p. 70) can be viewed as a **two-quadrant multiplier**. Its output current can be either positive or negative, but the bias current I_b can be only a positive current. V_b, which controls the current, can be only a positive voltage. So the circuit multiplies the positive part of the current I_b by the tanh of $(V_1 - V_2)$. If we plot $V_1 - V_2$ horizontally, and I vertically, then this circuit can work in only the first and second quadrants.

Four-Quadrant Multiplier

To multiply a signal of either sign by another signal of either sign, we need a **four-quadrant multiplier**. We can achieve all four quadrants of multiplication by using each of the output currents from the differential pair (I_1 or I_2) as the source for another differential pair. The principle is illustrated in Figure 6.7. The results for the two drain currents of the differential pair were derived in Equation 5.3 (p. 68)

$$I_1 = I_b \frac{e^{\kappa V_1}}{e^{\kappa V_1} + e^{\kappa V_2}}$$

$$= \frac{I_b}{2} \left(1 + \tanh \frac{\kappa(V_1 - V_2)}{2} \right) \tag{6.1}$$

and

$$I_2 = I_b \frac{e^{\kappa V_2}}{e^{\kappa V_1} + e^{\kappa V_2}}$$

$$= \frac{I_b}{2} \left(1 - \tanh \frac{\kappa(V_1 - V_2)}{2} \right) \tag{6.2}$$

Similar reasoning applied to the two upper differential pairs fed by I_1 and I_2

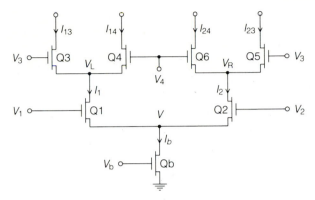

FIGURE 6.7 Partial schematic illustrating the use of the two outputs of a differential pair as current sources for two second-level differential pairs.

leads to expressions for the four upper drain currents.

$$I_{13} = \frac{I_1}{2}\left(1 + \tanh\frac{\kappa(V_3 - V_4)}{2}\right) \tag{6.3}$$

$$I_{14} = \frac{I_1}{2}\left(1 - \tanh\frac{\kappa(V_3 - V_4)}{2}\right) \tag{6.4}$$

$$I_{23} = \frac{I_2}{2}\left(1 + \tanh\frac{\kappa(V_3 - V_4)}{2}\right) \tag{6.5}$$

$$I_{24} = \frac{I_2}{2}\left(1 - \tanh\frac{\kappa(V_3 - V_4)}{2}\right) \tag{6.6}$$

When we had two quadrants, we had to have two wires: one for each quadrant. In other words, the wire on the right in Figure 5.3 (p. 70) carried I_2—the current that was subtracted from I_{out} (when V_1 is less than V_2); the wire on the left carried I_1—the current that was added to the output (when V_1 is greater than V_2). So, we can think of each wire as responsible for a quadrant in the multiplication. A four-quadrant multiplier can take the difference between two voltages (in this case V_3 and V_4), and multiply that difference by a difference between two other voltages (V_1 and V_2). Now we can use all four quadrants, because V_3 can be either less or greater than V_4, and V_1 can be either less or greater than V_2. We use the input voltage differences to generate currents, so we now have four wires, one to carry each current, which can be identified with each of the quadrants. In the small-signal range, where $V_1 - V_2$ and $V_3 - V_4$ are both less than $kT/(q\kappa)$, $\tanh x$ is approximately equal to x, and all four wires will carry information about the product. When the input voltage differences get large compared with $kT/(q\kappa)$, however, appreciable

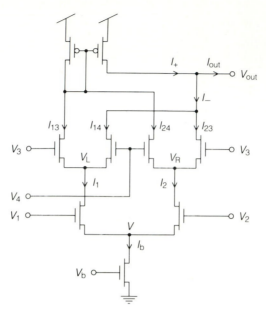

FIGURE 6.8 Schematic of the Gilbert multiplier. In the range where the tanh x is approximately equal to x, this circuit multiplies $V_1 - V_2$ by $V_3 - V_4$.

current will flow only in its respective wire. For example, if $V_3 - V_4$ is much larger than $kT/(q\kappa)$, and $V_1 - V_2$ is much larger than $kT/(q\kappa)$, then I_{13} will be nearly equal to I, and only the leftmost wire will carry any appreciable current.

We are now in a position to combine the four currents to generate the final product. The simplest approach to forming the product is shown in Figure 6.8. This circuit is known as the **Gilbert transconductance multiplier** [Gilbert, 1968], named for Barrie Gilbert, one of the great figures of analog integrated circuits. The original Gilbert multiplier was implemented with bipolar transistors, but was otherwise identical to the circuit of Figure 6.8.

We sum I_{13} and I_{24} to create I_+, the positive contribution to the output current. We can compute I_+ by adding Equations 6.3 and 6.6:

$$I_+ = \frac{I_1 + I_2}{2} + \frac{I_1 - I_2}{2} \tanh \frac{\kappa(V_3 - V_4)}{2} \tag{6.7}$$

Similarly, I_{14} and I_{23} are summed to create I_-, the negative contribution to the output current. We can compute I_- by adding Equations 6.4 and 6.5:

$$I_- = \frac{I_1 + I_2}{2} - \frac{I_1 - I_2}{2} \tanh \frac{\kappa(V_3 - V_4)}{2} \tag{6.8}$$

The output is formed by subtracting I_- from I_+. We can thus compute I_{out} by

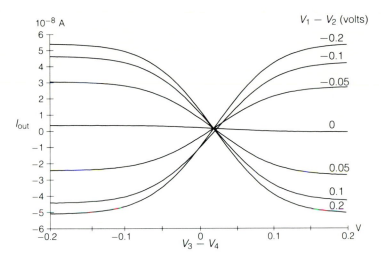

FIGURE 6.9 Output current of the basic Gilbert multiplier as a function of $V_3 - V_4$, for several values of $V_1 - V_2$. The tanh character of the output is readily apparent.

subtracting Equation 6.8 from Equation 6.7:

$$I_{out} = (I_1 - I_2) \tanh \frac{\kappa(V_3 - V_4)}{2} \tag{6.9}$$

Substituting Equations 6.1 and 6.2, we obtain:

$$I_{out} = I_b \tanh \frac{\kappa(V_1 - V_2)}{2} \tanh \frac{\kappa(V_3 - V_4)}{2} \tag{6.10}$$

The family of experimental curves taken from the circuit of Figure 6.8 is shown in Figure 6.9. The tanh behavior for both differential inputs is evident. For input voltage differences both less than $kT/(q\kappa)$, the tanh x is approximately equal to x, and the Gilbert circuit is indeed a multiplier, with the additional advantage that the output current saturates if one of the inputs gets stuck at some unseemly voltage. That is the good news; now let us look at the bad news.

Limits of Operation

The Gilbert circuit is even more constrained by the V_{min} problem than was the simple transconductance amplifier. In the multiplier, the output voltage is constrained by V_3 and V_4 rather than by V_1 and V_2:

$$V_{out} > V_{min} = \kappa\big(\min(V_3, V_4) - V_b\big)$$

The multiplier has the further limitation that source voltages V_L and V_R must satisfy the V_{min} condition for the bottom differential pair.

$$(V_L, V_R) = \kappa\big(\max(V_3, V_4) - V_b\big) > \kappa\big(\min(V_1, V_2) - V_b\big)$$

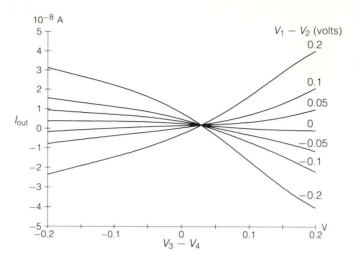

FIGURE 6.10 Output characteristics of the basic Gilbert multiplier. V_1 and V_2 are slightly greater than V_3 and V_4. The output current is limited by the V_{min} problem, caused by the low values of V_3 and V_4 on the first differential stage.

from which we conclude

$$\max(V_3, V_4) > \min(V_1, V_2) \tag{6.11}$$

We might be able to design a circuit for which Equation 6.11 is satisfied. A generally useful circuit, however, must be able to handle arbitrary inputs. In general, we cannot guarantee the relative range of the input voltages.

Figure 6.9 shows the circuit operating within its limits. Figure 6.10 shows how it looks when it starts to get into trouble. The V_2 input is set slightly above V_4, and the behavior is no longer acceptable. All input voltages are approximately 2 volts; we might very well want to use such voltage values. Once the limitation of Equation 6.11 is violated, the circuit is unusable.

Wide-Range Multiplier

If we need a multiplier that does not suffer from the limitations of Equation 6.11, we can use the same technique that allowed the output from the transconductance amplifier to cover a wider range. We use current mirrors to isolate the V_1–V_2 differential pair from the two V_3–V_4 pairs, as shown in Figure 6.11. The only unusual trick we have used is to run the V_3–V_4 stages upside down by using p-channel devices for Q7–Q9 and Q8–Q10. The layout of a typical implementation of the wide-range multiplier is shown in Plate 7(b).

The wide-range multiplier contains not quite twice as many transistors as the basic Gilbert circuit does, and has exactly the same output characteristic. The usable range of V_3 and V_4 is independent of V_1 and V_2. All voltages—input and output—work from very close to V_{DD} to very close to ground. The output current

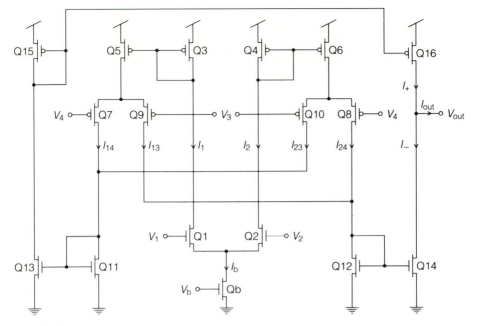

FIGURE 6.11 Wide-range version of the Gilbert multiplier. The ranges of V_1 and V_2 are independent of the values of V_3 and V_4, and vice versa.

measured over a wide range of V_3 for several fixed values of differential input $V_3 - V_4$ is shown in Figure 6.12. For input voltages more than about 1 volt below V_{DD}, the output current is relatively independent of the absolute input voltage level, as expected of a true differential amplifier. The ratio of the dependence of output current on the differential input voltage to its dependence on the absolute input voltage level is called the **common-mode rejection ratio (CMRR)**. For the top curve in Figure 6.12, the output current changes 3.9×10^{-9} amp for an extrapolated output voltage change of approximately 5 volts. In the steep part of the tanh, an input voltage change of approximately 35 millivolts is required to cause the same change in output current. For this set of inputs, the CMRR is thus 140 to 1.

Output current curves measured over a wide range of V_1 for several fixed values of differential input $V_1 - V_2$ are shown in Figure 6.13. For input voltages more than about 1 volt above ground, the output current is relatively independent of the absolute input-voltage level, as observed for the $V_3 - V_4$ inputs. From these data, the CMRR for the lower differential pair is about 87 to 1.

On the one hand, the wide-range multiplier has many things going for it. On the other hand, there are yet more transistors to be matched. So there are more ways this circuit can get unbalanced than there are in the simple Gilbert circuit. In practice, however, the wide-range multiplier does not seem to be any more adversely affected by transistor mismatch than the simple one is. We will see a system application of the multiplier in Chapter 14.

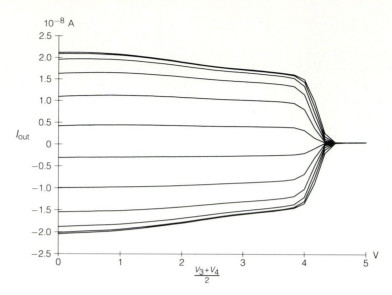

FIGURE 6.12 Dependence of the output current on the average (common-mode) upper input voltage. At input voltages near V_{DD}, the upper differential pair ceases to function. The data were taken for $V_3 - V_4$ equal to 0.05 volts, and $V_1 - V_2$ at 0.05-volt intervals.

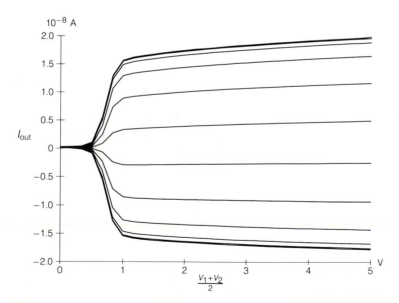

FIGURE 6.13 Dependence of the output current on the average (common-mode) lower input voltage. At input voltages near ground, the lower differential pair ceases to function. The data were taken for $V_1 - V_2$ equal to 0.05 volts, and $V_3 - V_4$ at 0.05-volt intervals. The output conductance of the lower differential pair is higher than that of the upper differential pair, because the doping of the substrate is less than that of the well (see Appendix A).

NONLINEAR FUNCTIONS

A large part of the nervous system deals with sensory input of one kind or another. Sensory signals can vary in intensity over many orders of magnitude. To deal with signals that have such a large **dynamic range**, it is essential that we have some method of compressing the range of signal values. Techniques that accomplish a reduction in the dynamic range of a signal generally are referred to as mechanisms for *automatic gain control*. We accomplish the simplest form of automatic gain control by applying a **compressive nonlinearity** to the signal. Examples of compressive functions are the logarithm, square root, and tanh.

Exponentials and Logarithms

We saw in Chapter 3 that a diode-connected transistor creates a voltage that is proportional to the logarithm of the input current. This voltage can be used to control the output currents of other transistors—a technique we used in Figure 6.1—but it is below the range of usable inputs for circuits such as transconductance amplifiers or multipliers. A voltage that is well within the operating range of these circuits can be generated by two diode-connected transistors in series, as shown in Figure 6.14(a). The inverse operation—creating a current proportional to the exponential of a voltage—is accomplished by the circuit of Figure 6.14(b). The relationship between voltage and current for these circuits is shown in Figure 6.14(c).

From Equation 3.15 (p. 39), we know that the saturated drain current I_{sat} is exponential in the gate–source voltage V_{gs}:

$$I_{\mathrm{sat}} = I_0 e^{\kappa V_{\mathrm{g}}} e^{-V_{\mathrm{s}}}$$

Applying this expression to Q1 and Q2, we obtain

$$I = I_0 e^{\kappa V_1} = I_0 e^{\kappa V_2 - V_1} \qquad (6.12)$$

Taking logarithms of the last two terms

$$V_2 = \frac{\kappa + 1}{\kappa} V_1$$

From which we conclude

$$\ln \frac{I}{I_0} = \frac{\kappa^2}{\kappa + 1} V_2 \qquad (6.13)$$

In the ideal case where κ is equal to one, Equation 6.12 has the solution

$$I = I_0 e^{V_2/2}$$

and we would expect the slope of the upper curve of Figure 6.14(c) to be twice that of the lower curve.

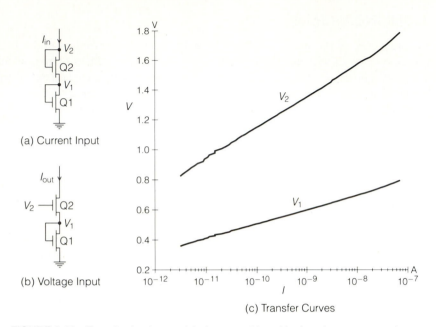

(a) Current Input

(b) Voltage Input

(c) Transfer Curves

FIGURE 6.14   Two circuits that exploit the natural logarithmic voltage–current characteristic of the MOS transistor. The voltage-input version (b) generates an output current
that is exponentially related to the input voltage. The current-input version (a) generates
an output voltage that is proportional to the logarithm of the input current. The advantage
of either arrangement over a single transistor is that the input voltage range is well
within the normal operating range of circuits such as the transconductance amplifier.
The measured transfer curve for V_2 (c) shows an *e*-fold increase in current for each
90-millivolt increase in V_2. This value corresponds to $\kappa \approx 0.7$.

Square Root

A variant of the circuit of Figure 6.14 can be used to implement a compressive
nonlinearity that is more gentle than the logarithm. One version of such a circuit
is shown in Figure 6.15. The voltage across Q1 can be written

$$\kappa V_3 = V_1 + \ln \frac{I_{\text{in}}}{I_0} \tag{6.14}$$

From Equation 6.13,

$$\ln \frac{I_{\text{out}}}{I_0} = \frac{\kappa^2}{\kappa + 1} V_3 \tag{6.15}$$

Substituting Equation 6.14 into Equation 6.15, we find the dependence of I_{out}
on I_{in}:

$$\frac{I_{\text{out}}}{I_0} = \left(\frac{I_{\text{in}}}{I_0} e^{V_1} \right)^{\frac{\kappa}{\kappa + 1}}$$

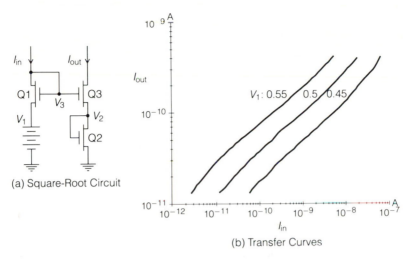

(a) Square-Root Circuit

(b) Transfer Curves

FIGURE 6.15   Compression circuit that generates an output current proportional to a fractional power of the input current. Ideally, the output would be the square root of the input; for the data shown, I_{out} is approximately equal to $I_{in}^{0.41}$, corresponding to $\kappa \approx 0.7$. The voltage V_1 can be used to set the scale of the output, as shown on the measured transfer curves.

The experimental dependence of I_{out} on I_{in} is shown in Figure 6.15(b), for several values of V_1. The dependence is between a square root and a cube root—this is a very nice compressive nonlinearity for many uses.

SUMMARY

We have seen how we can add and subtract currents using Kirchhoff's law, how we can subtract voltages using a differential amplifier, how we can multiply a voltage difference by a current in a transconductance amplifier, and how we can multiply two voltage differences using a Gilbert multiplier. Logarithms and exponentials are primitives provided by the Boltzmann relation, and we have pressed them into service to create a fractional-power compressive nonlinearity. Once again, physics has given us its own natural interpretation of certain mathematical functions. If we can use the primitives nature gives us, we can create formidable computations with physically simple structures. As we evolve the technology to the system level, we will see many applications of this opportunistic principle—the nervous system being the best example of all!

REFERENCES

Gilbert, B. A precise four-quadrant multiplier with subnanosecond response. *IEEE Journal of Solid-State Circuits*, SC-3:365, 1968.

7

AGGREGATING SIGNALS

There are enormous differences between biological systems and the kind of systems we find when we start digging inside a computer or looking at the schematic for a digital microprocessor chip. The most striking contrast between the two paradigms is the way in which signals are combined to form other signals. In a digital system, signals are combined by **logic elements** or **gates**. These elements take several inputs and form the logical AND, NOR, or similar functions. Each logic function can be thought of as making a *decision* about the inputs, and as reporting that decision as a binary signal at its output. We can construct any logic function by appropriately connecting two-input inverting gates of a single type— NOR, for example. We can think of a complex function as a decision about many inputs—we can always reach that decision by making partial decisions about a few inputs separately, and then combining these partial decisions into a more global decision. We can always subdivide the decision process in this way without increasing the complexity of the resulting circuit by more than a constant factor.

The nervous system combines inputs according to completely different principles. A very large number of inputs are brought together, or **aggregated,** in an analog manner. We can think of the simplest neuron as forming the analog sum of the inputs from the axons and dendrites of other neurons in a tree of passive dendritic processes, such as that shown in Figure 7.1 (see also Figure 4.1 (p. 44)). If enough current is injected into

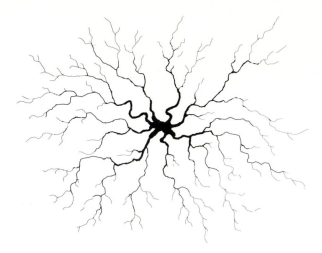

FIGURE 7.1   The dendritic tree of a neuron. This structure may or may not be used to generate action-potential outputs on an axon. Synapses on the tips of the tree provide outputs from, as well as inputs to, the dendritic processes.

the dendritic tree to bring the potential at the axon hillock to a *threshold* value, the nerve will initiate pulses (action potentials) in its axon. We can think of each branch of the dendritic tree as computing the sum of the currents in its two subtrees. Only when these partial sums have been fully aggregated into a total sum can the neuron make a decision to fire a pulse down the axon. In the aggregation process, analog information is preserved carefully. The nerve postpones the decision process until it has performed as much local aggregation as possible.

In addition to the analog aggregation of inputs, the nervous system differs markedly from digital systems in the sheer number of inputs that are factored into a given computation; this number is the **fan-in** of the neuron. The average circuit in a computer has a fan-in of two, three, or four. The fan-in of an average neuron is 1000 to 3000, or even 10,000. There are cells in the cerebellum with several hundred thousand inputs! The corresponding measure representing the number of distinct places to which the output of a computation goes is the **fan-out**. Considered over a system, the fan-in and fan-out must be the same—every input must be some other computation's output, and vice versa. Biologists use the term **convergence** for fan-in, and **divergence** for fan-out. We will use the biology and electrical engineering terms interchangeably.

Why do neurons have so many inputs? Each input synapse requires that an axonal process from another neuron be routed to the synaptic site. The more synapses there are, the more wiring is required. In the brain as in silicon, wire fills nearly the entire space. Economizing on wire is the single most important priority for both nerves and chips. At first sight, it would seem that the brain's profligate use of circuits with large fan-in and fan-out is horribly inefficient. As is usual in biological systems, however, there are a number of reasons that conspire to make the high–fan-in neuron a computing device of extraordinary power.

As an example, let us consider a population of neurons that recognize the presence of specific, reasonably complex objects in the visual field. Neuron A will fire if object A is present, neuron B will fire if object B is present, and so on. The excitatory synaptic inputs to any particular neuron represent the *features* that identify the corresponding object. These features have been computed by lower levels of the visual system. A crucial decision among nearly alike objects often is made on the basis of a single feature. The particular feature responsible for the decision is dependent on the circumstances: the viewing angle, what part of the object is obscured by intervening foliage, and so on. Each neuron therefore must have synaptic inputs representing *all features that might ever be used,* even though only a subset of them will contribute to any particular decision. No one has measured precisely the number of features needed to characterize a complex object; we will assume that several hundred is a reasonable estimate.

The nervous system represents a single feature not by the output of a single neuron, but rather by that of a population of neurons. The presence of a given feature is represented by the firing of, say, 100 neurons. Not all these neurons fire at the same rate—those best matched to the particular feature fire at a high rate, whereas those less well matched fire at a lower rate for this feature, but will fire at a higher rate for a similar but slightly different feature. When a target neuron requires information concerning the presence of a specific feature, its simplest strategy is to sum all or most of the 100 outputs, *weighting* each input by its firing rate for the desired feature. For several hundred features, this strategy would seem to require several tens of thousands of inputs to a target neuron. Because of the partial overlap of populations representing different features, however, the number of input synapses can be reduced to perhaps a few thousand.

We can think of the features characterizing a particular object as separate *dimensions* of the representation of the object. Any particular recognition task will have an **essential dimensionality** corresponding to the number of features that, under some circumstances, can become necessary to distinguish two objects. A unique recognition cannot be determined if the number of input synapses is less than the essential dimensionality of the task.

It is intuitive that the precision with which we treat inputs to a computation should be related to our confidence in those inputs. It does not pay to compute the cost of a proposed project to the penny when our estimates of the costs of several subtasks may be in error by many hundreds of dollars. The details of any two similar images seen by the visual system are never exactly alike. Even a familiar object is never seen twice in exactly the same way. We thus have little confidence in the details of any particular input. The major task of the nervous system is to make collective sense of sensory input. Under the conditions imposed by real input data, we can improve the reliability of a decision only by factoring a large number of inputs into the computation. In other words, when faced with a decision based on inputs in which it can place little confidence, the brain uses its resources to *increase the dimensionality* of the computational space, rather than to increase the precision with which each individual input is treated. Appendix D provides a formal treatment of several of the points we have mentioned here.

In the balance of this chapter, we will examine examples of networks that use large connectivity to compute interesting functions analogous to several of those computed in the brain.

STATISTICAL COMPUTATION

One important class of computation is the extraction of **statistical properties** of input data. For our purposes, statistical properties are interesting regularities or features that may be made evident by suitable computation on the input data. Statistics are imprecise for a small number of data points, so it is essential to perform the computation over many inputs. All of us who have done laboratory experiments are familiar with at least some rudimentary forms of data analysis. Historically, people were taught to *take* the data in the laboratory by repeated experiments, and then to *analyze* the data later. There are situations, however, in which we cannot make up for bad data by doing more experiments. The people who study earthquakes do not get to go back and collect more data. They can wait for the next earthquake, but it will be a different earthquake—a different experiment. A number of events associated with natural disasters cannot be replicated—the Mount St. Helen's eruption, for example. We can study what remains, but we do not get to do the experiment again.

Our sensory systems are perhaps the best example of sources of data that cannot be repeated. We never see the same scene twice—even if we try. We perceive familiar objects in a different position, with a different background, each time. The same predator is jumping on us from a different tree—there is no time to take a second look. Those animals that could extract the most information from a fleeting glance were most likely to survive, and to pass on that processing capability to their progeny.

Whenever we cannot replicate the conditions and collect several batches of data, the data that we do get are sure to contain some *bad data points*. Perhaps the voltmeter changed ranges and did not catch up with itself in time to take the reading correctly. Perhaps you walked across the room and zapped the experiment. Or, perhaps a cosmic ray came along. In the nervous system, neurons are dying all the time. We get not only good inputs from our visual and hearing systems—we get a lot of spurious inputs as well. No single input can be trusted completely. The system is designed to compute the most useful or informative result possible, in spite of inputs that are totally out of range.

Statisticians have various criteria by which, if a data point is sufficiently out of line, its effect may be reduced. A common procedure is to develop some notion of reasonable behavior. In an experiment, we often have sound theoretical reasons to believe that the output should be some smooth function of some independent variable (the input). The transistor curves in Chapter 3 and the amplifier transfer curves in Chapter 5 are examples. In both cases, there is a voltage scale given by $kT/(q\kappa)$. If we change the input less than this amount, we do not expect the output to change abruptly. Hence, if we take several data points within each $kT/(q\kappa)$ voltage interval, we have a great deal of *redundancy* in the input. If the distance from a single data point to a smooth curve passing through the average of other points in the neighborhood is relatively large, we should certainly check out that maverick data point. Any such scheme relies on four important features:

1. We know the size of a **region of smoothness** within which, for some fundamental reason, the data cannot change abruptly

2. Many data points are available within the region of smoothness

3. A method, consistent with the nature of the expected smoothness, is available for fitting a smooth function through the data points

4. Some method of estimating the average deviation of the data from the smooth function is available

Once we have formulated a computation with these attributes, we can use it to identify unexpected data points. These may be "bad" points, or they may be items of exceptional interest. Isolated points do not exist in a close-up visual image. It is desirable, however, to see stars in the night sky. One computation's bad datum is another computation's exceptional event. Sensory processing is replete with examples of spatially and temporally smoothed signals. These smooth functions are used to provide a reference for local computation. The most widely known example is the **center-surround** organization of many visual areas, from retina to cortex. The signal average in a central area is subtracted from an average over a much larger surrounding area; the resulting difference is reported as the output. A similar organization is found, in some form, in all known sensory pathways. In the following sections, we will discuss several ways to compute spatial averages of an ensemble of inputs.

FOLLOWER AGGREGATION

The simplest circuit for computing a smooth function is shown in Figure 7.2. It consists of n follower stages, all driving the single wire labeled V_{out}. A typical reaction to this **follower-aggregation circuit** might well be, "We are trying to make the V_{out} wire follow every input—and it obviously *cannot* follow every input. It is an n-way follower, but there can be only one output voltage." We have seen previously the importance of signal *types*. In the circuit of Figure 7.2, the output of each individual amplifier is a *current*, whereas the output of the entire aggregation is a *voltage*; that voltage is the outcome of a collective interaction of the entire set of amplifiers.

There are n amplifiers, each responsible for the contribution of its V_i input to the common output. Each amplifier has a transconductance: G_1 for A1, G_2 for A2, and so on to G_n for An. The Gs are set by the current controls on the transconductance amplifiers. We write Kirchhoff's law for the node V_{out}.

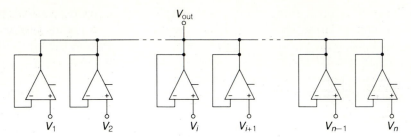

FIGURE 7.2   Schematic of the follower-aggregation circuit. Each follower supplies a current proportional to the difference between the input voltage and the output voltage. The contribution of each input to the output voltage is weighted by the transconductance of the associated amplifier.

The total current is the sum of the currents out of each amplifier. The current for the first amplifier is $G_1(V_1 - V_{\text{out}})$; that for the second is $G_2(V_2 - V_{\text{out}})$; that for the nth is $G_n(V_n - V_{\text{out}})$. Finally, the total has to be equal to zero:

$$\sum_{i=1}^{n} G_i(V_i - V_{\text{out}}) = 0$$

Transferring the V_{out} terms to the other side of the equation and rearranging, we obtain

$$V_{\text{out}} = \frac{\sum_{i=1}^{n} G_i V_i}{\sum_{i=1}^{n} G_i}$$

In other words, V_{out} is the average of the V_i inputs, each input weighted by its transconductance G_i.

Robustness

The follower-aggregation circuit computes the weighted average of the input voltages $V_1, \ldots, V_n$. Up to this point, our analysis has assumed a linear relation between input voltage and output current. This simplification has allowed us to write the solution, but has neglected what is probably the most charming attribute of the circuit and its relatives: The follower implementation of a neural network *has great* **robustness** *against bad data points*.

Transconductance amplifiers have a strictly limited current output. This limit is evident in their tanh transfer characteristics. The robustness of collective networks made with these circuits is a direct result of this current limitation. If any one input voltage is way off scale, it does not matter—the off-scale voltage will not pull any harder on the wire than would a voltage a few $kT/(q\kappa)$ different from the intended voltage of the wire. As long as all inputs are close to the average value, V_{out} will assume an average, with the inputs weighted by the current in their amplifier. The voltage V_{out} will not follow a few pathological inputs way off into left field.

Signals get stuck all the time, and biological wetware is even less reliable than silicon hardware. We have 1000 to 10,000 inputs to a neuron—we can be sure that some of them are going to be stuck on and some of them are going to be stuck off. If we have that many amplifiers with that kind of a fan-in, whether in a VLSI chip or in a neuron, some signals always will be stuck. There are just too many wires and too many amplifiers for all the components to be 100-percent reliable.

The follower-aggregation circuit shares with neural systems an exceptional level of reliability in the face of failure of individual components. In both cases, the robustness is a result of two factors: a large number of redundant inputs, and a limited current that can result from any given input.

From a statistical viewpoint, the tanh characteristic changes the computation done by the network. It implements what statisticians call a **resistant transformation**: The weighting assigned to outlying data points is reduced. For all signals close to V_{out}, we have seen that the circuit computes a weighted average, or *mean*. Signal values that are scattered by many $kT/(q\kappa)$ are treated as inputs to a weighted *median* calculation. In both cases, the data are weighted by the transconductances of their respective amplifiers. To ensure that no single amplifier contributes more than its share to the output, we use wide-range amplifiers to avoid the V_{min} problem described in Chapter 5.

RESISTIVE NETWORKS

The follower-aggregation circuit does a great job of computing an average that can be used as a reference against which to measure exceptional events. There is a problem, however, with this kind of average. The average is represented by the voltage on a single wire, and that wire is a single electrical node. The average, therefore, will be a *global* average: It will extend physically to the most remote location at which any input to it can originate. There are applications for which this kind of global average is desirable. In most systems, however, we will need a much more *local* average, one in which the contribution of spatially distant inputs is less than that of inputs in close proximity to the point at which the average is used.

An excellent example of local spatial averaging is found in the visual systems of all higher animals. The illumination level within a visual scene often varies from one point to another by several orders of magnitude. If the visual system used a global average as a reference, details in very bright and very dark areas would be invisible. A predator need only leap from the shadows—and such an arrangement would not make it into the next generation. For this reason, a locally weighted average signal level, from which local differences can be measured, is computed by a layer of *horizontal cells* in the retina. These cells are linked together by high-resistance connections called **gap junctions**, and form an electrically continuous *resistive network* just below the photoreceptors. The horizontal network is by no means the only place in the nervous system where this kind of a computation is used. As we mentioned in Chapter 4, the dendritic trees of all neurons are used to spread signals spatially, and the potential at any

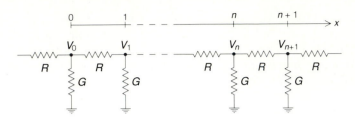

FIGURE 7.3   Resistive model of passive electrotonic spread in a neural process. The distance scale over which a signal dissipates is determined by the product RG.

given leaf of the tree is more affected by inputs in the immediate proximity than by those farther away. Propagation of signals in resistive networks is generically referred to as **electrotonic spread**.

Electrotonic Spread

The simplest example of electrotonic spread occurs in a long, straight, passive neural process of constant diameter. We can model the process as a resistive-ladder network, as shown in Figure 7.3. The R resistances correspond to the axial resistance per unit length of the cytoplasm, and the G conductances represent the leakage conductance per unit length through the membrane to the extracellular fluid. A potential V_0 is generated by an input at the left end of the process ($x = 0$). The voltage $V(x)$ generated by the input decreases with distance x from the input, because some of the current injected by the input is shunted to ground by the G conductances. We present a detailed analysis of continuous and discrete networks in one and two dimensions in Appendix C.

An important result, derived in Appendix C, is the rate at which signals die out with distance from the source. Intuitively, if the membrane-leakage conductance G is small compared with the conductance $1/R$ of the cytoplasm, the signal should propagate a large distance before it dies out. The greater the membrane conductance, the shorter the distance. For uniform, continuous networks, the voltage has the form

$$V = V_0 e^{-\alpha|x|} = V_0 e^{-\frac{1}{L}|x|} \tag{7.1}$$

where α is the **space constant** and L is the **characteristic length** or **diffusion length** of the process:

$$\alpha = \frac{1}{L} = \sqrt{RG} \tag{7.2}$$

A signal injected into a linear resistive ladder network decays exponentially with distance from the source. If a signal is injected into a node in the middle of a very long process, the influence of that input spreads out in both directions, not just in the $+x$ direction. For a one-dimensional model, the solution in the $-x$ direction is just the mirror image of the solution for the $+x$ direction. This observation is responsible for the absolute-value dependence on x in Equation 7.1.

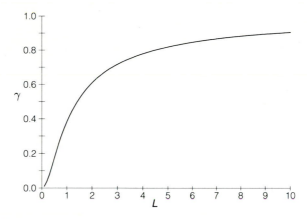

FIGURE 7.4   The exponent γ as a function of L, as computed from Equation 7.4.

For discrete networks, the decay also is exponential. For a node n sections away from the source, the voltage will be

$$V_n = \gamma^n V_0 \tag{7.3}$$

where

$$\gamma = \frac{V_1}{V_0} = 1 + \frac{1}{2L^2} - \frac{1}{L}\sqrt{1 + \frac{1}{4L^2}} \tag{7.4}$$

where $1/L$ is equal to $\sqrt{RG}$ as before, but in the discrete case the values of R and G are given per section rather than per unit length.

A plot of γ as a function of L is shown in Figure 7.4. For large values of L, γ approaches 1, and the continuous approximation of Equation 7.1 is valid. For values of L less than about 10, the magnitude of the decrement per stage given by the discrete solution differs markedly from that obtained from the continuous approximation. Later in this chapter, we will compare data from an experimental one-dimensional network with Equations 7.3 and 7.4.

A second important result derived in Appendix C is the **effective conductance** G_0 of the network. A voltage source V_0 driving one end of a semi-infinite network must supply a current $I = G_0 V_0$ into the network. From the point of view of a signal source, the network acts just like a single conductance G_0. For a continuous network, the effective conductance is given by

$$G_0 = \sqrt{\frac{G}{R}}$$

For discrete networks, the value of G_0 is somewhat different from that for continuous ones:

$$G_0 = \sqrt{\frac{G}{R}}\sqrt{1 + \frac{1}{4L^2}}$$

The G_0 values given here are for a terminated semi-infinite network. The effective

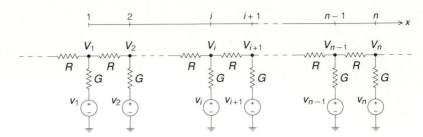

FIGURE 7.5 Electrotonic network in which input signals are supplied by voltage sources. This form of the network is equivalent to a current source in parallel with each G.

conductance at the center of a network that extends in both directions is $2G_0$, because a current $V_0 G_0$ must be supplied for each direction.

Multiple Inputs

Multiple signal inputs to a network can be provided in the form of either voltage- or current-type signals. If we inject currents at many places, the network performs an automatic weighted average: the farther away the inputs are, the less weight they are given, in accordance with Equation 7.3. The voltage at any given point k due to a number of inputs is just

$$V_k = \frac{1}{2G_0} \sum_n \gamma^{|n-k|} I_n$$

In other words, the voltage at any point due to a number of inputs is just the sum of the voltages that would have been measured at that point had each input been presented individually, with all other inputs held at zero. This great simplification is a result of the principle of linear superposition mentioned in Chapter 2. The superposition result is true for any linear system, and is not dependent on the one-dimensional nature of the network, or on the fact that G and R were constant, independent of x. We will use it for two-dimensional networks, such as the horizontal network in the retina, and for our treatment of electrotonic spread in the dendritic tree. In these cases, the weighting function is more complex than the simple γ^n form of the one-dimensional network.

A convenient way to generate inputs to the network is to connect voltage sources in series with the conductances, as shown in Figure 7.5. Because the principle of superposition will hold for this arrangement as well, we need compute only the node voltage due to a single input. In Appendix C, we will derive the node voltage V_i generated by a voltage source v_i in the middle of a very long, uniform, discrete, one-dimensional network:

$$\frac{V_i}{v_i} = \frac{1}{\sqrt{4L^2 + 1}}$$

As the effective length over which the network averages increases, the effect of any given input decreases. For large characteristic lengths, the voltage due to any particular input is proportional to $1/L$. The total effect of a set of uniformly spaced inputs included in one characteristic length is therefore constant, independent of the value of L, because the number of inputs is proportional to L. This conclusion is clear if we observe that, when the voltage at all inputs is the same, the output voltage anywhere in the network is equal to the input voltage. We will make extensive use of both one- and two-dimensional networks with many inputs to derive local averages.

DENDRITIC TREES

Inputs to one neuron from the axons and dendrites of other neurons are aggregated by a tree of passive dendritic processes. For many years, scientists believed that the primary function of the dendrites was to collect input current into the main body, or **soma**, of the cell from which an action potential was generated. It is certainly true that neurons with axons do generate action potentials, or *nerve pulses*, as a result of current collected by their dendrites. Researchers have discovered in recent years, however, that the role of the dendritic tree is considerably more complex than was previously supposed [Shepherd, 1972; Shepherd, 1978].

Many types of neurons have no axon whatsoever, so their primary role cannot be to produce action potentials. Many types of neurons—those with axons and those without—have been shown to have *synaptic outputs* as well as inputs on their dendrites. This remarkable finding implies that much of the lateral communication in the nervous system is extremely local, and is mediated by graded analog (electrotonic) potentials rather than by the more digital nerve pulses. The dendrites convey two-way information rather than merely collecting current into the soma. Sorting out the far-reaching implications of these findings will require many years.

Synaptic Inputs

If enough current is injected into the dendritic tree, then the neuron will release neurotransmitter from any output synapses it has on its dendrites. If the current into the cell as a whole reaches a high enough level, the nerve can initiate pulses in its axon (if it has one). *Depolarizing* inputs cause the release of neurotransmitter from dendritic synapses and, if sufficiently intense and prolonged, can cause the axon to fire as well. These inputs are called *excitatory*. Inputs that *hyperpolarize* the neuron act to cancel out the effect of excitatory inputs; they are therefore called *inhibitory*.

If the entire path from the leaves of the dendrites to the axon hillock is less than L in length, the neuron is said to be **electrically compact**. Such a cell can be assumed to be equipotential throughout its dendrites, and therefore can be modeled as a wire. A neuron with dendritic processes much longer than

L can have very different potentials at different locations in its dendritic tree. The dendrites of such a neuron can be modeled as linear resistive networks. We will derive the voltage–current relationships at branches in a tree network in Appendix C.

Shunting Inhibition

We have used the voltage sources of Figure 7.5 to model excitatory and inhibitory input synapses to the network. Inputs also may be injected as currents, of course, one sign of current being excitatory and the other inhibitory. There is a third class of inputs, often called **veto synapses**, that neither hyperpolarize nor depolarize the neuron, but instead partially short-circuit to ground any activity present in the process. This kind of inhibition is called **shunting inhibition**.

The simplest realization of shunting inhibition is implemented directly by the network of Figure 7.5; we merely make one conductance, G_{shunt}, very large compared with the others. This arrangement will attenuate a signal traveling in either direction in the process. We will derive the attenuation suffered by a signal as it passes such a shunt in Appendix C. The result is

$$V_{out} = \frac{V_0}{1 + \frac{G_{shunt}}{2G_0}}$$

where V_0 is the voltage that would have been present without the shunt. As G_{shunt} becomes large compared with the network effective conductance G_0, the operation performed by such a synapse resembles a division by G_{shunt}.

Shunting is one of those wonderful biological tricks by which an input can inhibit activity, but not create any activity of its own. In a complex biological system, it often is difficult to distinguish shunting inhibition from inhibitory synapses that contribute a net negative current to the tree. The same basic synaptic mechanisms are used in both cases. Release of neurotransmitter causes channels to open in the postsynaptic membrane. An inhibitory synapse causes an increase in conductance for an ion with a negative reversal potential. A shunting synapse causes an increase in conductance for an ion with a reversal potential near the resting potential of the membrane. From a system perspective, however, it makes a world of difference whether the operation is a subtraction or a division. For this reason, we must exercise care when we use the biological literature as a basis for electronic models. Biological distinctions that seem insignificant at the descriptive level may have profound effects on the performance characteristics of the neurobiological system.

TWO-DIMENSIONAL NETWORKS

The horizontal network in the retina is a flat mesh of dense processes that are highly interconnected by resistive gap junctions. These interconnections are somewhat random in number and direction. Any given cell is connected with

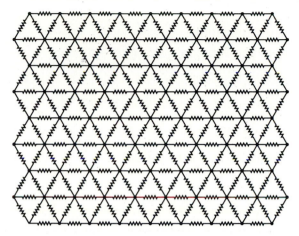

FIGURE 7.6 Topology of a hexagonal network. Because of its high degree of symmetry and redundancy, this network is the preferred form for two-dimensional applications.

many others, and there is a great deal of overlap among interconnected cells. In silicon, discrete two-dimensional networks are very useful, and generally are implemented in a regular array by interconnection of nearest neighbors. We have mentioned that this kind of network computes an average that is a nearly ideal way to derive a reference with which local signals can be compared. In Chapter 15, we describe a retina containing a hexagonal two-dimensional network, with six resistors coming into each node, as shown in Figure 7.6. A resistance R is connected between neighboring nodes, and a conductance G (not shown) is connected from each node to ground (as in Figure 7.3; in Figure 7.5, it is connected to a voltage source).

This network is particularly attractive, because it has the highest symmetry and connectivity of any regular, two-dimensional structure. If we inject a current into a node of the network (which we will call node 0), the resulting voltage decays exponentially with distance from that node. We can derive an approximate solution for the decay law in the following manner. As we progress outward from node 0 following a row of resistors, we encounter nodes that are vertices of larger and larger hexagons centered on node 0. The index of hexagon n (its "radius") is just the number of resistors we must pass through on the direct path from node 0 to a vertex. Our **circular approximation** assumes that all nodes on the perimeter of a given hexagon have the same voltage. Under this approximation, we can write a finite-difference equation for the current into hexagon n in terms of the voltage relative to that of hexagon $n - 1$ and to that of hexagon $n + 1$. We notice that there are $6n$ nodes on the perimeter of hexagon n, and that there are $12n - 6$ resistors from hexagon $n - 1$ to hexagon n, and $12n + 6$ resistors from hexagon n to hexagon $n + 1$. The current I into hexagon n is therefore

$$I = \frac{(12n - 6)(V_{n-1} - V_n) - (12n + 6)(V_n - V_{n+1})}{R} - 6nGV_n \qquad (7.5)$$

In steady state, this current must be zero. Simplifying Equation 7.5 for zero current, we obtain the finite-difference equation for the steady-state node voltage:

$$(2n + 1)V_{n+1} - n(RG + 4)V_n + (2n - 1)V_{n-1} = 0 \qquad (7.6)$$

Once again, we see our old friend RG (equal to $1/L^2$) appearing as the free parameter in Equation 7.6, as it did in the one-dimensional solution. The solution of this equation is the subject of the next section.

Solution for the Hexagonal Network
David Feinstein

Equation 7.6 relates the vertex voltages of three consecutive hexagons of the network. Solving for V_{n+1}, we obtain the forward-recursion relation

$$V_{n+1} = \frac{n(RG + 4)V_n - (2n - 1)V_{n-1}}{2n + 1} \qquad (7.7)$$

which produces the voltage on a given hexagon in terms of the voltages on the two smaller concentric hexagons. If we know V_0, the voltage at the center of the network, and V_1, the voltage at the first hexagon, we can solve for V_2. We can now iterate this procedure; given V_1 and V_2, we can determine V_3, and so on.

Determining V_1 for a given V_0 is the hard part of solving the network. The correct choice for V_1 leaves V_n finite as n approaches infinity. Any other choice for V_1 causes V_n to diverge as n approaches infinity. The exact expression for V_1 is given in [Feinstein, 1988]; it involves complete elliptic integrals, and is not especially illuminating. The values for V_1/V_0 as a function of L, computed by evaluating the exact expression, are shown in Figure 7.7. Once we know V_0 and V_1, we can use Equation 7.7 to evaluate the next few V_n. Knowing V_0 and V_1 also allows us to compute the current through the six resistors radiating from node 0, and hence to compute the input conductance of the network.

For n larger than about $2L$, the successive iteration of Equation 7.7 is subject to rapid erosion of numerical precision, and it is best to calculate V_n from the asymptotic relation

$$V_n \approx \gamma^n \frac{V}{\sqrt{n}} \qquad (7.8)$$

where

$$\gamma = 1 - \frac{2}{1 + \sqrt{1 + 8L^2}}$$

Equation 7.8 is the two-dimensional equivalent of the expressions given in Equations 7.3 and 7.4 for the one-dimensional network. The value of V in Equation 7.8 is a complicated function of L; it is derived in [Feinstein, 1988] and is plotted in Figure 7.8.

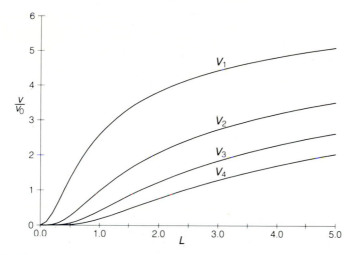

FIGURE 7.7   Voltages of the first few hexagons as a function of L. These curves were evaluated using the circular approximation. We can obtain the full solution using the procedure described in the text.

The relative error in the asymptotic relation of Equation 7.8 is approximately equal to $L/(5n)$. Application of Equation 7.7 in the forward direction loses about one significant digit per L iterations, but is stable when V_{n-1} is computed from V_n and V_{n+1}. We can compute accurately the full solution for any L by starting at large n with two values given by Equation 7.8, with an arbitrary value of V. We use the reverse form of Equation 7.7 to solve for successively smaller n until V_0 is obtained. Then we use this value of V_0 to normalize all the other values.

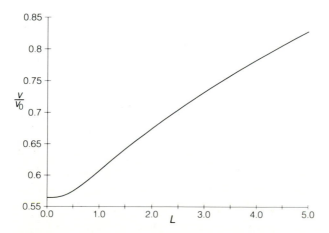

FIGURE 7.8   The value of V in Equation 7.8 as a function of L.

Wiring Complexity

We have discussed how a resistive network computes a smooth average over a number of neighbors, with the neighbors farther away contributing less to the average. If we were to replace this network with a set of circuits that did a completely separate computation at each location, the amount of wire required would proliferate enormously. For a computation centered at a given point, we would need to run a wire to every signal source that formed an input to the computation. A computation centered at a different location would require wires back to its sources also. By the time we were done, we would have duplicated many levels of wiring.

The secret to an efficient design is to share as many signal paths as possible. In that way, we avoid duplication of wire, and also share the maximum amount of processing circuitry. The resistive network is the ultimate example of a shared function. Every location can put signals into the network, read voltages off of the network, and use the same network to sense this weighted sum over its neighbors, including itself.

If we are willing to include the location itself in the average, letting it make the greatest contribution to the average, then we can use a resistive network to compute this kind of weighted average. There are many problems for which this solution is excellent. This trick may well be one of the most important ones played by neural circuitry. Because the computation is shared by every location, we need only one network, and every location gets taken into account.

THE HORIZONTAL RESISTOR (HRES) CIRCUIT

How do we build a resistive network? We could just lay down a resistive layer, such as polysilicon, everywhere. There are applications for which such a sheet is just what we would want. Certain fabrication processes include a layer of **undoped poly** that has a very high resistance. This material is used for pull-up resistors in static random-access memories. Such a layer is not defined in the process described in Appendix A, however, and is not available on many commercial processes. The resistance of ordinary poly or diffusion is much too low to be of any real value. We will describe a resistor with a control input that allows us to set the resistance electronically. We call the circuit the **horizontal resistor** (HRes), because we first developed it as a model of the horizontal cells in the retina described in Chapter 15. Alternative approaches to the resistive connection are described in [Gregorian et al., 1986].

The Resistive Connection

The most elementary resistive connection is implemented by two pass transistors in series, as shown in the shaded box in Figure 7.9. The gate voltage of each transistor is set at a fixed value V_q above the input voltage V_1 or V_2. This

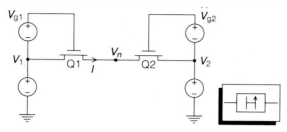

FIGURE 7.9   Schematic of the resistive connection (shaded area) of the horizontal resistor (HRes) circuit. Two pass transistors in series form a conducting path between the two nodes V_1 and V_2. When V_1 is greater than V_2, Q2 limits the current; when V_2 is greater than V_1, Q1 limits the current. The current is linear in $V_1 - V_2$ for small voltage differences, and saturates at high voltage differences at a value set by the gate bias. The symbol for the resistive connection is shown in the inset.

bias voltage controls the saturation current I_0 of the Q1 and Q2 pass transistors, and therefore sets the effective resistance of the connection.

From Chapter 3, we recall that the current I through a transistor is

$$I_0 e^{\kappa V_g} \left(e^{-V_s} - e^{-V_d} \right) = e^{\kappa V_g - V_s} \left(1 - e^{V_s - V_d} \right) \tag{7.9}$$

where all voltages are expressed in units of $kT/(q\kappa)$. This equation is completely antisymmetric under the interchange of source and drain terminals. For V_1 greater than V_2, V_1 acts as the drain of Q1, and the intermediate node V_n acts as the source of Q1 and the drain of Q2. The saturation current of Q1 is higher than that of Q2, because the gate–source voltage of Q1 is higher than that of Q2. The current I is limited by Q2, and saturates for $V_1 - V_2$ much greater than kT/q because the gate–source voltage of Q2 is set by the bias voltage. For V_2 greater than V_1, the roles of Q1 and Q2 are reversed, and I is negative. For V_1 approximately equal to V_2, the circuit acts like a resistor.

We can analyze the dependence of the current I on the voltage $V_1 - V_2$ across the resistor by assuming that the bias-generator adjusts both $\kappa V_{g1} - V_1$ and $\kappa V_{g2} - V_2$ to be equal to V_q. How we achieve this remarkable invariant is the subject of the next section. The current through Q1 must be the negative of that through Q2. Writing Equation 7.9 for Q1 and Q2, and setting the currents equal and opposite, we obtain

$$I = I_0 e^{V_q} \left(e^{V_1 - V_n} - 1 \right) = I_0 e^{V_q} \left(1 - e^{V_2 - V_n} \right) \tag{7.10}$$

From Equation 7.10, we can determine the voltage V_n at the junction between the two pass transistors:

$$2 e^{V_n} = e^{V_1} + e^{V_2} \tag{7.11}$$

Substituting Equation 7.11 into Equation 7.10, we obtain

$$\frac{I}{I_{sat}} = \frac{e^{V_1} - e^{V_2}}{e^{V_1} + e^{V_2}} \tag{7.12}$$

where

$$I_{\text{sat}} = I_0 e^{V_q}$$

Multiplying top and bottom of Equation 7.12 by $e^{-(V_1+V_2)/2}$ and simplifying, we obtain the final expression for the current:

$$I = I_{\text{sat}} \tanh \left(\frac{V_1 - V_2}{2} \right)$$

The slope of the tanh function at the origin is unity; therefore, the effective resistance R of this kind of resistive connection is

$$R = \frac{2kT/q}{I_{\text{sat}}}$$

Bias Circuit

For the kind of resistive connection shown in Figure 7.9 to be useful, we must find a way to implement the V_q bias voltage sources. The bias-voltage generator should adjust the value of V_q such that the saturation current of the resistive connection can be set by an external control, but not vary as the voltage level in the network changes.

A biasing circuit that achieves these properties with a minimum of components is shown in Figure 7.10. The node labeled V_{node} senses the network voltage at a network node—for example, V_1—and the circuit generates an output voltage V_g to bias the gates of all pass transistors connected to that node. We recognize the circuit as an ordinary transconductance amplifier connected as a follower, with the addition of the diode-connected transistor Qd. Because of the follower action described in Chapter 6, the voltage at the gate of Q2—which is connected to the source of Qd—follows the node voltage V_{node}. The output

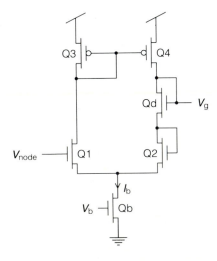

FIGURE 7.10 Schematic of the bias circuit for the horizontal resistor (HRes) circuit. The V_{node} input senses the voltage at one end of a resistive connection. Negative feedback to the gate of Q2 automatically adjusts the voltage at the source of Qd to equal V_{node}. The circuit generates an output V_g to bias the gates of any pass transistors connected to the node. This bias voltage is just sufficient to give the pass transistors a saturation current equal to the operating current through Qd. A separate bias circuit is required for each node of a resistive network.

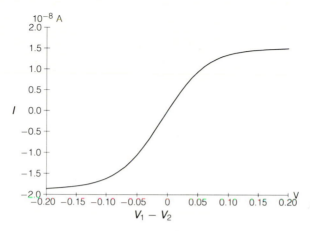

FIGURE 7.11   Measured current–voltage characteristics of the horizontal resistor (HRes) circuit. The current I is plotted as a function of $V_1 - V_2$, for V_2 equal to 2.5 volts. Note that the saturation current for a positive voltage difference is not equal to that for a negative voltage difference, due to transistor mismatch. In spite of the apparent mismatch, the current is zero at zero voltage difference. The leakage current to substrate is small compared with the saturation current of the circuit.

voltage V_g will follow the node voltage, but with a positive offset equal to the voltage across Qd. The diode-connected transistor Qd has both its source and gate voltages equal to those of the pass transistor. Half of the bias current I_b is flowing in Qd. Writing Equation 7.9 for Qd in each of the bias sources, we obtain

$$\frac{I_b}{2} = e^{\kappa V_{g1} - V_1} = e^{\kappa V_{g2} - V_2}$$

Thus, the saturation current of Qd will be the saturation current of the resistive connection, independent of the node voltage. We have accomplished this remarkable invariance without drawing any current out of the network. The bias current I_b serves two purposes in this circuit: It enables the follower to operate, and it biases the diode-connected transistor Qd. The voltage across Qd, and hence the gate–source voltage of the pass transistor, is set by the bias current. We therefore can use I_b to control the conductance of the resistive connection.

The measured current–voltage curve for the HRes circuit is shown in Figure 7.11. The current is linear with voltage across the resistor for differential voltages less than approximately ±100 millivolts, and saturates at I_{sat} for larger voltages. The negative saturation current is not equal to the positive saturation current, due to the mismatch between transistors in the bias circuit on the left and those in the bias circuit on the right. In spite of this mismatch, the current flowing from one circuit to the other, except for leakage current of the source and drain regions to substrate, is guaranteed to pass through zero at zero voltage. The leakage currents usually are negligible compared with I_{sat}.

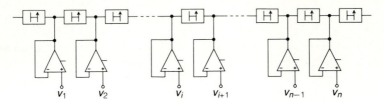

FIGURE 7.12 CMOS implementation of the abstract network of Figure 7.5. This network can be thought of as a generalization of Figure 7.2, where the output wire has been replaced by a network of horizontal resistor (HRes) circuits. There is a bias circuit (not shown) associated with each node in the network.

Networks in CMOS

The HRes circuit is the simplest element with which we can build an electronic analog of the neuron's dendritic tree. We will start by implementing a one-dimensional network analogous to the linear arrangement of Figure 7.5. Such a network is shown in Figure 7.12. Each local signal drives the network with a follower. The local current into the network is thus proportional to the difference between the signal and the local potential of the network.

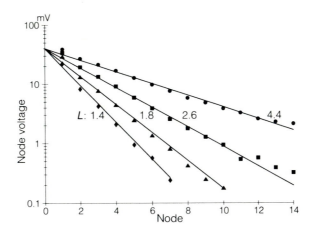

FIGURE 7.13 Measured (denoted by symbols) and theoretical signal decay in an experimental one-dimensional CMOS network constructed as shown in Figure 7.12. Inputs to the left half of the network (not shown) were held 100 millivolts higher than were inputs for the nodes shown. We determined the value of L for each curve from the ratio of the saturation current of the transconductance amplifier to the current through the resistor. We computed the slopes of the theoretical curves from Equation 7.3 using the value of γ given by Equation 7.4. We chose the common intercept for the best fit to the data. Each node was equipped with an individual follower, so that its voltage could be observed. We determined the offset voltages due to these followers by disconnecting the left half of the network. We subtracted these offset voltages from the node voltages to give the final values shown on the plot. The data for node 1 are higher than the curves predict because the end resistive connection is partially saturated.

The inputs to the transconductance amplifiers correspond to the voltage sources in Figure 7.5, the transconductance of the amplifiers corresponds to G in Figure 7.5, and the HRes circuits take the place of the resistors. The value of L is controlled by the ratio of the current in the bias circuit of the HRes circuits to the current in the transconductance amplifiers. Because the network voltage can be very different from the input voltage, it is desirable to use wide-range amplifiers for the followers in a network of this type. For small signals, the behavior of the circuit is the same as that of the linear resistive network, and we expect the same results. Data from an experimental one-dimensional network are compared with Equations 7.3 and 7.4 in Figure 7.13.

The structure shown in Figure 7.12 can be used to implement two-dimensional networks like the hexagonal topology shown in Figure 7.6. The HRes circuit is ideal for networks in which many resistive connections converge on each node. Only one biasing circuit is required per node; the node is connected to the voltage V_{node} of the biasing circuit. All pass transistors connected to that node have their gates connected to the V_{g} output of the biasing circuit. The larger connectivity required by the hexagonal network is thus achieved at low incremental cost: In addition to the bias circuit, each node requires only one pass transistor per connection.

SMOOTH AREAS

We saw that the follower-aggregation circuit computes node voltages that are a smooth approximation to the input data, as long as each element is operating within its linear range. The output of this computation is a single voltage.

The linear resistive network computes a set of node voltages from a set of input voltages. A given node voltage is a weighted sum of the inputs; the weight of each input decreases exponentially with distance from the node in accordance with Equation 7.3. If we view the inputs and outputs as functions in one dimension, the node voltages are a smooth approximation to the inputs. For small L, inputs within a small region around any given output node contribute to the output value, and the smoothing will be minimal. For larger L, proportionally more smoothing will occur.

Similarly, a two-dimensional resistive network computes node voltages that are a smooth approximation to a two-dimensional set of inputs [Hutchinson et al., 1986]. We can think of the network computing a smooth fit at each point to the data included in a region of diameter approximately equal to L.

Smoothing in two dimensions is an important computation in image processing. Often, objects in an image have some property, such as color or velocity, that is smooth over the object but changes discontinuously at the boundary of the object. A two-dimensional HRes network can smooth a signal over a large region in a visual image, even though a signal representing some property of the image changes by many $kT/(q\kappa)$ voltage units over that region. The voltage difference between any two neighboring nodes can be less than $kT/(q\kappa)$, even though the total difference across the smooth area of the image can be much greater. An abrupt discontinuity, however—as occurs when we try to put many kT/q voltage units across *one resistor*—will simply cause a discontinuity in the network voltage. The current out of the HRes circuits will limit at I_{sat}, no matter how large the voltage drop across the resistive connection is. So an HRes network computes a smooth approximation to the inputs as long as the drop across any one element is less than approximately kT/q. It allows larger voltage discontinuities by limiting the current through each element.

SEGMENTATION

For signals larger than approximately $kT/(q\kappa)$, both the followers and the resistors saturate; a small amount of saturation can be seen in the first data points in Figure 7.13. This saturation property leads to the same kind of robustness as that we noted for the follower-aggregation circuit. In addition, it has striking consequences for the kinds of computation that the circuit can accomplish.

In many situations, discontinuities are not only desirable but also necessary. An image is made up of smooth regions separated by discontinuities. The discontinuities carry the most information about the image. A network built of HRes circuits allows arbitrarily large discontinuities. Suppose, for example,

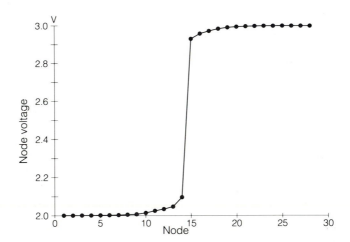

FIGURE 7.14   Segmentation due to saturation of resistive connections. When the input voltages to a horizontal resistor network have a discontinuity of many $kT/(q\kappa)$ units, the network naturally segments the image into smooth regions. The experimental data were taken on a one-dimensional network constructed as shown in Figure 7.12. The voltage at a number of nodes along the network is plotted as a function of node number n. Here, the inputs to all transconductance amplifiers for n less than or equal 14 were set to 2 volts; those for n greater than 14 were set to 3 volts. In spite of this very large discontinuity, no node voltage in either half of the network was driven more than 100 millivolts from its input potential.

we have a high-contrast edge in an image. There is a set of signals pulling *up* on one part of the network, and another set of signals pulling *down* on another part. Voltages at various positions in the network will look like Figure 7.14. A resistor on the high-contrast edge cannot supply enough current to keep the network within the linear range; there will be a big drop across that resistor, and then the network voltage will go off smoothly on the other side, as shown in the figure. That kind of discontinuity cannot occur in a network made of linear resistors, but it is a natural result of the nonlinear nature of a network of HRes circuits. The resulting image is *segmented* into regions over which the property represented by the input voltages $V(x,y)$ is smooth. We can easily identify the boundaries of these regions by finding the positions with voltage differences larger than $kT/(q\kappa)$. Computation of the natural boundaries in an image is called **segmentation**, and is considered to be a difficult problem [Geman et al., 1984]. Once again, the physics of a simple nonlinear circuit enables us to perform a complex computation in a simple way.

SUMMARY

In this and the previous two chapters, we have developed a respectable repertoire of analog computations on steady signals. Perhaps the most rewarding aspect of this endeavor is the extent to which important primitives are a direct consequence of fundamental laws of physics.

In Chapter 3, we saw that a single transistor takes on its gate a voltage-type signal and produces at its drain a current-type signal that is exponential in the input voltage. This exponential function was a direct result of the Boltzmann distribution. In Chapter 6, we saw how addition and subtraction of currents follow directly from the conservation of charge. In this chapter, we saw how the average of many inputs was computed by a simple resistive network. We are able to sense discontinuities by allowing the network to saturate, and then finding the boundaries at which saturation occurred.

Neural systems evolved with access to a vast array of physical phenomena that implemented useful functions. They have never been constrained by the traditional notions of mathematics or engineering analysis. In subsequent chapters, we will explore computations in which *time* is an explicit variable. Once again, we will find that the physical laws inherent in electronic and neural devices implement key primitives naturally and efficiently.

REFERENCES

Feinstein, D. The hexagonal resistive network and the circular approximation. *Caltech Computer Science Technical Report,* Caltech-CS-TR-88-7, California Institute of Technology, Pasadena, CA, 1988.

Geman, S. and Geman, D. Stochastic relaxation, Gibbs distributions, and the Bayesian restoration of images. *IEEE Transactions on Pattern Analysis and Machine Intelligence,* PAMI-6:721, 1984.

Gregorian, R. and Temes, G.C. *Analog MOS Integrated Circuits for Signal Processing.* New York: Wiley, 1986.

Hutchinson, J.M. and Koch, C. Simple analog and hybrid networks for surface interpolation. In Denker, J.S. (ed), *Neural Networks for Computing.* New York: American Institute of Physics, 1986, p. 235.

Shepherd, G.M. The neuron doctrine: A revision of functional concepts. *Yale Journal of Biology and Medicine,* 45:584, 1972.

Shepherd, G.M. Microcircuits in the nervous system. *Scientific American,* 238(2):93, February 1978.

DYNAMIC FUNCTIONS

For the natural inquirer, determinations of time are merely abbreviated statements of the dependence of one event upon another, and nothing more.
— Ernst Mach   *Popular Scientific Lectures* (1943)

CHAPTER

8

TIME-VARYING SIGNALS

Circuits that work with time-dependent signals allow us to do operations such as integration and differentiation *with respect to time.* The nervous system makes incredibly effective use of the fact that there are numerous events happening in the world that are functions of time; that they are functions of time is *the* important thing. If *sound*, for example, did not vary with time, it would not be sound. Your ear responds to derivative signals; the time variation of the signal contains all the information your ear needs. The steady (DC) part carries no information whatsoever.

People doing vision research take a picture out of the *New York Times* or *Life* magazine and throw it at a computer. They try to get the computer to determine whether there is a tree in that picture. That is a hard job; it is so hard that researchers are still arguing about how to do it, and will be for years. It is one of those classic problems in vision.

The reason such problems are intractable is that they start with only a small fraction of the information your eye uses to do the same job. Most of the input to our sensory systems is actively generated by our body movements. In fact, it is fair to view all sensory information as being generated either by the movement of objects in the world around us, or by our movements relative to those objects.

The retina is an excellent example of time-domain processing. The retina does not recognize trees at all. Except for the tiny fovea in the middle (with which we see acutely and which we use for activities such as reading), the vast majority of the area of the retina is devoted to the *periphery*. Peripheral vision is not concerned with the precise representation of shapes. It is overwhelmingly concerned with *motion*. For that reason, most of the bandwidth in the optic nerve is used for time-derivative information.

The reason for this preoccupation with motion is that animals that noticed something was jumping on them were able to jump out of the way, and they did not get eaten. The ones that did not notice leaping predators got eaten. So the ones that have survived have good peripheral vision. Peripheral vision is almost totally concerned with detecting time derivatives, because nobody ever got jumped on by something that was not moving.

An example of information generated by our natural body movements is the visual cues about depth. For objects more than about 6 feet away from us, most depth information comes from motion rather than from binocular disparity. If we are in the woods, it is important to know which tree is nearest to us. We move our bodies back and forth, and the shape (tree) that moves most, relative to the background, is the closest. We use this technique to detect depth out to great distances. People who navigate in the woods do it regularly without being conscious of what they are doing. Motion cues are built into our sense of the three-dimensionality of space. The derivative machinery in our peripheral vision gives us a great deal of information about what is in the world. It is only when we use our *attentive system*, when we fasten on tiny details and try to figure out what they are, that we use the shape-determining machinery in the fovea.

In this and the next few chapters, we will discuss time-varying signals and the kind of time-domain processing that comes naturally in silicon. In Chapter 9, we will do *integration* with respect to time. Then, we will be in a position to discuss *differentiation* with respect to time in Chapter 10. At that point, we will build several important system components.

LINEAR SYSTEMS

By definition, a **linear system** is one for which the size of the output is proportional to the size of the input. Because all real systems have upper limits on the size of the signals they can handle, no such system is linear over an arbitrary range of input level. Many systems, however, are *close enough* to linear that the viewpoint that comes from linear systems provides a basis from which we can analyze the nonlinearity.

For example, many people listen to their car radios while they drive. The radio-receiver systems in all cars are equipped with **automatic gain control**. Automatic gain control is a technique for maintaining a steady output amplitude, independent of the input signal strength, so that, for example, the music does not fade out when we drive under an overpass. In a linear system, if we cut the size of the input in half, then the response at the output also will be cut in half. So, by its very nature, a radio that has automatic gain control is a highly *nonlinear* system. On the other hand, when we receive music from the local radio station, the program is broadcast without a lot of distortion. Absence of distortion is one characteristic of a linear system. The people who designed the radio were clever. They did not ask *how loud the music was* when they built the automatic gain control; they asked *how much signal* they were getting from the radio station—and they decreased the gain proportionally. So, if the signal strength stays relatively constant over the period of oscillation of the sound waveform, the receiver acts like a linear system even though it is, in another sense, extremely nonlinear.

This mixed linear and nonlinear behavior is characteristic of many living systems. Your ear, for example, acts in many ways like the radio receiver: It has an automatic-gain-control system that allows it to work over a factor of 10^{12} in sound amplitude. In spite of this tremendous *dynamic range*, a particular waveform is perceived as being essentially the same at any amplitude; a very faint voice is just as intelligible as a very loud voice. The same comments hold for the visual system.

In summary, although many sensory systems are decidedly nonlinear overall, *the way they are actually used* allows much of their behavior to be represented, at least to first order, by linear-system terminology. We use this terminology as a language in which we can discuss any system that deals with signals, even nonlinear systems. The language is a useful underlying representation.

THE RESISTOR–CAPACITOR (RC) CIRCUIT

We will illustrate the linear-system viewpoint with the specific electrical circuit shown in Figure 8.1. We write Kirchhoff's law for the node labeled V:

$$\frac{V}{R} = -C\frac{dV}{dt} \tag{8.1}$$

Any current that goes through the resistor necessarily originates from charge stored on the capacitor; there is nowhere else from which that current can come. The current that flows through the resistor is V/R, and the current through the capacitor is $-C\,dV/dt$.

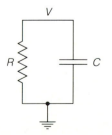

FIGURE 8.1   Schematic diagram of the simple resistor–capacitor (RC) circuit. Because there is no input, any current through the resistor must come from charge stored on the capacitor.

We can rewrite Equation 8.1 as

$$V + RC\frac{dV}{dt} = 0 \tag{8.2}$$

Notice that the first term has the units of voltage and the second term contains dV/dt, so the units would not be correct if the term in front of dV/dt did not have the units of *time*. The RC combination is called the **time constant** of the circuit, τ, which has units of time. We can develop an intuition for this relation from the hydraulic analogy in Figure 2.1 (p. 14). There the water tank represents a capacitor, and the friction in the pipe represents the resistor. The time it takes to empty the tank is proportional to the volume of water in the tank. It is also inversely proportional to the flow rate through the pipe. Because the flow rate is inversely proportional to the friction in the pipe, the emptying time will be proportional to the pipe resistance times the tank capacity.

We thus rewrite Equation 8.2 as

$$V + \tau\frac{dV}{dt} = 0 \tag{8.3}$$

There is only one function that has a derivative equal to itself: the exponential. So the solution to Equation 8.3 is

$$V = V_0 e^{-t/\tau} \tag{8.4}$$

Because this is a linear system, the constant V_0 can be any size; it is just the voltage on the capacitor at $t = 0$. The circuit behaves in the same way whether we start with 1 volt or 10 volts.

Equation 8.3 is a **linear** differential equation because it contains no terms such as V^2 or $V\,dV/dt$. It is **time invariant** because none of the coefficients are explicit functions of t. It is a **homogeneous** equation because its **driving term** on the right-hand side is zero. It is a **first-order** equation because it contains no higher-order derivatives than dV/dt. In most equations representing real circuits, the right-hand side is not equal to zero. A typical circuit is *driven by* one circuit, and *drives* another: The output signal of one circuit is the input signal of the next. The response of the circuit depends on what the driving term is. The most important defining characteristic of any linear system is its **natural response**— the way the circuit responds when it is out of equilibrium and is returning to equilibrium with time. The natural response is a property of the circuit itself, if you just leave that circuit alone; it does not have anything to do with what is driving the circuit. Equation 8.4 is the natural response of Figure 8.1.

HIGHER-ORDER EQUATIONS

Of course, not all linear differential equations are first-order, as Equation 8.3 is. Circuits with second-order equations are common; we will study one in Chapter 11. A simple form of such a second-order equation is

$$\frac{d^2 V}{dt^2} + \beta V = 0 \tag{8.5}$$

We can substitute Equation 8.4 into Equation 8.5, to obtain

$$\frac{1}{\tau^2} + \beta = 0$$

independent of the sign of the exponent. If β is negative, the solution is, indeed, an exponential. For positive β, we recall the derivatives of trigonometric functions:

$$\frac{d}{dx}(\sin x) = \cos x \tag{8.6}$$

$$\frac{d}{dx}(\cos x) = -\sin x \tag{8.7}$$

Substituting Equation 8.6 into Equation 8.7, and comparing with Equation 8.5, we obtain

$$V = \cos \sqrt{\beta}\, t$$

Similarly, $\sin \sqrt{\beta}\, t$ also is a solution.

The solutions of Equation 8.5 thus will be sines and cosines when β is positive, and exponentials when β is negative. In both cases, $1/\sqrt{\beta}$ has the units of time. The annoying property of higher-order equations is that we get a solution of a completely different kind when we change one parameter of the system by a small amount. It would be nice to have a unified representation in which any solution to a linear system could be expressed. The key to such a representation is to use exponentials with *complex arguments*.

We will first review the nature of complex numbers. Then we will develop the use of complex exponentials as a universal language for describing and analyzing time-varying signals.

COMPLEX NUMBERS

A complex number $N = x + jy$ has a **real part** Re(N), x, and an **imaginary part** Im(N), y, where both x and y are real numbers. In all complex-number notation, we will use the electrical-engineering convention $j = \sqrt{-1}$. Most other fields use i for the unit imaginary number, but such usage prevents i from being used as the current variable in electrical circuits. Such a loss is too great a price for electrical engineers to pay.

Any complex number can be visualized as a point in a two-dimensional **complex plane**, as shown in Figure 8.2. Mathematically, we have only redefined the set of points in the familiar x, y plane, and have packaged them so that

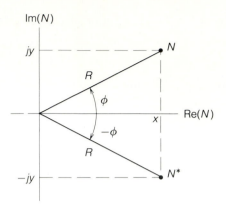

FIGURE 8.2   Graphical representation of a complex number N. Any number can be represented as a point in the plane. The x coordinate of the point is the real part of the number; the y coordinate is the imaginary part. Alternately, we can think of the number as a vector from the origin to the point. The complex conjugate N^* has the same real part, but its imaginary part is of the opposite sign.

any point can be dealt with as a single entity. This repackaging underlies a beautiful *representation* of signals, as we will see shortly—that representation is dependent on several *operations* on complex numbers. The first operation of note is **addition**; the sum of two complex numbers $A = x_1 + jy_1$ and $B = x_2 + jy_2$ is just the familiar form for the addition of ordinary vectors:

$$A + B = (x_1 + x_2) + j(y_1 + y_2)$$

In other words, the real and imaginary parts of the numbers are simply added separately.

Multiplication of two complex numbers also is defined by the rules of ordinary algebra, where j^2 has the value -1:

$$A \times B = x_1x_2 + jx_1y_2 + jx_2y_1 + j^2y_1y_2$$

$$= x_1x_2 - y_1y_2 + j(x_1y_2 + x_2y_1)$$

The product of complex numbers is much more simply expressed when the numbers are represented in *polar form*.

Polar Form

A natural alternate but completely equivalent form for specifying a point in the complex plane is to use the **polar form**. In the polar form, we give the point's radius R from the origin, and the angle ϕ between the horizontal axis and a line from the origin to the point. In the engineering community, R is called the **magnitude** of the complex number, and ϕ is the **phase angle**, or simply the *phase*. The key observation is that an expression for each unique point N in the plane can be written as

$$N = x + jy = Re^{j\phi} \tag{8.8}$$

Because $e^{j\phi_1} \times e^{j\phi_2}$ is equal to $e^{j(\phi_1+\phi_2)}$, multiplication by an exponential with an imaginary argument is equivalent to a rotation in the complex plane. The polar form allows us to develop a natural definition of the **multiplication** operation on complex numbers. The product of $A = R_1 e^{j\phi_1}$ and $B = R_2 e^{j\phi_2}$ is

$$A \times B = (R_1 \times R_2)e^{j(\phi_1 + \phi_2)}$$

Complex Conjugate

We can verify these relations and develop insight into complex numbers in the following way. The **complex conjugate** N^* of the complex number N has the same magnitude as N does, but has the opposite phase angle:

$$N^* = x - jy = Re^{-j\phi} \tag{8.9}$$

The product $N \times N^*$ will have an angle of zero, so it is a real number equal to the square of the magnitude of N:

$$N \times N^* = Re^{j\phi} \times Re^{-j\phi} = R^2 = (x + jy) \times (x - jy) = x^2 + y^2$$

The magnitude R of the number N (also called its **length, modulus,** or **absolute value**) is given by the square root of $N \times N^*$:

$$R = \sqrt{x^2 + y^2}$$

From Figure 8.2, it is clear that the real part x is just the projection of the vector onto the horizontal axis:

$$x = \mathrm{Re}(N) = R\cos\phi \tag{8.10}$$

Similarly, the imaginary part y is just the projection of the vector onto the vertical axis:

$$y = \mathrm{Im}(N) = R\sin\phi \tag{8.11}$$

Substituting Equations 8.10 and 8.11 into Equations 8.8 and 8.9, we obtain definitions of the exponentials of imaginary arguments in terms of ordinary trigonometric functions:

$$\cos\phi + j\sin\phi = e^{j\phi} \tag{8.12}$$

$$\cos\phi - j\sin\phi = e^{-j\phi} \tag{8.13}$$

Addition and subtraction of Equations 8.12 and 8.13 lead to the well-known identities that define ordinary trigonometric functions in terms of exponentials of imaginary arguments:

$$\sin\phi = \frac{e^{j\phi} - e^{-j\phi}}{2j}$$

$$\cos\phi = \frac{e^{j\phi} + e^{-j\phi}}{2}$$

We have seen that there is a direct connection between exponentials with imaginary arguments and the sine and cosine functions of ordinary trigonometry. We might suspect that using exponentials with complex arguments would give us a way of representing functions with properties intermediate between the oscillatory behavior of sine waves and the monotonically growing or decaying behavior of exponentials. That suspicion will be confirmed.

COMPLEX EXPONENTIALS

Exponentials with complex arguments are unique in the world of mathematical functions. They form the vocabulary of a language that has evolved over the years for representing *signals* that vary as a function of time. The complete formalism is called the *s*-plane; it is a beautiful example of *representation*. Its elegance stems in large measure from the fundamental mathematics that lies behind it. The formal derivations are beyond the scope of our discussion; they can be found in any text on complex variables, or in any text on linear system theory [Siebert, 1986; Oppenheim et al., 1983]. The complex variable $s = \sigma + j\omega$ will be the new central player of our drama. As the plot unfolds, we will find this complex variable multiplying the time t in every problem formulation involving the time response of linear systems.

We can illustrate the complex-exponential approach by considering the general second-order equation

$$\frac{d^2V}{dt^2} + \alpha\frac{dV}{dt} + \beta V = 0 \tag{8.14}$$

This equation can have solutions that are sine waves, or exponentials, or some combination of the two. The observation was made a long time ago that, if we use exponentials with a complex argument, we can always get a solution. We therefore substitute e^{st} for V into Equation 8.14. Because

$$\frac{d}{dt}(e^{st}) = se^{st} \qquad \text{and} \qquad \frac{d^2}{dt^2}(e^{st}) = s^2e^{st}$$

Equation 8.14 becomes

$$s^2e^{st} + \alpha se^{st} + \beta e^{st} = 0 \tag{8.15}$$

The complex exponential term e^{st} appears in every term of Equation 8.15, and therefore can be canceled out, leaving the expression for s that must be satisfied if e^{st} is to be a solution to the original differential equation:

$$s^2 + \alpha s + \beta = 0 \tag{8.16}$$

The fact that derivatives of any order give back the original function e^{st} is a special case of a much more general body of theory. If some operation on a function gives a result that has the same form as the original function (differing by only a constant factor), the function is said to be an **eigenfunction** of that operation. Complex exponentials are eigenfunctions of any linear, time-invariant operation, of which differentiation with respect to time is but one example.

Equation 8.16 is a quadratic in s, with solutions

$$s = \frac{-\alpha \pm \sqrt{\alpha^2 - 4\beta}}{2} \tag{8.17}$$

Depending on the (real) values of α and β, the two values of s given by Equation 8.17 may be real, imaginary, or complex. If $\alpha^2 - 4\beta$ is positive, both roots will be real. If $\alpha^2 - 4\beta$ is negative, the roots will be complex conjugates of each other. That complex roots come in conjugate pairs turns out to be a general result, although we have shown it for only the second-order system.

So what does it mean to have a *complex waveform* when we have to take the measurement on a real oscilloscope? As we might guess, a real instrument can measure only the *real part* of the signal. Real differential equations for real physical systems must have real solutions. Simply looking at the real part of a complex solution yields a solution also, because

$$\mathrm{Re}(f(t)) = \frac{f(t) + f^*(t)}{2}$$

and the roots come in conjugate pairs.

So, if our signal voltage is $V = e^{st}$, we will measure

$$V_{\mathrm{meas}} = \mathrm{Re}\left(e^{st}\right) = \mathrm{Re}\left(e^{(\sigma + j\omega)t}\right) = e^{\sigma t}\,\mathrm{Re}\left(e^{j\omega t}\right) = e^{\sigma t}\cos\left(\omega t\right)$$

For most signals, σ will be negative, and the response will be a **damped sinusoidal response**. If σ is equal to zero, the signal is a pure sinusoid, neither decaying or growing. If σ is greater than zero, the signal is an exponentially growing sinusoid. If ω is equal to zero, the signal is a growing or decaying exponential, with no oscillating component. If we wish to represent a sinusoid with a different phase ϕ—for example, a sine instead of a cosine—the signal multiplied by $e^{j\phi}$ still will be a solution:

$$\mathrm{Re}(e^{j\phi} \times e^{st}) = \mathrm{Re}(e^{j\phi} \times e^{(\sigma+j\omega)t}) = e^{\sigma t}\cos(\omega t + \phi)$$

The procedure we carried out on the second-order equation can be generalized to linear differential equations of higher order. No matter what the order of the differential equation is, we can always substitute in e^{st} as a solution, and get an equation in which the e^{st} appears in all the terms. Then we can go through and cancel out the e^{st} from every term, which leaves us with an equation involving only the coefficients. For a differential equation of *any* order, we get a polynomial in s with coefficients that are *real numbers*. They are real numbers because they come from the values of real circuit elements, such as resistors and capacitors.

We thus have a formal trick that we use with any time-invariant linear differential equation. We convert the manipulation of a *differential equation* into the manipulation of an *algebraic equation* in powers of the complex variable s. We achieved this simplification by using a clever representation for signals.

If a term is differentiated once, we get an s. If a term contains a second derivative, we get an s^2. (After a while, you will find that you can do this operation in your head.) What the procedure allows us to do is to treat s as an *operator*, that operator meaning *derivative with respect to time*. If we apply the s operator once, it means d/dt. If we take the derivative with respect to time twice, that means we apply the operator s, and then apply it again, so we write the composition of the operator with itself as s^2. In general,

$$s^n \Leftrightarrow \frac{d^n}{dt^n}$$

Similarly, we can view $1/s$ as the operator signifying *integration with respect to time*. This way of thinking about s as an operator was first noticed by a man by the name of Oliver Heaviside [Josephs, 1950].

THE HEAVISIDE STORY

Oliver Heaviside was the person who discovered that the ionosphere would reflect radio waves; there is a *Heaviside layer* [van der Pol, 1950] in the ionosphere that is named after him. He was thinking about the transient response of electronic circuits, and he noticed that, if he was careful, he could treat the variable s as the operator d/dt. He could perform the substitution and instantly convert differential equations into algebraic equations. He derived a unified way of treating circuits that involved only algebraic manipulations on these operators. It became known as the *Heaviside operator calculus* [van der Pol, 1950]. This was back in the old days, when the only thing most engineers worked with was sine waves. Heaviside had the whole method worked out to the point that, by multiplying and dividing by polynomials in s, he could actually predict the response due to step functions, impulses, and other kinds of transient inputs—it was beautiful stuff. It was a generalization of the behavior of linear systems in response to signals other than sine waves.

Heaviside operator calculus is a bit like the Mendeleev periodic table. Mendeleev figured out that different elements were related systematically by simple reasoning from special cases. Heaviside was smart enough to see that there *had to be* a general method, and he was able to determine what it was, even though he did not understand the deep mathematical basis for it. Ten years after he developed his calculus and was able to predict the behavior of many circuits, mathematicians started to notice that his method was successful and started wondering *what it really represented*. Finally, somebody else said, "Ah! you mean the *Laplace transform*."

So, it turns out that these polynomials in s are Laplace transforms; they are covered in all the first courses in complex variables. All the books about linear systems are full of them now—they have become the standard lore. Notice, however, that the technique was *invented* by someone who did not work out the mathematical details; he just went ahead and started working real problems that were very difficult to solve by any other approach. When he perfected the method and made it useful, somebody noticed that Laplace had written down the mathematics in abstract form 100 years before. So the Laplace transform should be called the Heaviside–Laplace transform. But formalism often is viewed as standing on its own, without regard for the applications insight that breathes life into it.

DRIVEN SYSTEMS

Systems that are not being driven are not very interesting—like your eye when it is perfectly dark or your ear when it is perfectly quiet. Real systems do not just decay away to nothing—they are *driven* by some input. The right-hand side of a differential equation for a driven system is not equal to zero; rather, it is some *driving function* that is a function of time. A differential equation for the output voltage has the input voltage as its right-hand side. The input voltage drives the system.

Now we need more than the homogeneous solution. Instead, we will examine the **driven solution** to the equation. We apply some input waveform, and observe the output waveform. Most physical systems have the property that, if we stop driving them, their output eventually dies away. Such systems are said to be **stable**. Because the system is linear, no matter what shape of input waveform we apply, the size of the output signal is proportional to the size of the input signal. So the output voltage can be expressed in terms of the input voltage by what electrical engineers call a **transfer function**, V_{out}/V_{in}. For a linear system, V_{out}/V_{in} will be independent of the magnitude of V_{in}. If we double V_{in}, we double V_{out}. That is why a transfer function has meaning—because it is independent of the size of the input signal.

Consider the driven RC circuit of Figure 8.3. The output voltage satisfies the circuit equation

$$C\frac{dV_{out}}{dt} = \frac{1}{R}(V_{in} - V_{out}) \tag{8.18}$$

In s-notation, Equation 8.18 can be written as

$$V_{out}(\tau s + 1) = V_{in} \tag{8.19}$$

where, as before, τ is equal to RC. If the input voltage is zero, Equation 8.19 is identical to Equation 8.3. Rearranging Equation 8.19 into transfer function form, we obtain

$$\frac{V_{out}}{V_{in}} = \frac{1}{\tau s + 1} \tag{8.20}$$

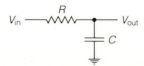

FIGURE 8.3 Simple RC circuit driven by a voltage V_{in}. The homogeneous response of this circuit is the same as that of Figure 8.1.

The term $1/(\tau s + 1)$ in Equation 8.20 is the s-plane transfer function $H(s)$ of the circuit of Figure 8.3. In general, for any time-invariant linear system,

$$V_{\text{out}} = H(s)V_{\text{in}}$$

As we noted, there is a form of input waveform $V_{\text{in}} = e^{st}$ that has a special place in the theory of linear systems, because it is an eigenfunction of any linear, time-invariant operation. The response $r_s(t)$ of a system with transfer function $H(s)$ to the input e^{st} is

$$r_s(t) = H(s)e^{st} \tag{8.21}$$

We will use the transfer function $H(s)$ in two ways: to derive the circuit's frequency response when the circuit is driven by a sine-wave input, and to derive the response of a circuit to any general input waveform. Equation 8.21 will allow us to derive a fundamental relationship between the system's impulse response and its s-plane transfer function.

The reason we have devoted most of this chapter to developing s-notation is that we wish to avoid re-deriving the response of each circuit for each kind of input. Heaviside undoubtedly had the same motivation.

SINE-WAVE RESPONSE

Even in today's world of digital electronics, people do apply sine waves to circuits, and it is useful to understand what happens under these conditions. This is what happens to your ear when you listen to an oboe. We use the transfer function in s-notation to derive the response when a system is driven by a sine wave.

Transfer Function

We saw how the complex exponential e^{st} can be used to represent both transient and sinusoidal waveforms. This approach allows us to use the s-notation for derivatives, as described earlier. It also illustrates clearly how a linear circuit driven by a single-frequency sinusoidal input will have an output at that frequency and at no other, as we will now show.

We can determine the system response to a cosine-wave input by evaluating the system response when V_{in} is equal to $e^{j\omega t}$. We notice that this form of input is a special case of the more general form $V_{\text{in}} = e^{st}$ used in Equation 8.21, with $s = j\omega$. The real part of the response of a linear system to the input $e^{j\omega t}$ carries exactly the same information as does the response to a cosine. Hence, by merely setting s equal to $j\omega$ in the transfer function, we can evaluate the amplitude and phase of the response.

To understand what is going on, we will return to our derivation of the response of a linear differential equation, starting with Equation 8.21. Because the equation is linear, the exponential $e^{j\omega t}$ will appear in every term. No matter how many derivatives we take, we cannot generate a signal with any other frequency. The $e^{j\omega t}$ will cancel out of every term, leaving the output voltage equal to the input voltage multiplied by some function of ω. That function is just the transfer function with $s = j\omega$. For any given frequency, the transfer function, in general, will be a complex number. It often is convenient to express the number in polar form:

$$\frac{V_{\text{out}}(\omega)}{V_{\text{in}}(\omega)} = R(\omega)e^{j\phi(\omega)}$$

$R(\omega)$ is the magnitude $|V_{\text{out}}/V_{\text{in}}|$ of the transfer function, and ϕ is the phase.

RC-Circuit Example

We will, once again, use the RC circuit of Equation 8.19 as an example:

$$\frac{V_{\text{out}}}{V_{\text{in}}} = \frac{1}{\tau s + 1} = \frac{1}{j\omega\tau + 1}$$

At very low frequencies, $\omega\tau$ is much less than 1 and V_{out} is very nearly equal to V_{in}. For very high frequencies, $\omega\tau$ is much greater than 1, and

$$\frac{V_{\text{out}}}{V_{\text{in}}} \approx \frac{1}{j\omega\tau} = \frac{-j}{\omega\tau} \tag{8.22}$$

The $-j$ indicates a *phase lag* of 90 degrees. The $1/\omega$ dependence indicates that in this range the circuit functions as an integrator.

The most convenient format for plotting the frequency response of a circuit is shown in Figure 8.4. The horizontal axis is log frequency, the vertical axis is $\log|V_{\text{out}}/V_{\text{in}}|$. Logarithms are strange; zero is $-\infty$ on a log scale. When we plot $\log\omega$, zero frequency is way off the left edge of the world. By the time we ever see it on a piece of graph paper, ω is not anywhere near zero anymore—it may be three orders of magnitude below $1/\tau$. While we are crawling up out of the

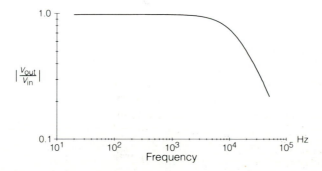

FIGURE 8.4 Response of the circuit of Figure 8.3 to a sine-wave input. The log of the magnitude of $V_{\text{out}}/V_{\text{in}}$ is plotted as a function of the log of the frequency. Because the circuit is linear, the frequency of the output must be the same as that of the input.

hole near zero, we are going through orders and orders of magnitude in ω, and nothing is happening to the response of the system. As a result, the response on a log plot is absolutely dead flat for decades, because $-\infty$ is a long way away.

Eventually, we will get up to where ω is on the same scale as $1/\tau$ is, so there will be one order of magnitude at which the scale of frequency is the same as the scale of $1/\tau$. Above that, ω will be very large compared with the scale of $1/\tau$. When we get to the order of magnitude at which $\omega\tau$ is near 1, the denominator starts to increase and the response starts to decrease. At frequencies much higher than $1/\tau$, the response decreases with a slope equal to -1, corresponding to the limit given in Equation 8.22.

At low frequencies, the response is constant; at high frequencies, it varies as $1/\omega$; in between, it rounds off gracefully. At $\omega = 1/\tau$,

$$\frac{V_{\text{out}}}{V_{\text{in}}} = \frac{1}{j+1} \tag{8.23}$$

Because the magnitude of a complex number N is $\sqrt{(\text{Re}(N))^2 + (\text{Im}(N))^2}$, the magnitude of Equation 8.23 is $1/\sqrt{2}$. So, at that frequency, the amplitude is decreased by $\sqrt{2}$.

The plot makes sense when we look at the circuit. The capacitor stores charge when everything is DC (nothing is changing with respect to time); it charges up to the input voltage and does not draw any more current. If there is no current, there is no voltage drop across the resistor, so everything remains static, and V_{out} is equal to V_{in}. If we suddenly change V_{in}, the output will exponentially approach the new value with time constant τ.

As the input frequency increases, the imaginary part of the response becomes more negative. This condition is called *phase lag*; the output waveform lags behind the input waveform. The lag occurs because the capacitor takes time to catch up! Another way of looking at it is that the capacitor is integrating the input, and the integral of a cosine is a sine, which lags behind the cosine by 90 degrees. If the input starts up instantly, it still takes a while for the output to catch up—it is *lagging*. By convention, we refer to the lagging phase angle ϕ as negative.

RESPONSE TO ARBITRARY INPUTS

We can derive the response of any stable, linear, time-invariant system to an arbitrary input waveform in the following manner. Let us suppose that we apply an input $f(t)$ to our system, starting at $t = 0$, as shown in Figure 8.5(a). We can think of making up that waveform out of narrow pulses, like the one shown in Figure 8.5(b); this pulse, which we will call $p_\epsilon(t)$, has width ϵ and unit amplitude. In other words, $p_\epsilon(t)$ is equal to 1 in the narrow interval between $t = 0$ and $t = \epsilon$, and is zero for all other t. We can build up an approximation to the arbitrary waveform $f(t)$ starting at $t = 0$ by placing a pulse of height $f(0)$ at $t = 0$, followed by a pulse of height $f(\epsilon)$ at $t = \epsilon$, followed by a pulse of

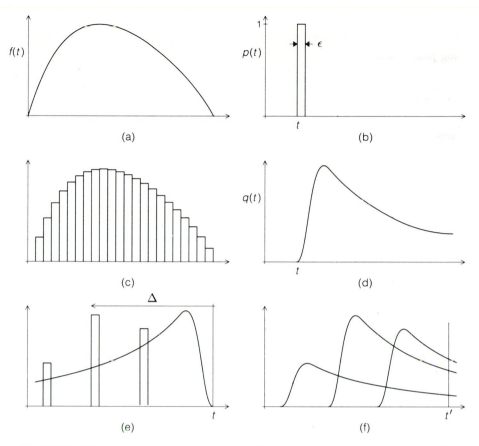

FIGURE 8.5 This sequence of graphs illustrates how an arbitrary waveform can be built up from pulses, and how the response of a system to the waveform can be built up from the responses to the individual pulses. The horizontal axis of all graphs is time; the vertical axis is amplitude.

The arbitrary waveform (a) is the input to a linear, time-invariant system. We can approximate the input waveform as a sum of narrow pulses, as shown in (c). In (b), the pulse $p(t)$ starts at time t, and has unit amplitude, and width ϵ. The input waveform is approximated by a sum of these pulses, each weighted by the value of the function at the time t, as shown in (c). The response of the linear system to the pulse $p(t)$ is shown in (d). To illustrate the summation process, we choose three individual pulses, as shown in (e). The individual responses of the system to these three pulses are shown in (f). At any measurement time t', the response of the system is just the sum of the individual values where the curves cross the time t'. This picture is a literal interpretation of Equation 8.25.

A more elegant formulation of the result is suggested by the response curve in (e), which runs backward from the measurement time. The value of this curve at any time Δ before the measurement is taken can be used as a weighting function, determining the contribution to the result of the pulse starting at that time. This interpretation is given in mathematical form in Equation 8.26. In the limit of small ϵ, the shape of the system response $q(t)$ becomes independent of ϵ, and its amplitude becomes directly proportional to ϵ. That limit allows us to define the *impulse response* $h(t)$ in Equation 8.27. A continuous version of the sum shown graphically in (e) can then be carried out; it is called the *convolution* of the waveform with the impulse response, as given in Equation 8.28.

height $f(2\epsilon)$ at $t = 2\epsilon$, and so on, as shown in Figure 8.5(c). Because the function $f(t)$ does not change appreciably over the time ϵ, we can express the pulse with amplitude $f(n\epsilon)$ occurring at time $t = n\epsilon$ as $f(n\epsilon)\, p_\epsilon(n\epsilon)$. Because the pulses do not overlap, we can express the discrete approximation of Figure 8.5(c) as

$$f(t) \approx \sum_{n=0}^{\infty} f(n\epsilon) p_\epsilon(n\epsilon) \tag{8.24}$$

The response of our system to the pulse $p_\epsilon(t)$ will be some function $q_\epsilon(t)$; a typical response is shown in Figure 8.5(d). Because the system is linear, its response to a pulse $A\, p_\epsilon(t)$ will be $A\, q_\epsilon(t)$; this property is, in fact, the definition of a linear system—the *form* of the response does not depend on the amplitude of the input, and the *amplitude* of the response is directly proportional to the amplitude of the input. Because the system is time invariant, its response to a pulse identical to $p_\epsilon(t)$ but starting at a later time $t + n\epsilon$ is simply $q_\epsilon(t + n\epsilon)$. By the principle of *linear superposition* mentioned in Chapter 2, we can approximate the response of the system to the input $f(t)$ as the sum of the responses to each of the individual input pulses of Equation 8.24. Each pulse initiates a response starting at its initiation time t. The measurement time t' occurs a period $t' - t$ later, and the response at t' is therefore $q_\epsilon(t' - t)$. For the pulse train shown in Figure 8.5(c), the response $r(t')$ of the system at measurement time $t' = N\epsilon$ to a pulse occurring at time $t = n\epsilon$ is therefore $q_\epsilon((N - n)\epsilon)$.

Real physical systems, linear or nonlinear, are **causal**—inputs arriving after the measurement time cannot affect the output at that time. Causality is expressed for our linear system by the fact that $q_\epsilon(t)$ is zero for t less than zero. For this reason, terms in Equation 8.25 with values of n greater than N will make no contribution to the sum. We can therefore approximate the response of our system to the input $f(t)$ as a sum up to $n = N$:

$$r(N\epsilon) \approx \sum_{n=0}^{N} f(n\epsilon)\, q_\epsilon((N - n)\epsilon) \tag{8.25}$$

We can develop an intuition for the sum in Equation 8.25 by plotting a few of the individual terms, as shown in Figure 8.5(f).

The time-invariant property of our system allows us to interpret this result in a much more elegant way than is expressed by Equation 8.25. We notice that the argument of q represents the interval between the time f is evaluated and the time the measurement is taken. We can thus view q as a weighting function that determines the contribution of f to the response as a function of time *into the past*. By making a change of variables, we can express the result of Equation 8.25 in terms of the time-before-measurement $\Delta = (N - n)\epsilon$:

$$r(t') \approx \sum_{\Delta=0}^{N\epsilon} f(t' - \Delta)\, q_\epsilon(\Delta) \tag{8.26}$$

This interpretation of the result is shown pictorially in Figure 8.5(e). Notice that our original time scale has disappeared from the problem; it has been replaced by the relevant variables associated with the time when the output is measured, and with the time before the measurement was taken.

We can derive a continuous version of Equation 8.26 by noticing that no physical system can follow an arbitrarily rapid change in input—a mechanical system has mass, and an electronic system has capacitance. A finite current flowing into a finite capacitor for an infinitesimal time can make only an infinitesimal change in the voltage across that capacitor. For that reason, there is a lower limit to the width ϵ of our pulses, below which the *form* of the response does not change. As the width ϵ of each pulse becomes smaller, the pulse amplitude stays the same in order to match the curve ever more closely, and the number of pulses N increases to fill the duration of the observation.

We can reason about the behavior in that limit by considering the response to two pulses of equal amplitude that are adjacent in time. Because ϵ is very small compared to the time course of the response $q_\epsilon(t)$, the response due to each of the pulses will be nearly indistinguishable. The response when both pulses are applied therefore will be nearly identical in form, and will be twice the amplitude of the response to either pulse individually. In other words, in the limit of very narrow pulses, the *shape* of the response becomes independent of pulse width, and the amplitude of the response becomes directly proportional to the pulse width. This limit allows us to define the **impulse response** $h(t)$ of the system:

$$h(t) = \lim_{\epsilon \to 0} \frac{1}{\epsilon} q_\epsilon(t) \tag{8.27}$$

The impulse response $h(t)$ of any stable, linear, time-invariant analog system must approach zero for infinite time. This property of **finite impulse response** allows us to write Equation 8.26 as an integral in the continuous variables t and Δ, including the effect of inputs into the indefinite past. Because the original time scale does not appear in the formulation, we use the variable t for the time of measurement; we use Δ for the time before measurement.

$$r(t) = \int_0^\infty f(t - \Delta)\, h(\Delta)\, d\Delta \tag{8.28}$$

Notice that $d\Delta$ is the limit of ϵ, canceling the $1/\epsilon$ behavior of $h(\Delta)$ given by Equation 8.27.

Equation 8.28 is called the **convolution** of f with h, and it often is written $r = f * h$. It is the most fundamental result in the theory of linear systems. In practical terms, it means that we can fully characterize a circuit operating in its linear range by measuring the circuit's impulse response in the manner we have described. We then can compute the response of the system to any other input waveform, as long as the circuit stays in its linear range. We will have many occasions to apply this principle in later chapters.

Relationship of *H(s)* to the Impulse Response

We are now in a position to derive one of the truly deep results in linear system theory by applying an input e^{st} to our system. From Equation 8.28, the response $r_s(t)$ of the system to this input is

$$r_s(t) = \int_0^\infty e^{s(t-\Delta)}\, h(\Delta)\, d\Delta \tag{8.29}$$

In Equation 8.21, we derived the response to this same input in terms of $H(s)$:

$$r_s(t) = H(s)e^{st} \tag{8.21}$$

But these two expressions represent the *same* response. Equating Equations 8.29 and 8.21, we find that

$$H(s)e^{st} = \int_0^\infty e^{s(t-\Delta)}\, h(\Delta)\, d\Delta$$

Or, multiplying both sides by e^{-st}, we conclude that

$$H(s) = \int_0^\infty e^{-s\Delta}\, h(\Delta)\, d\Delta \tag{8.30}$$

Because Δ is just a dummy variable of integration, it could be any other variable as well. The impulse response is specified with respect to the time t, so we will write Equation 8.30 using t as our variable of integration:

$$H(s) = \int_0^\infty e^{-st}\, h(t)\, dt$$

The s-plane transfer function is the product of e^{-st} and the impulse response $h(t)$, integrated over time. This integral is known as the **Laplace transform** of the transfer function. The use of such transforms to determine the properties of linear systems is a beautiful topic of study, and is highly recommended to those readers who are not already familiar with the material [Seibert, 1986].

Impulse Response

In general, the transfer function of any circuit formed of discrete components will be a quotient of two polynomials in s:

$$\frac{V_{\text{out}}}{V_{\text{in}}} = \frac{N(s)}{D(s)}.$$

We can always rewrite such a transfer function as

$$V_{\text{out}}\, D(s) = V_{\text{in}}\, N(s)$$

The homogeneous response of the system is the solution when V_{in} is equal to 0:

$$V_{\text{out}}\, D(s) = 0 \tag{8.31}$$

In other words, the homogeneous response of the system is made up of signals corresponding to the roots of the denominator of the transfer function. These roots are called the **poles** of the transfer function. Each root, or complex-conjugate pair of roots, will represent one way in which the system can respond. The response function always is e^{st}, with the value of s corresponding to the particular root. Each such function is called a **natural mode** of the system.

We can illustrate the procedure with the simple RC circuit of Figure 8.3. The denominator $D(s)$ of the transfer function of Equation 8.19 was $\tau s + 1$. The solution of Equation 8.31 is $s = -1/\tau$. We obtain the corresponding mode by substituting this value of s into $V = e^{st}$; the result is

$$V = V_0 e^{-t/\tau}$$

This is the same result as the one we found by direct solution of the differential equation in Equation 8.4.

The homogeneous response itself is sufficient to answer the most important questions about a system—in particular, whether it is stable, and by what margin. The poles of a stable system must have a negative real part—those of an unstable system have a positive real part. Questions of stability therefore are related not to the form of the input waveform, but rather to only the nature of the natural modes.

The total homogeneous response of the system always is the sum of the individual modes, each of which has a certain amplitude determined by the initial conditions—the voltages stored on capacitors at $t = 0$. If we know the initial values of all voltages and currents in the network, we have enough information to determine uniquely the amplitude of each of the natural modes that sum together to make up the response of the system. An impulse and a step function are examples of two common input waveforms that do not change after $t = 0$, so the response to either of these inputs will be special cases of the natural response of the system. The amplitudes of the natural modes can be determined from the values of the voltages and currents just after $t = 0$. These initial values can, in turn, be determined from the values of the voltages and currents just before $t = 0$, and from the amplitude of the input waveform. Using this approach, we can derive the impulse response of a circuit, and we can use that response in Equation 8.28 to predict the behavior of the circuit to any input waveform.

Although the application of these techniques gives us a powerful and useful method for deriving system properties, we must avoid the temptation to apply this approach blindly to a new situation. All physical circuits are inherently nonlinear. Over a suitably limited range of signal excursions, it usually is possible to make a linear approximation and to apply the results of linear system theory. Normal operation of a circuit, however, may extend well beyond the range of linear approximation. We must always check the conditions under which a linear approximation is valid before we apply that approximation to a specific circuit.

SUMMARY

We have seen by the example of a simple RC circuit how the complex exponential notation can give us information about the response of the circuit to both transient and sinusoidal inputs. We will use the s-notation in all discussions of the time response of our systems to small signals. Once the systems are driven into their nonlinear range, the results of linear system theory no longer apply. Nonetheless, these results still provide a useful guide to help us determine the large-signal response.

REFERENCES

Josephs, H.J. *Heaviside's Electric Circuit Theory.* London: Methuen, 1950.

Oppenheim, A.V., Willsky, A.S., and Young, I.T. *Signals and Systems.* Englewood Cliffs, NJ: Prentice-Hall, 1983.

Siebert, W.M. *Circuits, Signals and Systems.* Cambridge, MA: MIT Press 1986.

van der Pol, B. Heaviside's operational calculus. *The Heaviside Centenary Volume.* London: The Institution of Electrical Engineers, 1950, p. 70.

FOLLOWER–INTEGRATOR CIRCUIT

In Chapter 4, we noted that neural processes are insulated from the extra-cellular fluid by a membrane only approximately 50 angstroms thick. The capacitance of this nerve membrane serves to integrate charge injected into the dendritic tree by synaptic inputs. Much of the real-time nature of neural computation is vastly simplified because this integrating capability is used as a way of storing information for short time periods—from less than 1 millisecond to more than 1 second. There is an important lesson to be learned here, an insight that would not follow naturally from the standard lore of either computer science or electrical engineering. Like the spatial smoothing performed by resistive networks in Chapter 7, temporal smoothing is an essential and generally useful form of computation.

In CMOS technology, the elementary temporal-smoothing circuit is the **follower–integrator circuit** shown in Figure 9.1. It is the most universally useful of all time-dependent circuits.

The circuit consists of a transconductance amplifier connected as a follower, with its output driving a capacitor. As usual, we set the transconductance G with the bias voltage V_b. The rate at which the capacitor charges is proportional to the output current of the follower:

$$C\frac{dV_{out}}{dt} = I_b \tanh\left(\frac{\kappa(V_{in} - V_{out})}{2}\right) \qquad (9.1)$$

where the voltages are measured in units of kT/q.

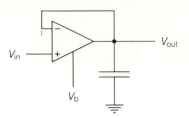

FIGURE 9.1 Schematic of the follower–integrator circuit. The current into the capacitor is proportional to the difference between V_{in} and V_{out}. The rate at which V_{out} is able to respond to changes in V_{in} is set by the transconductance of the amplifier.

First, we will examine the behavior of this circuit for signals that have small time-dependent deviations from some steady (quiescent) value. We will restrict the quiescent input voltage to the range within which the amplifier is well behaved, as described in Chapter 5. Under these conditions, we can analyze the circuit using the linear-systems-theory approach of Chapter 8. We will then compare the results with those we obtained for the RC integrator of Chapter 8. We will consider the large-signal behavior of the circuit at the end of the chapter.

SMALL-SIGNAL BEHAVIOR

For small signals, the tanh can be approximated by its argument, and Equation 9.1 becomes

$$C\frac{dV_{out}}{dt} = G(V_{in} - V_{out}) \tag{9.2}$$

Equation 9.2 can be rewritten in s-notation as

$$\frac{V_{out}}{V_{in}} = \frac{1}{\tau s + 1} \quad \text{where} \quad \tau = \frac{C}{G} \tag{9.3}$$

The response of the circuit of Figure 9.1 to a step input is shown in Figure 9.2. It can be compared with that of the RC integrator, which is shown in Figure 9.3. The two responses are not distinguishably different for the small (approximately 40-millivolt) signals used.

Using the principle of linear superposition of Equation 8.28 (p. 143), we can define precisely the temporal-smoothing properties of a single time-constant integration such as Equation 9.3

$$V_{out}(t) = \int_0^\infty V_{in}(t - \Delta)e^{-\Delta/\tau}\, d\Delta$$

The output at any time t is made up of the input for all previous times; the contribution of the input to the present output decreases exponentially with time into the past. In other words, the output is a moving average of the input, exponentially weighted by its timeliness. One could hardly ask for a more biologically relevant single measure of history—which is, no doubt, why this is the most ubiquitous computation in neural systems.

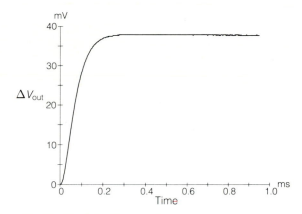

FIGURE 9.2   Measured response of the follower–integrator circuit to an approximately 40-millivolt step change in input voltage. The quiescent input voltage was approximately $V_{DD}/2$. The output is a temporally smoothed version of the input. Because the circuit is not linear, the form of the response will be different for large inputs (see Figure 9.12). We can adjust the time constant of the response over many orders of magnitude by setting the transconductance of the amplifier.

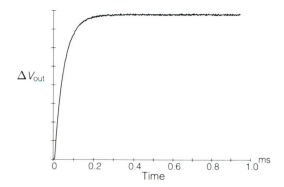

FIGURE 9.3   Measured response of the RC circuit of Figure 8.3 (p. 137) to step change in input voltage. Because the circuit is linear, the form of the response is independent of the size of the input.

COMPOSITION

The transfer function V_{out}/V_{in} of the follower–integrator circuit is identical to that of the RC integrator of Chapter 8. You might think, therefore, that we have used a very difficult solution to a simple problem: We have replaced a simple resistor by a complicated transconductance amplifier. From the point of view of the transfer function, that is indeed what we have done; but a system has more properties than just its transfer function. There are important differences between the RC circuit and the follower–integrator circuit, which we can best

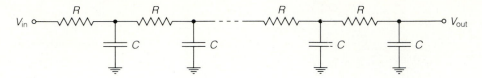

FIGURE 9.4 Delay line made up of a large number of RC-integrator sections in cascade.

appreciate by conducting an experiment. Let us take the RC integrator of Figure 8.3 (p. 137) and say, "If one is good, a lot more are better." We connect the output of one section to the input of another to form the RC delay line shown in Figure 9.4.

The response measured at the output of the first section of the line is shown in Figure 9.5. It is clear that the response of the first RC section has been changed from that of Figure 9.3 by the addition of the rest of the line. The reason is obvious: There is current flowing out of the first output through the second resistor, to charge up the rest of the line. This current must come from the input, and no particular node capacitance can get charged up until the capacitors between that node and the input get charged up. The waveform at the output of the first section of the line is much more sluggish than that out of the same single section with the rest of the line disconnected.

Transfer functions are most useful when their form is not changed by the environment in which they are used. Assume we have two circuit building blocks, the output of the first one feeding the input of the second. If we want to know the transfer function of this combined circuit, we just multiply the two transfer functions of the two individual circuits. The transfer functions are algebraic functions of s, and their product is the transfer function for the whole cir-

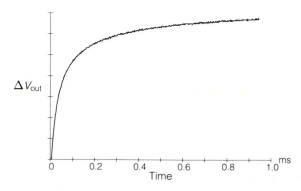

FIGURE 9.5 Measured response of the output of the first section of the RC delay line of Figure 9.4. The addition of subsequent stages has drastically changed the form of the response from that of a single RC integrator (Figure 9.3).

cuit. For a circuit to be an independent *module*, it must have this composition property.

The RC circuit does not have this important property. Although that circuit *is* linear, it is *not* an independent module. The RC circuit looks simple, but in a system context it is actually extremely complicated; whenever we hook up one to another, we change what the first one does. So we cannot just multiply the transfer functions. The transfer function of the *composition* of the two circuits is not the composition of their individual transfer functions. In other words, the RC circuit does not have a simple *abstraction*.

Each input of the follower–integrator circuit is the gate of a transistor. The gate is isolated from the rest of the circuit by the gate oxide, which for all practical purposes is a perfect insulator. We can hook the input of such an amplifier to the output of any other circuit without drawing any current. We can obtain the transfer function of the composition by multiplying the two transfer functions, because we have not disturbed the first one by hooking up the second one. Using the amplifier instead of a resistor has bought us a clean abstraction of the smoothing function.

By throwing away the amplifier voltage gain A, we have obtained unity gain at very low frequencies to a high accuracy. We also have got much better control over the value of G, because G is directly related to the bias current in the amplifier, which we can control with a current mirror. The time constants are useful up to about 10 seconds. The follower–integrator first-order section works just like the RC integrator would have done had we put unity-gain amplifiers between every stage.

IMPLEMENTATION

The layout of a typical follower–integrator circuit is shown in Plate 8(a). The circuit consists of a wide-range amplifier driving a capacitor structure. In CMOS technology, the only excellent capacitor material we have available is the gate oxide. Unfortunately, the p- and n-type diffused areas do not extend under the polysilicon gate material, and hence we do not have a structure with good conductors on both sides of the thin gate oxide. Instead, we use a p-type transistor with its source tied to V_{DD}, and an n-type transistor with its source tied to ground. Because each transistor is biased above its threshold voltage, its capacitance is very nearly equal to the *oxide capacitance*—the same value as that of an ideal capacitor employing the gate oxide as its dielectric. If the gate voltage falls below the transistor threshold voltage, the capacitance falls rapidly. For the structure shown in Plate 8(a) to maintain a relatively constant capacitance, the voltage on the common polysilicon gate area should be kept away from both rails by at least the threshold voltage of the relevant transistor. This limitation is not much more severe than are the voltage limitations imposed by other circuits in a system.

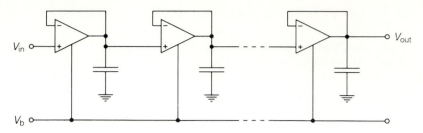

FIGURE 9.6   Delay line formed by connection of a large number of follower–integrator circuits in cascade.

DELAY LINES

We can create a delay line using follower–integrator first-order sections, as shown in Figure 9.6. The step response at the first few taps is shown in Figure 9.7. We can compare this figure with a similar plot for the RC line of Figure 9.4, shown in Figure 9.8. It is clear that the signal decays much faster in the RC line, because current must flow all the way from the input to the point at which the capacitor is being charged. In the follower–integrator line, the current required for charging each capacitor is supplied from the power supply, mediated by the transconductance amplifier.

Follower–Integrator Delay Line

Because of the modular nature of the sections, we can write the transfer function of the line up to the nth section as the product of the transfer functions of each of the individual sections:

$$\frac{V_{\text{out}}}{V_{\text{in}}} = \left(\frac{1}{\tau s + 1}\right)^n \tag{9.4}$$

To understand how Equation 9.4 represents a signal propagating along the line, we will pick a particular form for the input—a sine wave. We represent a sinusoidal signal of angular frequency ω by setting s equal to $j\omega$ in the transfer function. We need to understand what the nth power of a complex number represents, and how to take the inverse of a complex number. We can delay worrying about the inverse by considering $V_{\text{in}}/V_{\text{out}}$ instead of $V_{\text{out}}/V_{\text{in}}$. We therefore write the inverse of Equation 9.4 for $s = j\omega$:

$$\frac{V_{\text{in}}}{V_{\text{out}}} = (j\omega\tau + 1)^n \tag{9.5}$$

We will be interested in lines with many sections. For such lines, the response at high frequency will decrease very steeply, falling with increasing frequency as $(1/\omega\tau)^n$. We are concerned with frequencies for which the line has measurable output, so we can safely assume that $\omega\tau$ is much less than 1. In Chapter 8, we

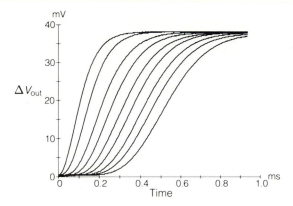

FIGURE 9.7   Measured response at the outputs of the first nine taps of the delay line of Figure 9.6. The spacing between any two curves is the delay of a particular section. The delay varies randomly due to transistor mismatch, as discussed in Chapter 3.

noted that the polar form of a complex number was the representation in which multiplication is a simple operation. In this regime, each term in Equation 9.5 can be approximated by the polar form

$$1 + j\omega\tau \approx \left(1 + \tfrac{1}{2}(\omega\tau)^2\right)e^{j\omega\tau} \tag{9.6}$$

Using Equation 9.6 and the rule for multiplying complex numbers given in Chapter 8, we can approximate Equation 9.5 for $j\omega\tau$ much less than 1:

$$\frac{V_{\text{in}}}{V_{\text{out}}} = \left(1 + \tfrac{n}{2}(\omega\tau)^2\right)e^{nj\omega\tau} \tag{9.7}$$

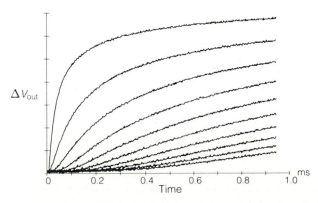

FIGURE 9.8   Measured response at the outputs of the first 10 sections of the RC delay line of Figure 9.4. The rise time of the waveforms increases rapidly with distance through the line.

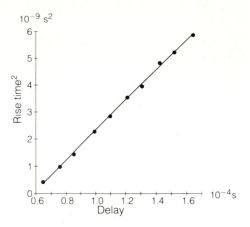

FIGURE 9.9   Linear relationship between the delay at several taps along a follower–integrator line and the square of the rise time at the same taps. The data were obtained from Figure 9.7 by the procedure described in the text.

Equation 9.7 leads to the following approximate form for the transfer function:

$$\frac{V_{\text{out}}}{V_{\text{in}}} \approx \frac{1}{1 + \frac{n}{2}(\omega\tau)^2} e^{-jn\omega\tau} \tag{9.8}$$

The line acts as a phase delay of $n\omega\tau$ radians, corresponding to a time delay of $n\tau$ seconds—τ seconds per section. The signal magnitude is attenuated by $\frac{1}{2}(\omega\tau)^2$ per section. We can estimate the **bandwidth** of the line by finding the frequency where the response has decreased to one-half of the input amplitude. To the level of approximation used in Equation 9.8, the cutoff frequency ω_c is given by

$$\omega_c\tau = \sqrt{\tfrac{2}{n}} \tag{9.9}$$

The bandwidth of the line thus decreases as the square root of the number of sections, whereas the delay is linear with the number of sections.

The **rise time** to a step input is approximately the reciprocal of the bandwidth. We can measure the rise time of the curves of Figure 9.7 by extrapolating the steep part of the signal upward to its upper steady-state value, and downward to its initial value. The delay is the time when the output crosses the level midway between the two limiting values. The square of the rise time is plotted as a function of the delay in Figure 9.9. The result is an excellent straight line, as predicted by Equation 9.9. Note that the delay of the individual sections varies considerably, due to the mismatch among the bias transistors in the individual amplifiers. In spite of this variation, the relationship between delay and bandwidth is in excellent qualitative agreement with our analysis. We will see in Chapter 16 that the form of the behavior of much more sophisticated delay lines also is preserved despite a wide variation among the individual delay elements.

RC Delay Line

In Chapter 7, we analyzed the propagation of steady (DC) signals in a passive dendritic process. The signals were not varying with time, and hence we could neglect the membrane capacitance. We will now derive the behavior of such a process, including the effects of membrane capacitance on time-dependent signals.

We model the process by adding capacitors at every node, as shown in Figure 9.10. We can analyze the line by using the same approach by which we derived Equation C.5 (p. 340). The differential equations for current and voltage are

$$-\frac{\partial V}{\partial x} = IR \tag{9.10}$$

and

$$-\frac{\partial I}{\partial x} = C\frac{\partial V}{\partial t} + VG \tag{9.11}$$

where R is the axial resistance, G is the conductance to ground, and C is the capacitance, all given per unit length of line. Both x and I are taken to be positive pointing to the right. Differentiating Equation 9.10 with respect to x, and substituting into Equation 9.11, we can eliminate I, and thus we obtain the equation for $V(x,t)$:

$$\frac{\partial^2 V}{\partial x^2} = RGV + RC\frac{\partial V}{\partial t} \tag{9.12}$$

We recognize our old friend $RG = \alpha^2 = 1/L^2$, where α is the *space constant* and L is the *diffusion length* of the line, as defined in Equation 7.2 (p. 108).

Equation 9.12 is called the **diffusion equation**; it governs the time course of signal propagation in a dissipative passive medium where the stuff out of which the signal is made is stored in the medium, and the fraction lost as the signal propagates is proportional to the amount present. The passive dendrites of a neuron obey this equation: V is the voltage across the membrane, C is the capacitance of the membrane, R is the axial resistance of the cytoplasm, and G is the conductance to the extracellular fluid, all given per unit length. The flow of

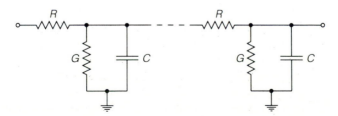

FIGURE 9.10 Network model of a dendritic process. The *R*s represent the axial resistance of the cytoplasm, the *C*s represent the membrane capacitance, and the *G*s represent the membrane conductance.

heat in a medium also is governed by Equation 9.12: R is the thermal resistance, C is the heat capacity, and V is the temperature. The diffusion of minority carriers in a semiconductor follow Equation 9.12 as well; in that medium, G models the recombination process with the majority carriers. All these applications are rich sources both of mathematical treatments of the problem and of intuition concerning the nature of particular solutions. Treatments of the diffusion equation in one, two, and three dimensions, under various boundary conditions in time and space, are the subject of entire books [Carslaw et al., 1959]. Time-dependent electrotonic spread in neural processes was first discussed by Wilfrid Rall [Rall, 1960], and is treated at length in Jack, Noble, and Tsien [Jack et al., 1983]. We will derive only certain solutions of the one-dimensional problem of Equation 9.12, and will compare them with those for the follower–integrator line.

We use the method of separation of variables, assuming $V(x,t)$ can be expressed as

$$V(x,t) = X(x)\,T(t) \tag{9.13}$$

where X is a function of x alone, and T is a function of t alone. Substituting Equation 9.13 into Equation 9.12, we obtain

$$T\frac{\partial^2 X}{\partial x^2} = RGXT + RCX\frac{\partial T}{\partial t}$$

Dividing by XT, we obtain

$$\frac{1}{X}\frac{\partial^2 X}{\partial x^2} = RG + \frac{RC}{T}\frac{\partial T}{\partial t} = -\lambda^2$$

Because one side of the equation is a function of x alone, and the other is a function of t alone, both sides of the equation must be independent of x and t. Therefore, λ^2 must be a constant. The left-hand side then becomes

$$\frac{\partial^2 X}{\partial x^2} = -\lambda^2 X \tag{9.14}$$

and the right-hand side becomes

$$\frac{\partial T}{\partial t} = -\left(\frac{1}{\tau} + D\lambda^2\right)T \tag{9.15}$$

where $\tau = C/G$ is the **time constant** of the line, and $D = 1/(RC)$ is called the **diffusion constant** of the line. Because R and C are the values per unit length, the units of D are length^2/time. We have encountered Equation 9.15 before; it is of the same form as Equation 8.3 (p. 130). We know that its solutions are

$$T = e^{st} \tag{9.16}$$

Both λ and s are, in general, complex. Substituting Equation 9.16 into Equation 9.15, we obtain

$$s = -\left(\frac{1}{\tau} + \lambda^2 D\right) \tag{9.17}$$

Similarly, the solutions to Equation 9.14 can be written

$$X = e^{j\lambda x} \tag{9.18}$$

There are two special cases in which physically meaningful solutions can be obtained trivially: one when X is constant, and the other when T is constant. The first is obtained by setting λ equal to 0, in which case

$$T = e^{-t/\tau}$$

As we expect, when the voltage on the line is independent of x, it dies away exponentially with time constant τ.

The second case is obtained by setting s equal to 0 in Equation 9.17:

$$\lambda^2 = -\frac{1}{D\tau} \qquad \text{or} \qquad \lambda = \pm j\alpha \tag{9.19}$$

where $\alpha = \sqrt{RG} = 1/\sqrt{D\tau}$ is the space constant of the line, as defined in Equation 7.2 (p. 108). As we found in that analysis, when the line is driven by a DC source at the origin $(x = 0)$, the voltage dies away exponentially with space constant α:

$$X = e^{-\alpha|x|} \tag{9.20}$$

The $+j$ root in Equation 9.19 corresponds to a signal dying out in the $+x$ direction, and the $-j$ root in Equation 9.19 represents a signal dying out in the $-x$ direction. These two roots give rise to the absolute value of x in Equation 9.20; the signal dies out as it propagates in either direction away from the source.

Now that we have a sanity check on the solutions of Equations 9.18 and 9.16, we can derive the response of the line to a sine-wave input. To compare the results directly with those for the follower–integrator line, we will treat the case where G is 0. Substituting $j\omega$ for s into Equation 9.17, we obtain

$$\lambda^2 = -\frac{j\omega}{D} \tag{9.21}$$

The square root of a complex number N has magnitude $\sqrt{|N|}$ and angle one-half that of N. In Equation 9.21, the magnitude of λ^2 is ω/D and the angle is 270 degrees; λ therefore will have magnitude $\sqrt{\omega/D}$ and angle 135 degrees. In terms of real and imaginary parts,

$$\lambda = (j - 1)\sqrt{\frac{\omega}{2D}}$$

The solution for $V(x,t)$ can thus be written[1]

$$V = e^{j\lambda x} e^{j\omega t} = e^{-kx} e^{j\omega(t - x/v)} \tag{9.22}$$

---

[1]   Equation 9.21 also has a $1 - j$ solution, it is a wave propagating in the $-x$ direction.

where

$$k = \sqrt{\frac{\omega}{2D}} \qquad \text{and} \qquad v = \sqrt{2D\omega} \qquad (9.23)$$

Equation 9.22 is the classic form for a wave traveling at velocity v, attenuated with space constant k. For any given point x along the line, the bandwidth can be defined as the **cutoff frequency** ω_c at which kx is equal to 1. From Equation 9.23,

$$\text{bandwidth} = \omega_c = \frac{2D}{x^2}$$

The delay is x/v, which at the cutoff frequency is $1/kv$.[2] From Equation 9.23,

$$\text{delay} = \frac{1}{kv} = \frac{1}{\omega_c} = \frac{x^2}{2D}$$

We can compare these results directly with those for the follower–integrator line given in Equations 9.9 and 9.8. In that case, the delay was linear in x, and the bandwidth decreased as $1/\sqrt{x}$. The delay of the RC line is quadratic in x, and the bandwidth is the inverse of the delay.

The rise time to a step input is approximately the inverse of the bandwidth at any point x. Thus, for the RC line, *the rise time is equal to the delay.* This behavior can be seen in the plots of Figure 9.8. The response curves become slower, but they still extrapolate back to near the origin; they never develop the delay-line behavior exhibited in Figure 9.7.

LARGE-SIGNAL BEHAVIOR

The large-signal response of the follower–integrator circuit is either not so nice or quite nice, depending on our point of view. We will look at the large-signal behavior of the circuit both in the time domain and in the frequency domain.

Transient Response

If we put a small step function of amplitude Δv into this circuit (Figure 9.11), the output responds as

$$V_{\text{out}} = \Delta v(1 - e^{-t/\tau})$$

The $e^{-t/\tau}$ term is the homogeneous solution. The "1" occurs because the DC value after the step is different from that before the step.

---

[2] A rigorous treatment of this problem is beyond the scope of this book. An excellent treatment of time-domain solutions to various forms of the diffusion equation is given in Carslaw and Jaeger [Carslaw et al., 1959].

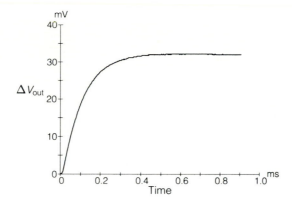

FIGURE 9.11 Response of the follower–integrator circuit to a small (approximately 30-millivolt) step-function input.

If we put in a big step (Figure 9.12), we get *tanh-ed*. Remember, these circuits can supply only a certain amount of current—the bias current I_b. Once the difference in the input voltages is larger than about 100 millivolts, the output is just a current source; the current I charges the capacitor C at a constant rate. Eventually, when the output gets close enough to its final value, the response approaches its final value as $e^{-t/\tau}$.

One way of looking at this behavior is with horror—there is no linear system anymore! If we double the input, we certainly do not get an output that is just scaled up by a factor of two. On the other hand, as the output gets close to its final value, the approach is just like the small signal response. The voltage just does not get there as fast because there is a limit to the maximum rate at which the output can charge its capacitor.

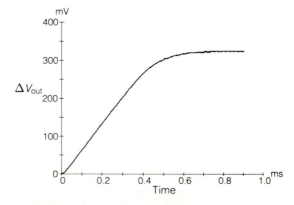

FIGURE 9.12 Response of the follower–integrator circuit to a large (approximately 300-millivolt) step-function input. The constant slope of the initial response is due to the current-limiting behavior of the transconductance amplifier.

If you have ever watched a plotter plot with a pen, you may have noticed that this system has the same property. There is a maximum speed at which the servo system that runs the pen can drive the motors. When the plotter is programmed to draw a shape in one corner of the page, and then to draw the next shape in the opposite corner, it goes zzzZZZZZZ.... There is a maximum tone the plotter makes when it tries to get to the other side; that tone represents the device's **slew-rate limit**.

Our amplifier is slew-rate limited, just like the plotter; in fact, every physical system has a slew-rate limit. There is an inevitable capacitance associated with any electrical node—in particular, with the output of our amplifier—and we can draw only a finite current out of any power supply. There are finite energy resources we can devote to getting from here to there. When a system reaches its slew-rate limit, it cannot accelerate beyond this speed. An automobile has a velocity limit at which the horsepower of the engine matches the drag due to the friction of the air; that is the car's cruising speed on a straight, deserted road. When you start a car from a stop light, it is acceleration limited. But when you are driving it across the desert, it is the slew-rate limit you are up against.

So every physical system has a slew-rate limit, but the follower–integrator circuit has it in spades—at 100 millivolts. That might seem to be a problem. The circuit is not a linear system even in the voltage range in which we are going to use it. Alternately, we can look at the low slew-rate limit as a fortunate factor—because we are going to build VLSI systems. If anything goes wrong somewhere (which it certainly will—somewhere), the amount of damage any one of these amplifiers can do is restricted. If one input gets stuck on, or if something at one spot is driving the system crazy, the magnitude of the damage one amplifier can cause is limited. So the slew-rate limit can be either a blessing or a curse, depending on how you look at it.

Frequency Response

Of course, the slew-rate limit also affects the time scale of the response. In a strict sense, a bandwidth is defined for only a linear system. On the other hand, if we think about bandwidth in a looser sense, it is reasonable to define one for the real system, but that bandwidth will be a function of the amplitude of the input. For small signals, we saw that the rise time for a step input was inversely proportional to the bandwidth. We can define an amplitude-dependent bandwidth that is the inverse of the rise time, for any input amplitude.

When the circuit is slew-rate limited,

$$C\frac{dV}{dt} = I$$

where I is the current that is set by the transconductance control. The solution under these conditions is just a straight line. The input step has amplitude Δv, so the time t it would take the output to get to Δv if it kept going at its maximum rate is

$$t = \frac{C}{I}\Delta v \qquad (9.24)$$

That peculiar rise time depends on the size of the input signal—of course! The larger the signal, the longer it takes the output to reach its final value. If you go from Los Angeles to New York, it takes longer than if you go from Los Angeles to Las Vegas. That is not a big surprise. In the small-signal case, $t = \tau$. We can compute the fraction of the small-signal bandwidth we have available for any size signal. We recall from Figure 5.5 (p. 71) that the tanh function has unity slope at the origin, and the point at which the tangent intersects the asymptote I is $2kT/(q\kappa)$, which is 90 millivolts or so. We can thus relate the slew rate to the small-signal parameters: $G = I/(2kT/(q\kappa))$ and $\tau = C/G$. So, from Equation 9.24, the time for a large-signal response is

$$\frac{t}{\tau} = \Delta v/\left(2kT/(q\kappa)\right)$$

What else could it be? It is the size of the output signal in the natural voltage units of the technology. If we make the output signal many times larger, then we get a frequency response that is that many times lower. Or a time response that is that many times longer. Another way of looking at it is that, for large signals, this device is a perfect integrator; it turns into a single time-constant circuit for small signals.

STAYING LINEAR

We can always make sure the follower–integrator circuit acts like a linear system; we just do not allow the input to change by more than approximately 1 $kT/(q\kappa)$ in 1 time-constant τ. In that way, the dV/dt of the input is always less than the slew-rate limit, and the system is always linear. The signal range can be as large as we want if the rate of change of the input is less than the slope of the large-signal response waveform. Under those conditions, the *difference* between the output and the input of the amplifier never gets very big, even though the signal may be huge. The circuit will stay linear nearly up to V_{DD} and nearly down to ground, provided we use one of the wide-range amplifiers, and do not put large step functions into it. If we increase dV/dt past $\left(kT/(q\kappa)\right)/\tau$, the circuit still works well, but it is slew-rate limited.

That is a graceful way for a computation to degrade; it does not give you a floating exception or an integer overflow or any dumb thing like that, it just follows as fast as it can. Such a nice gentle way to behave itself. In Chapter 16, we will study a system in which we can guarantee, by the way the system is arranged, that the input never varies so quickly that the circuit becomes nonlinear. Because the follower–integrator circuit responds only up to a maximum rate, it automatically limits the rate any subsequent device will have to follow. We use the slew-rate limit of the first to control the rise time of the input to the second.

If staying linear is important to us, we organize the system so that it will not be subjected to rise times that are embarrassingly short, and we thus ensure that it will be a linear system. And because it is a follower, it will try very hard to keep in the linear range if we just give it half a chance.

SUMMARY

We have introduced our first explicitly time-dependent computational metaphor. The follower–integrator circuit allows us to perform the same kind of smoothing in the *time domain* that resistive networks achieved in the *space domain*. Integration in one domain or the other (or in both) is the basis on which a large (but unknown) fraction of neural computation is built. The balance of this part of the book is devoted to the more elaborate computations that can be derived from this humble beginning.

REFERENCES

Carslaw, H.S. and Jaeger, J.C. *Conduction of Heat in Solids.* 2nd ed., Oxford, Oxfordshire: Clarendon Press, 1959.

Jack, J.J.B., Noble, D., and Tsien, R.W. *Electric Current Flow in Excitable Cells.* Oxford, England: Claredon Press, 1983.

Rall, W. Membrane potential transients and membrane time constant of motoneurons. *Experimental Neurology,* 2:503, 1960.

10

DIFFERENTIATORS

All known sensory input channels emphasize temporal changes in the pattern of input signals. The simplest mathematical operation that has this property is differentiation with respect to time. Differentiation is a high-pass filtering operation: It passes rapidly varying signal components and ignores slowly varying ones. In this chapter, we take a rather broad view of the enhancement of temporal changes, and show several alternative circuit implementations.

DIFFERENTIATION

The classical electrical-engineering method for taking derivatives is to measure the current through a *capacitor*. The current into a capacitor is the derivative with respect to time of the voltage across the capacitor, multiplied by the capacitance:

$$I = C\frac{dV}{dt}$$

So a capacitor is a perfect differentiator. We just measure the current.

One way to develop an intuition for the behavior of a differentiator is to consider the response to a sine-wave input:

$$I = j\omega CV$$

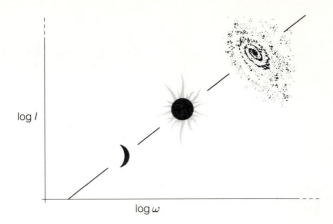

FIGURE 10.1 Frequency dependence of the current through an ideal capacitor. This figure emphasizes the unrealizable nature of a mathematically perfect derivative operation.

We can plot $\log I$ versus ω, as shown in Figure 10.1. The bigger ω is, the bigger the response is. It starts somewhere and goes up, up, and up; somewhere up there is the moon, and somewhere farther up is a star. Even when it has gone so far that it passes the galaxy level, the frequency response keeps climbing. *At infinite frequency, the current is infinite.*

That is really awkward. There is no source in the world that can supply infinite current. What is wrong with differentiators in general is that they are *physically unrealizable*, because nothing has infinite gain and nothing has infinite frequency response. So there is no such thing as a perfect differentiator, in the same sense that there is no perfect integrator. Every system has some leakage, some friction, some flaw that causes it to be imperfect. In the case of a capacitor, there will always be some resistance that will limit the current.

REALIZABLE DIFFERENTIATOR

Even if we could use the capacitor to differentiate, we would need some way to turn the current-type signal back into a voltage, so that it could be used in the next step of processing. The simplest way to turn the current back into a voltage is to put a small resistor in series with the capacitor, and to measure the voltage across the resistor, as shown in Figure 10.2. As long as the output voltage is small compared to the input voltage, we will not disturb the capacitor very much, and V_{out} will be a good approximation to the derivative of V_{in}.

We can write the differential equation for the circuit by equating the current through the capacitor to that through the resistor:

$$C\frac{d}{dt}(V_{\text{in}} - V_{\text{out}}) = \frac{V_{\text{out}}}{R} \tag{10.1}$$

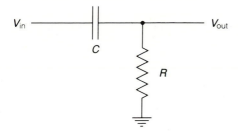

FIGURE 10.2 A physical circuit that realizes an approximation to the time-derivative operation. If the output voltage is small compared with the input voltage, the voltage across the resistor will be a good approximation to the derivative of the input voltage.

Using the s operator for d/dt, Equation 10.1 can be written in transfer-function form:

$$\frac{V_{\text{out}}}{V_{\text{in}}} = \frac{\tau s}{\tau s + 1} \tag{10.2}$$

where, as before, $\tau = RC$.

The frequency response of the circuit is shown in Figure 10.3. We can compare it directly with Figure 10.1. At low frequencies, the form of the curve is the same. At high frequencies, the response of the RC circuit levels off.

We can compute the form of the response as follows: For a sine-wave input, $s = j\omega$, Equation 10.2 becomes

$$\frac{V_{\text{out}}}{V_{\text{in}}} = \frac{j\omega\tau}{j\omega\tau + 1}$$

At low frequencies, where $\omega\tau$ is much less than 1, $V_{\text{out}}/V_{\text{in}}$ is very nearly equal to $j\omega\tau$, just as before, but we no longer have unlimited response at high frequen-

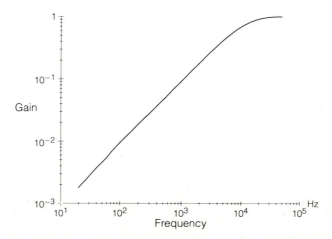

FIGURE 10.3 Measured response of the circuit of Figure 10.2. At low frequencies, the circuit acts as a differentiator. At high frequencies, the current through the capacitor is limited by the resistor. For this plot, R is 1000 ohms and C is 0.01 microfarads.

cies. In fact, when $\omega\tau$ is much greater than 1, the gain of the circuit will be 1. So we have made a *physically realizable differentiator* by limiting the current through the capacitor.

TRANSIENT RESPONSE

We can reason about the differentiator's behavior in the following way. Suppose we change the input voltage abruptly from 0 to V_0. In zero time, we would need infinite current to accumulate a finite charge on the capacitor. The resistor, however, limits the current to a finite value. Just after we change the input voltage by some amount ΔV, the output voltage will also change by ΔV, because the voltage across the capacitor cannot change in zero time. As time passes, current flows through the resistor and charges the capacitor until the circuit reaches its final steady-state condition in which V_{out} is equal to 0. By direct substitution in Equation 10.1, we can verify that the solution is

$$V_{\mathrm{out}} = V_0 e^{-t/\tau}$$

The true derivative of the step input would be an δ-function "spike" having an area proportional to V_0 and a width of zero. The actual response of the RC circuit is shown in Figure 10.4. It is an approximation to the ideal response. We can always make τ short enough that the output will look very spikey on any time scale we choose. In this sense, the first-order differentiator abstracted by Equation 10.2 can be a workable approximation to a true derivative.

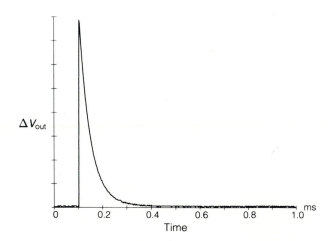

FIGURE 10.4 Transient response of the circuit of Figure 10.2 to a step increase in input voltage. The time constant of the decay is *RC*. The values of the circuit elements were the same as those for the frequency response shown in Figure 10.3.

FOLLOWER-BASED DIFFERENTIATION

The mathematical definition of a **derivative** is

$$\frac{dV}{dt} = \lim_{\delta t \to 0} \frac{V(t) - V(t - \delta t)}{\delta t} \tag{10.3}$$

A finite approximation to a derivative can be computed by subtracting the value of the signal at some time in the past from that signal's current value. How do we compute the value some time in the past?

We have seen that the follower–integrator circuit computes a moving-window average. The weight given any input value decreases exponentially with time into the past. We can view the process of differentiation in a less rigid way by using a computable approximation for $V(t-\delta t)$ in Equation 10.3. The output of a single–time-constant integration is such an approximation. If we subtract the output of the follower–integrator circuit from its input, we derive the same approximation for the derivative given in Equation 10.2.

THE DIFF1 CIRCUIT

The simplest form of such a differentiator is shown in Figure 10.5. From Equation 9.3 (p. 148), the response of the first amplifier, A1, is

$$\frac{v}{V_{\text{in}}} = \frac{1}{\tau s + 1}$$

The second amplifier, A2, has an open-circuit output, so it will have some voltage gain A:

$$V_{\text{out}} = A(V_{\text{in}} - v) = A V_{\text{in}}\left(1 - \frac{1}{\tau s + 1}\right) = \frac{A \tau s}{\tau s + 1} V_{\text{in}}$$

So, the circuit is a differentiator, just like the RC circuit of Figure 10.2 is. The sign of the output depends on how we hook up the two inputs of A2—we can get either plus or minus derivatives. In Figure 10.5, we chose to hook V_{in} to the plus input of that amplifier and v to the minus input, so we got a positive derivative. If we need a negative derivative, we can just interchange the inputs.

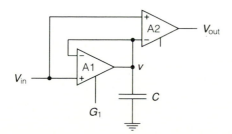

FIGURE 10.5 The diff1 circuit—a simple form of the follower-based differentiator. A delayed version of the input is subtracted from the input to compute an approximation to the time derivative.

The theoretical response of the diff1 circuit to a step input is identical to that in Figure 10.4, except that it is multiplied by a gain A. If the input step is one unit high, V_{out} goes up to A units high and then it dies away with the time constant of the follower–integrator circuit.

In a sense, the diff1 circuit is A times as ideal as the RC differentiator. The output goes up to A (not quite infinity), and it comes back down such that the area under the response to a unit-step transient is $A\tau\Delta V$.

Input Offset

In practice, the diff1 circuit has a severe drawback: the output voltage has a large offset, equal to the gain A times the difference δV between the offset voltages of the two amplifiers:

$$V_{out} = AV_{in}\frac{\tau s}{\tau s + 1} + A\delta V$$

For the amplifiers we are using, A is about 2000, so an offset of a few millivolts is enough to drive the output into one of the rails. The effect can be seen clearly in Figure 10.6. The output is against the lower rail; a positive excursion of more than approximately 20 millivolts is required before the output can come unstuck from the rail. Negative excursions of the input generate no output whatsoever.

Mathematically, the system is ideal: substantial gain at high frequencies, zero gain at zero frequency. Because of the offset voltage, however, the circuit normally will be against one stop or the other. We have no control over the

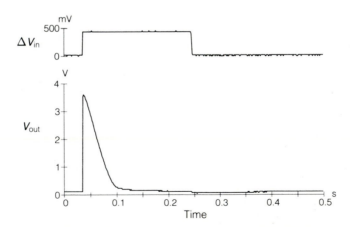

FIGURE 10.6   Measured response of the circuit of Figure 10.5 to the waveform shown. Due to the input offset voltage between the two amplifiers, the output is against the lower rail, and cannot respond to negative excursions of the input. For another identical circuit on the same chip, the input offset was of the opposite sign, and the output was stuck against the upper rail.

steady-state output voltage. This is a problem typical of real-life engineering. The mathematical description works perfectly. When we build the real circuit, however, small practical details dominate the system's behavior.

THE DIFF2 CIRCUIT

Another circuit that has derivativelike properties is shown in Figure 10.7. It also uses two amplifiers (A1 and A2). We will use the transconductance control on A2 to adjust τ. Provided the current in A1 is high enough, A1 will have a time response that is much faster than that of A2. If we do not keep the A1 response faster than that of A2 by several orders of magnitude, the circuit will have stability problems, as we will discuss later.

The idea behind this circuit is to have feedback from the capacitor to the negative inputs of *both amplifiers*. A1, with a gain of A, takes any difference between inputs V_1 and V_3 and creates a current that charges the capacitor C in the direction to reduce the input voltage difference. In that sense, the circuit is just a glorified follower. In effect, we add an amplifier to make a follower follow better. So, for DC signals, this circuit is just a follower; if V_3 is different from V_1, then A1 amplifies the difference. The second follower just provides a gain of 1 for long times. This may seem to be a dumb way to make a follower—we use two amplifiers instead of one. Remember, however, that the second follower (A2) is the slow one. So, if we put in a time-varying waveform, the output of A1 will vary greatly; A1 is driven by the difference between the input and the smoothed version of the input. In that sense, this differentiator is a lot like the diff1 circuit; it responds to the difference between the actual input and a smoothed version of the input, and that difference always is a derivative of sorts.

Effect of Input Offset

The difference between the original diff1 circuit and the diff2 circuit of Figure 10.7 is that the latter has an extra feedback loop to the negative input of A1. For steady signals, that feedback will drive the output voltage V_2 to a value very

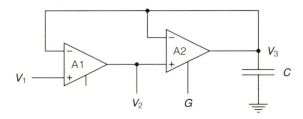

FIGURE 10.7 Schematic diagram of the diff2 circuit. The smoothed output of A2 is fed back to the negative inputs of both amplifiers, thereby greatly reducing the effect of input offset voltages. The output of the circuit is V_2.

near the input voltage. If there is an offset voltage in A1, eventually V_2 will go around through the follower and charge V_3 until the difference in input voltages is just equal to the offset voltage. The offset voltages are well within the range of the tanh, so this circuit always will respond to high- and low-going transients. We put negative feedback around all the gain elements, so that, if we have differences in offset voltages, the amplifiers will still have enough gain to drive the negative inputs back to where they cancel out the input offset voltage. We thus eliminate the blind spot that our simple differentiator had—that the actual offset could be well outside the range of the amplifier.

The output voltage V_2 of the diff2 differentiator may be off by 20 to 30 millivolts, but it will not be up at V_{DD} or down at ground. The diff1 offset voltage is multiplied by the gain A to give us the steady-state output voltage. The diff2 offset is multiplied by 1, because there is a feedback loop that drives the negative input to within an offset voltage of the positive input.

Transfer Function

Now we can derive the diff2 transfer function for small voltage differences between the amplifier inputs. A1 has an open-circuit output, so its output voltage can be written

$$V_2 = A(V_1 - V_3) \tag{10.4}$$

A2 is just a follower–integrator circuit with transconductance G, so

$$V_3 = \frac{V_2}{\tau s + 1} \qquad \text{where} \qquad \tau = C/G \tag{10.5}$$

Substituting Equation 10.5 into Equation 10.4, we obtain

$$V_2 = A\left(V_1 - \frac{V_2}{\tau s + 1}\right)$$

which can be simplified to give the transfer function

$$\frac{V_2}{V_1} = \frac{A}{A+1} \frac{\tau s + 1}{(\tau/(A+1))\, s + 1} \tag{10.6}$$

We can see immediately that the natural response, given by the denominator of Equation 10.6, has a time constant $\tau/(A+1)$, whereas the diff1 response had a time constant τ. The faster response of the diff2 circuit results from the fact that the signal excursions at the input of the A2 follower are amplified by the gain of A1, so the current into the capacitor is A times larger.

Frequency Response

Let us first look at the frequency response of the circuit by setting $s = j\omega$. We can see immediately that the response does not go to zero at zero frequency. We can plot $\log|V_2/V_1|$ versus $\log \omega$, as shown in Figure 10.8. At zero frequency,

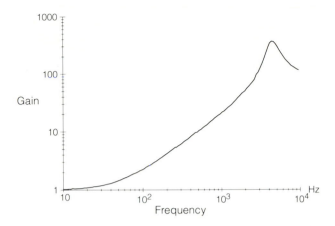

FIGURE 10.8   Frequency response of the diff2 circuit of Figure 10.7. The gain is close to unity at low frequencies, guaranteeing that the output will not be against the rails for a steady input. The distinct resonant peak in the response around 4.5 kilohertz is due to parasitic capacitance on the V_2 output node.

the gain is $A/(A+1)$—a little bit less than 1. It is exactly the gain of a follower. The gain remains at slightly less than 1 until the frequency approaches $1/\tau$, which is about 50 hertz in Figure 10.8. As the frequency is increased above $1/\tau$, the gain is proportional to frequency for nearly two orders of magnitude. In this range, $j\omega\tau$ is much greater than 1, but much less than $A+1$, and hence the s term in the denominator can be neglected. So the circuit is a good differentiator for about two orders of magnitude in frequency. When the frequency is increased still further, we observe a resonant peak in the frequency response at about 5 kilohertz in Figure 10.8. This behavior is due to parasitic capacitance on the V_2 node, an effect that we neglected in the preceding simple analysis. Above the resonant peak, the gain of the circuit is well below the known DC gain of the amplifier, and is limited by parasitic capacitance. Parasitic effects are apparent in the transient response of the circuit as well, as we will soon see.

The diff2 circuit thus differentiates over two orders of magnitude in frequency. It has a little bit less than unity gain at DC, so it still has some DC response. That DC response ensures that the output will not get driven into the stops by the offset voltages.

Transient Response

Perhaps the easiest way to see the difference between the behavior of the diff1 and diff2 circuits is to look at the response to a step-function input, as shown in Figure 10.9. The DC output level is midway between V_{DD} and ground; it has followed the input to that DC value. The output signal has sharp triangular spikes on both edges of the input waveform. So the diff2 circuit is a much better differentiator than the diff1 circuit is.

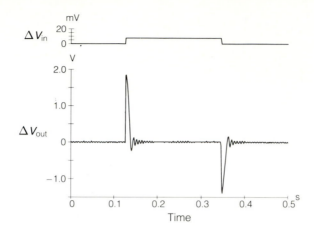

FIGURE 10.9   Measured response of the diff2 circuit of Figure 10.7 to the input waveform shown. The input step size was approximately 8 millivolts, so the effective gain of the amplifier was approximately 250. The ringing in the output waveform corresponds to the resonant peak in Figure 10.8, and is due to the capacitance of the V_2 output node. The analysis of circuits with second-order behavior of this sort will be discussed in Chapter 11. Both amplifiers in this example were wide-range amplifiers.

We can describe the circuit's qualitative behavior simply. For very short times and small signals, the output step is A times as large as the input step. Even for small inputs, the output voltage V_2 is well outside of the range of the tanh, so A2 will be slew-rate limited. V_3 is driven toward the new input level as fast as the current control on A2 will let it be. The result is the triangular spike shown in Figure 10.9. As the output gets within $kT/(q\kappa)$ of the input, we observe some oscillation. This behavior is due to the same parasitic capacitance on the V_2 node that caused the resonant peak in the frequency response of the circuit.

Another deviation from ideality is not so readily apparent from the waveforms. The magnitude of the step input in Figure 10.9 was 8 millivolts. The peak of the output spike is about 2 volts. Hence, the effective gain in this circuit is only about 250. A gain A of 2000 was measured on an identical amplifier on the same chip. The transient gain of the circuit is thus well below the DC gain. The analysis of these second-order effects is quite technical, but is important for readers who wish to design their own circuits. We will be in a much better position to discuss such questions after we have analyzed second-order phenomena in Chapter 11.

Large-Signal Response

With a gain A of several hundred, we can increase V_{in} a few millivolts, and the output will go from ground all the way up to V_{DD}. So the circuit behaves linearly only for steps that are less than 10 millivolts. Figure 10.10 shows how

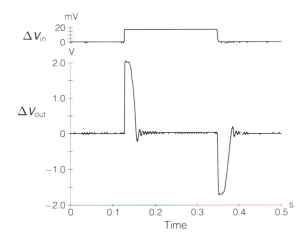

FIGURE 10.10   Measured response of the diff2 circuit to the input waveform shown. The output limits against the upper and lower power-supply rails, but the area under each transient gives an indication of the magnitude of the input step size.

the output looks when a 20-millivolt step is applied to the input. The output increases to V_{DD}, stays at V_{DD} until V_3 approaches V_{in}, and then decreases back to its initial value. The circuit lops off the top of the waveform whenever A times the input voltage is greater than V_{DD}.

Decapitating the derivative is not a real problem; any circuit that takes the derivative with a lot of gain will clip at both the top and the bottom if we put in a large derivative. We have asked the differentiator to generate a signal that represents a derivative. If we put in a signal that is changing faster than can be represented with V_{out} equal to V_{DD}, the output just stops at V_{DD}. We can compare this civilized behavior of the analog system with that of a digital system, in which a numeric overflow may cause the whole program to come to a halt. In a real-time system, halting the program is not one of the alternatives. Instead, the output of the follower–differentiator circuit just limits at V_{DD}, and then decreases gracefully when the rate of change of the input waveform decreases.

HYSTERETIC DIFFERENTIATOR

Both diff1 and diff2 in the previous section were derived from the follower–integrator circuit; the time derivative was approximated by the difference between the input and a delayed (and smoothed) version of the input. The diff1 circuit was subject to problems caused by mismatch between the offset voltages of two amplifiers, and the response of the diff2 circuit had damped oscillatory behavior because the feedback path included two time-delay stages. Both circuits required two amplifiers, with two bias controls. At this point, we might ask whether there is another view of the differentiation process that produces a

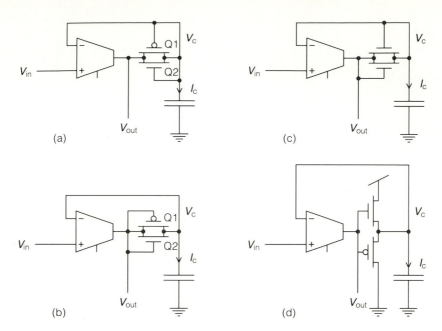

FIGURE 10.11 Schematic diagrams of four versions of the hysteretic differentiator. In the first version of the circuit (a), the capacitor is charged through the *p*-channel transistor, and is discharged through the *n*-channel transistor. In the second version (b), the capacitor is charged through the *n*-channel transistor, and is discharged through the *p*-channel transistor. The characteristics of these two implementations are only slightly different, as shown in Figure 10.12. The third implementation (c) sometimes is a bit more compact, because it uses only *n*-type transistors. The fourth version (d) has the distinct advantage that it uses none of the output current of the wide-range amplifier to charge the capacitor, and hence will be the preferred form in applications where the fastest possible output response is desired.

simpler and more natural implementation. Such an alternate view emerges immediately when we abandon the linear-systems view of the world that underlies the conceptualization of our follower-based differentiators.

The most basic property of any approximation to a time derivative is that *changes* in the input signal are amplified, whereas the *steady value* of the input signal is not. This property can be achieved by a single amplifier with a nonlinear element in its feedback path, as shown in Figure 10.11.

Small-Signal Behavior

We can understand the operation of the circuit Figure 10.11(a) in the following way. Imagine an irregular waveform input with average value $V_{DD}/2$, and assume that the bias current in the amplifier has been set at a high enough value that the amplifier never uses all of its current-driving capability. Under these conditions, the amplifier will act as a differential-input voltage amplifier with

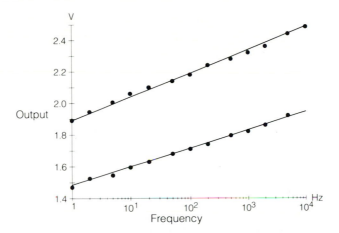

FIGURE 10.12 Measured peak-to-peak amplitude of the output waveform of the hysteretic differentiator for a constant 20-millivolt amplitude triangle-wave input. As the frequency of the input is increased, the magnitude of the time derivative increases, and more current is required to charge and discharge the capacitor. Because the current in the diode-connected transistors increases exponentially with voltage, the output voltage is proportional to the logarithm of the frequency. Data from the lower curve were taken from the first version of the circuit (Figure 10.11a); those of the upper curve were taken from the second version (Figure 10.11b).

gain A. Assume also that the voltage on the capacitor C is $V_{\mathrm{DD}}/2$. If the peak amplitude of the input waveform is small, the amplifier output will be simply a replica of the input waveform, with amplitude multiplied by the gain A. Because the current through the diode-connected transistors Q1 and Q2 is an exponential function of the voltage across them, the current will be negligible for sufficiently small outputs, and the capacitor voltage will remain at $V_{\mathrm{DD}}/2$.

Large-Signal Behavior

Because the gain of the amplifier is high (typically 50 to 300), the situation just described will apply for only those signal amplitudes less than a few millivolts. For larger signals, the output voltage will cause nonnegligible currents to flow in Q1 and Q2. Under large output-voltage conditions, the voltage V_{C} follows the input with some lag due to the integrating effect of the capacitor. As the input voltage increases, Q1 is saturated and conducts according to the following equation:

$$I = I_0 e^{V_{\mathrm{out}} - \kappa V_{\mathrm{C}}}$$

Similarly, as the input voltage decreases, the saturation current through Q2 is given by

$$I = -I_0 e^{\kappa V_{\mathrm{C}} - V_{\mathrm{out}}}$$

where all voltages are expressed in units of kT/q. For increasing input voltages,

$$V_{\text{out}} - \kappa V_C \approx \ln\left(\frac{C\,dV_C/dt}{I_0}\right) \tag{10.7}$$

and for decreasing voltages,

$$V_{\text{out}} - \kappa V_C \approx -\ln\left(\frac{-C\,dV_C/dt}{I_0}\right) \tag{10.8}$$

Equations 10.7 and 10.8 can be interpreted in the following way. If we could wait for infinite time, the circuit would act just like a follower; the capacitor voltage V_C would charge up to the output voltage, and both voltages would become equal to the input voltage. So the circuit must be understood in the context of time-varying signals. The capacitor voltage always lags behind the input voltage enough to generate an input differential, which, when run through the gain A of the amplifier, generates the output voltage required to cause a current $C\,dV_{\text{in}}/dt$ in the appropriate diode-connected transistor. At points in the waveform where there are major changes in the sign of the derivative, there will be a large, very fast change in the output of the amplifier, as the solution will change from that of Equation 10.7 to that of Equation 10.8.

An example of the operation of the circuit is shown in Figure 10.13. For small-amplitude input signals, the output is just an amplified version of the input, as expected. For larger inputs, there is about a 1.5-volt change in the output voltage at the time when the slope of the input waveform changes sign. During the time when either Q1 or Q2 is conducting, the output waveform is a replica of the input waveform offset by the voltage drop across Q1 or Q2 required to charge or discharge the capacitor.

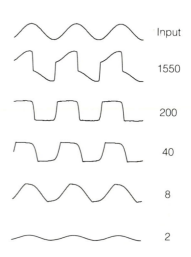

FIGURE 10.13 Measured response of the hysteretic differentiator to sine-wave input of different amplitudes. The top trace is the input waveform, which has a DC value of about 2 volts. The numbers opposite each output waveform are the peak-to-peak amplitude of the input in millivolts. All output waveforms are plotted on the same vertical scale, and are displaced vertically for clarity. At 2 millivolts input amplitude, the excursion of the output is insufficient to cause appreciable current to flow through the diode-connected transistors, and the voltage on the capacitor remains essentially constant. Under these conditions, the output is just an amplified version of the input; the gain of the amplifier is about 250. As the input amplitude is increased, the output signal excursion is sufficient to cause appreciable current to flow through the transistors, and the capacitor voltage begins to follow the input voltage. A rapid transition in output voltage occurs when the derivative of the input voltage changes sign.

Logarithmic Compression

If we apply a waveform of a fixed shape to the input of the circuit, we can change the magnitude of the time derivative by changing the frequency of the wave, while maintaining the input amplitude constant. Because the current into the capacitor is proportional to the charging rate $I_C = C\,dV/dt$, from Equations 10.7 and 10.8 we expect the amplitude of the output to vary as the logarithm of the frequency. A plot of the peak-to-peak output amplitude as a function of frequency for a 20-millivolt triangle-wave input is shown in Figure 10.12. The dependence is logarithmic, as expected, with a slope of 50 millivolts per e-fold increase in frequency. Because one diode-connected transistor is responsible for the positive peak, and the other is responsible for the negative peak, we can attribute 25 millivolts per factor of e to each transistor. We recall from Chapter 2 that 25 millivolts is equal to kT/q. In other words, the current in both the n- and p-channel transistors increases by a factor of e for each kT/q increase in V_{out}, as expected from Equations 10.7 and 10.8.

At the positive peak of the output waveform, both the input voltage and the capacitor voltage V_C are equal to the peak amplitude of the input waveform. Current is flowing through the p-channel transistor. The amplifier output is acting as the source of the transistor, and the V_C node is acting as the drain. As the frequency of the input waveform is increased, the source voltage must increase to supply the additional current, but the gate voltage is unchanged. The potential of the channel with respect to the substrate for the p-channel transistor therefore is not affected by the magnitude of the output voltage. As the peak current is increased, the source voltage is increased relative to a fixed energy barrier. Under these conditions, we expect the current to increase by a factor of e for every kT/q increase in output voltage, as observed.

In the version of the circuit shown in Figure 10.11(b), the capacitor is charged through the n-channel transistor Q2, and discharged through the p-channel transistor Q1. For this circuit, the charging current is given by $I = I_0 \ln(\kappa V_{\text{out}} - V_C)$ and the discharging current is given by $I = -I_0 \ln(V_C - \kappa V_{\text{out}})$. Thus, κ appears in the output voltage term, and we should be able to observe its effect on the circuit behavior. Data from this alternate implementation are shown in Figure 10.12(b). We notice that the slope of this curve is considerably steeper, corresponding to 65 millivolts for an e-fold increase in current. This value is approximately equal to the sum of the $kT/(q\kappa)$ values from the two types of transistors on this particular fabrication batch.

Noise Immunity

The utility of the hysteretic differentiator is that its output is primarily responsive to major changes in the sign of the derivative of the input voltage. Minor changes in slope cause almost no change in output voltage, due to the logarithmic nature of the response (Equation 10.7). Even changes in the sign of the derivative, if they occur and disappear before V_C has caught up with V_{in}, do not perturb the output much. We can enhance this noise-immune behavior by reducing the transconductance of the amplifier, to cause V_C to lag even farther behind V_{in}. Noise immunity achieved in this way comes at the cost of reduced output-driving capability.

In any case, the hysteretic differentiator has many desirable properties reminiscent of those found in biological systems. It generates large excursions in output voltage when the derivative of the input waveform changes sign. The magnitude of these excursions is a logarithmic function of the input amplitude for large inputs, but is linear with input amplitude for small inputs. The time derivative of the output waveform continues to increase with input amplitude, resulting in increasingly crisp time resolution as the quality of the input signal is improved. All told, these properties are remarkable for a simple, one-amplifier circuit—they come as a direct result of the blatant application of gross nonlinearities.

SUMMARY

In Chapter 7, we saw that a spatial average could be computed by a resistive network, and that such an average could serve as a nearly ideal *reference* against which spatially varying patterns could be compared. In the present chapter, we have used a similar approach to time-varying signals. The follower–integrator circuit and its kin have computed a temporal average—and that average has provided us with a reference against which the temporal variation of signals can be compared. Subtracting the input signal from some time-averaged version of that input has given us several well-defined methods for generating an output that emphasizes temporal changes in the input.

CHAPTER

11

SECOND-ORDER SECTION

We have done integration and differentiation with simple, single–time-constant circuits that had $\tau s + 1$ in the denominator of their transfer functions. These systems gave an exponentially damped response to step or impulse inputs. In Chapter 8, we showed how a second-order system can give rise to a sinusoidal response. In this chapter, we will discuss a simple circuit that can generate a sinusoidal response. We call this circuit the **second-order section**; we can use it to generate any response that can be represented by two poles in the complex plane, where the two poles have both real and imaginary parts. With this circuit, we can adjust the positions of the complex-conjugate poles anywhere in the plane.

The second-order circuit is shown in Figure 11.1; it contains two cascaded follower–integrator circuits and an extra amplifier. The capacitance C is the same for both stages ($C_1 = C_2 = C$), and the transconductance of the two feed-forward amplifiers, A1 and A2, are the same: $G_1 = G_2 = G$ (approximately—if G is defined as the average of G_1 and G_2, small differences will have no first-order effect on the parameters of the response). We obtain an oscillatory response by adding the *feedback amplifier* A3. This amplifier has transconductance G_3, and its output current is proportional to the difference between V_2 and V_3, but the sign of the feedback is *positive*; for small signals, I_3 is equal to $G_3(V_2 - V_3)$.

If we reduce the feedback to zero by shutting off the bias current in A3, each follower–integrator circuit will have the transfer function given

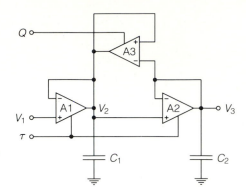

FIGURE 11.1   Circuit diagram of the second-order section. The amplifier A3 tends to keep V_2 ahead of V_1, once V_2 has gained the lead. For that reason, A3 has a destabilizing effect on the circuit behavior.

in Equation 9.3 (p. 148). Two follower–integrator circuits in cascade give an overall transfer function that is the product of the individual transfer functions, so there are two poles at $s = -1/\tau$:

$$\frac{V_3}{V_1} = \left(\frac{1}{\tau s + 1}\right)^2 = \frac{1}{\tau^2 s^2 + 2\tau s + 1}$$

We can understand the contribution of A3 to the response by following through the dynamics of the system when a perturbation is applied to the input. Suppose we begin with the input biased to some quiescent voltage level. In the steady state, all three voltages will settle down, and V_2 and V_3 will both be equal to V_1. If we apply to V_1 a small step function on top of this DC level, V_2 starts increasing, because we are charging up the first capacitor C1. Eventually, V_2 gets a little ahead of V_3, and then amplifier A3 makes V_2 increase even faster. Once V_2 is increasing, the action of A3 is to keep it increasing; the feedback around the loop is positive. If we set the transconductance G_3 of amplifier A3 high enough, V_2 will increase too fast, and the circuit will become unstable.

SMALL-SIGNAL ANALYSIS

A2 is a follower–integrator circuit, so, from Equation 9.3 (p. 148),

$$V_3 = \frac{V_2}{\tau s + 1} \tag{11.1}$$

where $\tau = C/G_2$. The current I_1 coming out of amplifier A1 is proportional to the difference between V_1 and V_2, its two inputs:

$$I_1 = G_1(V_1 - V_2) \tag{11.2}$$

We can describe I_3, the output of A3, in the same way:

$$I_3 = G_3(V_2 - V_3) \tag{11.3}$$

We need an equation for V_3 in terms of V_1. Combining the two currents into the capacitor (Equations 11.2 and 11.3), we obtain

$$C\frac{dV_2}{dt} = G_1(V_1 - V_2) + G_3(V_2 - V_3)$$

Using $s = d/dt$ and collecting terms,

$$V_2(sC + G_1 - G_3) = G_1V_1 - G_3V_3$$

Substituting V_2 from Equation 11.1, and simplifying using $\tau = C/G_1 = C/G_2$ and $\alpha = G_3/(G_1 + G_2)$,

$$H(s) = \frac{V_3}{V_1} = \frac{1}{\tau^2 s^2 + 2\tau s(1 - \alpha) + 1} \tag{11.4}$$

Equation 11.4 is the transfer function for the circuit; as we expected, it is a second-order expression in τs. The parameter α is the ratio of the feedback transconductance G_3 to the total forward transconductance $G_1 + G_2$. If α is equal to 0, Equation 11.4 should give the response of two first-order sections. The denominator is $(\tau s + 1)^2$, just as we expected.

We also can see that, when α is equal to 1, the center term in the denominator becomes 0, and we get

$$\frac{V_3}{V_1} = \frac{1}{\tau^2 s^2 + 1}$$

Under these conditions, the roots of the natural system response are thus

$$\tau^2 s^2 = -1 \qquad \text{or} \qquad \tau s = \pm j$$

Complex Roots

We can put the poles on the imaginary axis when α is equal to 1, or right down on the real axis when α is equal to 0. Now our job is to determine

1. Where the poles are located when α is neither 0 nor 1
2. How the system responds under such conditions

We can write the transfer function

$$\frac{V_3}{V_1} = \frac{1}{(\tau s - \tau R_1)(\tau s - \tau R_2)} \tag{11.5}$$

where R_1 and R_2 are the roots of the denominator in the s-plane. We can define the position of any root as $Re^{j\theta}$, where R is the distance to the root from the origin and θ is the angle from the positive real axis to the root; that is just the polar form of a complex number. As we discussed in Chapter 8, complex roots of real polynomials must occur as complex-conjugate pairs:

$$R_1 = Re^{j\theta} \qquad \text{and} \qquad R_2 = Re^{-j\theta} \tag{11.6}$$

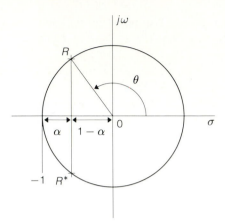

FIGURE 11.2 Complex-plane representation of small-signal behavior of the second-order section. The effect of $\alpha = G_3/(G_1 + G_2)$ is to move the poles toward the $j\omega$ axis. For α greater than 1, the circuit is unstable.

We will solve for R and θ in terms of α and τ by comparing the denominator of Equation 11.5 with that of Equation 11.4. Substituting Equation 11.6 into Equation 11.5, we obtain

$$\tau^2 s^2 + 2\tau s(1 - \alpha) + 1 = \tau^2 s^2 - \tau^2 sR\left(e^{j\theta} + e^{-j\theta}\right) + \tau^2 R^2$$

Using the identity $2\cos\theta = e^{j\theta} + e^{-j\theta}$, we arrive at an important result:

$$\tau = \frac{1}{R} \qquad \text{and} \qquad -\cos\theta = 1 - \alpha$$

The roots are located on a circle of radius $1/\tau$; they move to the right from the negative real axis as we increase the transconductance of the feedback amplifier. The angle of the roots is determined by the ratio of feedback transconductance to forward transconductance, and is independent of the absolute value of τ.

We can normalize the plot, so the roots lie on the unit circle, by expressing all distances in the plane in units of $1/\tau$, as shown in Figure 11.2. From this construction, we have the following important relation between the major circuit variables:

$$(\omega\tau)^2 + (\sigma\tau)^2 = 1 \tag{11.7}$$

We can see from Figure 11.2 that $\cos\theta$ is the projection of either root onto the σ axis. The poles are $1 - \alpha$ to the left of the origin. The real part σ of both roots is given by

$$-\sigma\tau = 1 - \alpha \tag{11.8}$$

When α is 1, the real part is 0, and we are left with a pair of roots on the $\pm j\omega$ axis. When α is 0, the root pair is at the point -1 on the negative real axis; for α greater than 0, the distance between that point and the real part of the roots is just α.

We now have a way to visualize the effect of the feedback ratio α on the location of the roots: α is the horizontal distance from the roots to their original position when there was no feedback in the circuit. The roots start at -1 on the real axis; as we increase G_3, we push them to the right, decreasing the magnitude of the damping constant σ. Eventually, we push them across the $j\omega$ axis and the circuit begins to oscillate. We have shown that we have an independent control on the location of the roots on the circle. The radius of the circle is determined by G. By changing α to be equal to $G_3/(2G)$, we can locate the roots anywhere on the circle. As we change the location of the roots, we change the response of the circuit. That is why the second-order section is such a useful device.

Second-order systems often are characterized in terms of a Q parameter, defined by $Q = -1/(2\sigma\tau)$, or by the transfer function expression

$$H(s) = \frac{1}{\tau^2 s^2 + \frac{1}{Q}\tau s + 1}$$

By comparing this expression with Equation 11.4 or Equation 11.8, we find that

$$Q = \frac{1}{2(1-\alpha)}$$

Note that Q starts from 0.5 with no feedback ($\alpha = 0$), and grows without bound as the feedback gain approaches the total forward gain ($\alpha = 1$ or $G_3 = G_1 + G_2$); beyond this point, small signals grow exponentially—the circuit is unstable.

Transient Response

In Chapter 8, we saw that the natural response of a linear system always could be written

$$V(t) = e^{st} = e^{\sigma t} e^{j\omega t}$$

where the value of s is given by the root or conjugate pair of roots of the denominator of the transfer function. The impulse response of the circuit, for positive t, is of the same form as this natural response.

Depending on the value of α, the behavior of the second-order section may be best described in either the time domain or the frequency domain. The impulse response of the circuit when the roots are on the real axis is just an exponential; the response does not oscillate at all, and there is therefore no frequency associated with it. It is simply a dying exponential. When the roots are on the imaginary axis, the circuit is an oscillator—it just sits there and oscillates, on and on and on. For α between 0 and 1, the impulse response is a damped sine wave, as shown in Figure 11.3, because s has both a real and an imaginary component. The $e^{j\omega t}$ is an oscillating response, composed of sines and cosines. The $e^{\sigma t}$ is the damping term, as long as σ is negative.

The values of ω and σ can be determined directly from Figure 11.3. The duration of one cycle is 460 microseconds. A cycle is 2π radians; ω is thus equal to 1.37×10^4 radians per second, which is about $1/\tau$. The wave damps by a factor of $1/e$ in 2.6 milliseconds. The damping constant σ is thus -3.85×10^2 per second.

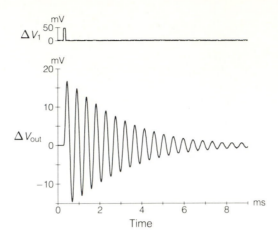

FIGURE 11.3   Measured impulse response of the second-order section for $\alpha \approx 0.97$.

The value of α from Equation 11.8 is

$$\alpha = 1 + \sigma\tau = 0.97$$

The circuit becomes unstable when G_3 is greater than $2G$. We can think about the onset of instability in the following way. There are two amplifiers (A1 and A2) with negative feedback, but there is only one amplifier (A3) with positive feedback. Negative feedback damps the response, and positive feedback reduces the damping. To make the circuit unstable, A3 must provide as much current as do the two amplifiers, A1 and A2, that provide the damping. When the two effects are equal, the circuit is just marginally damped. As we increase G_3 above $2G$, the damping becomes negative, and the response becomes an exponentially *growing* sine wave. Exponential growth is an explosive kind of thing, so the second-order section rapidly leaves the small-signal regime, and becomes dominated by large-signal effects, as we discuss later in this chapter.

Frequency Response

When the damping of the circuit is low, we find it natural to view the response as a function of frequency. The frequency response of the second-order section of Figure 11.1 is shown in Figure 11.4 for a number of values of α. The highest peak corresponds to the setting used for the transient response shown in Figure 11.3.

We can evaluate the frequency response by substituting $j\omega$ for s into Equation 11.4:

$$\frac{V_3}{V_1} = \frac{1}{-\omega^2\tau^2 + j2\omega\tau(1 - \alpha) + 1}$$

We can simplify the algebra by computing D, the magnitude of the denominator of the transfer function, in terms of a normalized frequency $f = \omega\tau$ and

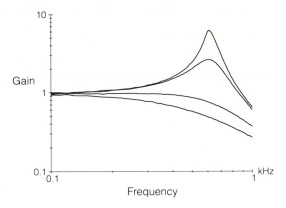

FIGURE 11.4   Measured frequency response of the second-order section for several values of α. The highest curve is for $\alpha \approx 0.94$, slightly lower than the value used for the transient behavior shown in Figure 11.3. The lowest curve is for $\alpha = 0$, and the second curve is very near $Q^2 = 1/2$.

$2(1 - \alpha) = 1/Q$. Using the fact that the magnitude of a complex number can be computed from the Pythagorean theorem, we have

$$D^2 = \left(1 - f^2\right)^2 + \frac{f^2}{Q^2} = f^4 - f^2\left(2 - \frac{1}{Q^2}\right) + 1 \qquad (11.9)$$

It is convenient to plot the log of the magnitude of the transfer function as a function of $\log f$. But

$$\log\left|\frac{V_3}{V_1}\right| = -\tfrac{1}{2}\log(D^2)$$

Hence, we can reason about the response directly from the behavior of D^2. When f is small, the f^4 term is much smaller than is the f^2 term, so

$$\log\left|\frac{V_3}{V_1}\right| = -\tfrac{1}{2}\log\left(1 - f^2\left(2 - \frac{1}{Q^2}\right)\right) \approx f^2\left(1 - \frac{1}{2Q^2}\right)$$

At low frequencies (f much less than 1), the response grows larger as f is increased, provided Q^2 is greater than $1/2$ or Q is greater than 0.707. At some frequency, the f^4 term is no longer negligible, and it starts canceling the effect of the f^2 term. Above that frequency, f^4 increases much faster than f^2 does, so the response decreases. Eventually, the f^4 term is much larger than the other terms are, so the response decreases as $1/f^2$, because

$$-\tfrac{1}{2}\log\left(f^4\right) = -2\log f$$

The plot decreases with a slope of -2 when f is much greater than 1.

So we know the asymptotes. Near zero frequency, the gain is 1 and the response is flat (independent of frequency); at very high frequencies, the slope on a log scale approaches -2, because the response is proportional to $1/f^2$; between the two extremes, there is a maximum. The f^2 term increases before the f^4 term does; as f^2 increases, so does the response. Eventually, the f^4 term becomes large enough to dominate the f^2 term, and then the response begins to decrease.

The response will be a maximum where D^2 is a minimum—that is, where the derivative is zero:

$$\frac{dD^2}{df} = 4f^3 - 2f\left(2 - \frac{1}{Q^2}\right) = 0$$

$$f^2_{\max} = 1 - \frac{1}{2Q^2} \tag{11.10}$$

Equation 11.10 tells us *where* the peak in the response curve is. Now we can take that maximum frequency from Equation 11.10 and put it back into the transfer function Equation 11.9 to find the *value* of the denominator at the peak:

$$D^2_{\max} = \frac{1}{Q^2}\left(1 - \frac{1}{4Q^2}\right) \tag{11.11}$$

Equation 11.11 gives a maximum value of the transfer function

$$\left.\frac{V_3}{V_1}\right|_{\max} = \frac{Q}{\sqrt{1 - \frac{1}{4Q^2}}}$$

So, as Q becomes large, the height of the peak approaches Q, and the peak frequency approaches $1/\tau$.

When Q^2 is equal to $1/2$, the peak gain is 1 at zero frequency and the response is maximally flat (that is, the lowest-order frequency dependence is f^4). For lower Q values, the gain drops off quadratically with frequency.

LARGE-SIGNAL BEHAVIOR

Thus far, we have been concerned with the second-order section as a linear system. The linear approximation is valid for small amplitudes of oscillation. As we might expect, the circuit has all the slew-rate limitations we saw for first-order filters. When the second-order section becomes slew-rate limited, however, its behavior is much more exciting than that of its first-order cousins. When the circuit that generated the small-signal impulse response of Figure 11.3 is subjected to a large impulse input, it breaks into a sustained **limit-cycle os-cillation**, as shown in Figure 11.5. The amplitude of the oscillation is the full range of the power supply. Thus, the circuit that is perfectly stable for small signals becomes wildly unstable for large signals. We need a little imagination to visualize a system controlled by such a circuit, gripped by recurring seizures of this violent electronic epilepsy. As with any pathology, we must understand the etiology, and take precautions against any possible onset of the disease.

We can analyze this grotesque behavior by realizing that the input voltages to all three amplifiers are many $kT/(q\kappa)$ units apart over almost all parts of the waveform. Under these conditions, the currents out of the amplifiers are constant,

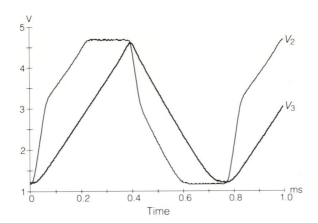

FIGURE 11.5 Limit-cycle oscillation of the second-order section for $\alpha \approx 0.97$, the same setting under which the small-signal response of Figure 11.3 was obtained. The output traverses the entire range from ground to V_{DD}.

equal to plus or minus the value of the bias current in the differential-pair current source. This current was called I_b in Chapter 5. We designate the bias currents in amplifiers A1, A2, and A3 as I_1, I_2, and I_3, respectively. The small-signal transconductances of the amplifiers are directly proportional to these currents. We should thus be able to relate the large-signal instability to the small-signal properties of the second-order section.

Recall what the feedback amplifier A3 is doing: It is sensing the difference between V_2 and V_3 and feeding a current back into V_2 to increase dV_2/dt. In the slew-rate limit, V_3 does not have the benefit of positive feedback, and thus it is lagging behind V_2. As long as V_2 is less than V_1, both A1 and A3 are feeding their maximum current into C_1. The steep ascent of V_2 thus has the slope

$$\frac{dV_2}{dt} = \frac{I_3 + I_1}{C_1} \qquad \text{where} \qquad V_3 \ll V_2 \ll V_1$$

Once V_2 passes through V_1, the current out of A1 changes sign, and

$$\frac{dV_2}{dt} = \frac{I_3 - I_1}{C_1} \qquad \text{where} \qquad V_3 \ll V_2 \gg V_1$$

For the entire first half of the oscillation cycle, V_2 is well ahead of V_3, and the output current from A2 is just I_2:

$$\frac{dV_3}{dt} = \frac{I_2}{C_2} \qquad \text{where} \qquad V_3 \ll V_2$$

Stability Limit

The large-signal oscillation is sustained if V_2 reaches the rail before V_3 catches up to V_2. As the feedback current I_3 is decreased, there is a point at which V_2 and V_3 reach the rail at virtually the same time. The oscillation waveform under

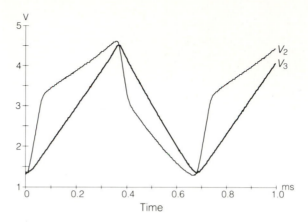

FIGURE 11.6   Minimum limit-cycle oscillation of the second-order section for $\alpha \approx 0.81$. Lower settings of α lead to a damped response for all amplitudes of input signals.

those conditions is shown in Figure 11.6. If I_3 is decreased below the value shown in the figure, oscillation ceases. We can solve for the value of I_3 that will just sustain a large-signal limit cycle by equating the time required for V_2 to reach V_{DD} with that required for V_3 to do so.

The time t_0 required for the output voltage to ramp from zero to V_{DD} is the total voltage excursion divided by the rate at which the voltage increases:

$$t_0 = \frac{C_2 V_{DD}}{I_2}$$

Similarly, the time t_l for V_2 to reach V_1 is

$$t_l = \frac{C_1 V_1}{I_3 + I_1}$$

and the time t_h for V_2 to ramp from V_1 to V_{DD} is

$$t_h = \frac{C_1 (V_{DD} - V_1)}{I_3 - I_1}$$

Marginal oscillation occurs when

$$t_l + t_h = t_0 \tag{11.12}$$

For the example shown in Figure 11.6, V_1 is approximately $V_{DD}/2$, and the result is independent of the value of V_{DD}. We assume that $I_1 = I_2 = I$ and that $C_1 = C_2$, and we divide all terms by I to obtain a dimensionless form of Equation 11.12:

$$\frac{1}{2\alpha + 1} + \frac{1}{2\alpha - 1} = 2 \tag{11.13}$$

where, as before, α is equal to $I_3/(2I)$.

Equation 11.13 can be simplified to

$$4\alpha^2 - 2\alpha - 1 = 0 \qquad (11.14)$$

The solution of Equation 11.14 is

$$\alpha = \frac{1 + \sqrt{5}}{4} = 0.809$$

The astute observer will immediately recognize that this number is one-half of the **golden ratio** of classical Greek antiquity.

What a quaint result! We cannot allow current in the feedback amplifier to exceed 0.809 times the sum of the currents in the forward amplifiers if we wish the circuit to be stable for all possible inputs. In the realm of small signals, we could increase that ratio to nearly 1. But small-signal linear behavior is not limiting us here. We are strictly at the mercy of the nonlinearities.

Small-Signal Behavior at Stability Limit

We have found the maximum value of α at which it is safe to operate the second-order section. If we adjust the current in amplifier A3 such that large-signal oscillations are just marginally stable, we can examine how the section will operate in its small-signal regime. The small-signal response to a step input with $\alpha = 0.809$ is shown in Figure 11.7. From Equation 11.8 we can determine that $\sigma\tau = 0.191$ is the damping constant expected under these conditions.

The natural period of the oscillation is $2\pi/\omega$. From Equation 11.7, we find that $\omega\tau$ is equal to 0.9816 for the present conditions. In one cycle of oscillation, we expect the waveform to have been damped by

$$\frac{V(t=0)}{V(t=2\pi/\omega)} = e^{2\pi\sigma/\omega} \qquad (11.15)$$

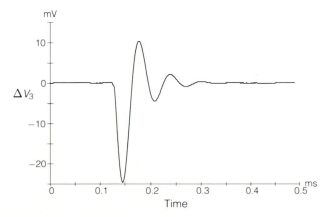

FIGURE 11.7 Small-signal response of the second-order section measured for $\alpha \approx$ 0.81. This setting gave the minimum large-signal limit-cycle shown in Figure 11.6.

For operation at the large-signal stability limit, Equation 11.15 predicts a factor of 3.4 decay in the waveform per cycle of oscillation. The measured damping of the waveform of Figure 11.7 is a factor of between four and five per cycle. This discrepancy between prediction and measurement may be due to the substantial mismatch between real transistors—a problem that has been completely neglected in the preceding analysis.

Recovery from Large Transients

When the feedback current is set below the stability limit, the circuit will recover from large transient inputs. The waveforms for V_2 and V_3 observed during such a recovery are shown in Figure 11.8. They are similar to those observed in the marginal-stability case (Figure 11.6). We can analyze the dynamics of the recovery using the construction shown in Figure 11.9. The slopes of all waveforms have been normalized to that for V_3. While V_2 is below the input voltage V_1, it rises with a slope of $2\alpha + 1$. After V_2 exceeds V_1, its slope is $2\alpha - 1$. The analysis is similar to that used to obtain the stability limit, except the excursion of V_h above V_1 is smaller than the initial deviation V_l below V_1. Because we have normalized all slopes to the slope of V_3, the total time will be $V_l + V_h$:

$$t_l + t_h = \frac{V_l}{2\alpha + 1} + \frac{V_h}{2\alpha - 1} = V_l + V_h \tag{11.16}$$

The decrement by which the amplitude decreases during each half-period is $\Delta V = V_l - V_h$. We can express that decrement in terms of the total peak-to-peak amplitude $V_l + V_h$. Solving Equation 11.16, we obtain

$$\frac{V_l - V_h}{V_l + V_h} = 4\alpha^2 - 2\alpha - 1 \tag{11.17}$$

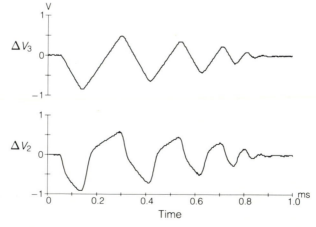

FIGURE 11.8 Recovery of the second-order section from a large-signal input. The response was measured for $\alpha < 0.8$.

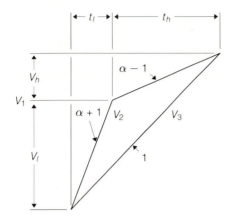

FIGURE 11.9 Idealized waveform of large-signal response for $\alpha < 0.809$. The amplitude of the oscillation decreases at each half-cycle because V_3 intersects V_2 slightly earlier on each excursion.

Setting this expression equal to 0 gives the value of α for marginal stability (Equation 11.14); larger values of α lead to growing solutions, smaller values lead to decaying solutions. Recognizing that the time for the half-period Δt is $V_l + V_h$, we see that the expression of Equation 11.17 is the *decrease in amplitude per unit time*:

$$\frac{\Delta V}{\Delta t} = 4\alpha^2 - 2\alpha - 1 \qquad (11.18)$$

Equation 11.18 is the large-signal equivalent of a differential equation: It relates the amplitude at one time to that at a later time. Because the amplifiers are slew-rate limited, the value of the signal does not affect the rate, as it would in the "linear" regime. For this reason, the decay is linear instead of exponential; the large-signal behavior is simpler than the corresponding small-signal behavior. The approximately linear decay can be seen in Figure 11.8.

SUMMARY

We have derived the properties of second-order systems by way of a specific example. Second-order behavior can arise out of any complex system with feedback. We encountered a precursor to the matter in Chapter 10, when we observed damped oscillations in the response of the follower–differentiator circuit. It is common knowledge in the engineering community that feedback-control systems usually oscillate; getting these systems to be stable is the hardest part of designing them. This difficulty is the origin of the old electrical-engineering saying, "If you want an oscillator, design an amplifier."

Neural systems are notorious for generating large-signal limit-cycle behavior, either as part of their normal behavior pattern (as in a heartbeat) or as a pathology (as in an epileptic seizure). The deep mystery of large-scale neural systems is how they manage to stay stable at all! A hint can be gleaned from a comment by Gordon Shepherd "There is the impression from these experiments of a broad curtain of inhibition drawn across the olfactory bulb, through which excitation pierces, carrying specific information about the stimulating molecules." [Shepherd, 1979, p. 173] A similar comment could be made about any of the sensory systems, as well as about many other parts of the brain.

Inhibition as applied in biological systems is concerned with the magnitude of activity, not with the sign. A dark edge moving across the visual field excites as much response as a light edge would. The auditory system has a hard time distinguishing a negative pressure pulse from a positive one. It could be that the nonlinear nature of inhibitory feedback is the key to building a complex analog-processing system with a great deal of gain and time delay, and to keeping the entire mess stable. We will know that we understand these matters only when we can build such a system—and can keep it stable.

REFERENCES

Shepherd, G.M. *The Synaptic Organization of the Brain.* 2nd ed., New York: Oxford University Press, 1979.

12

AXONS

In Chapter 4, we described the computation done in the dendritic trees of real neurons, and we discussed some of the properties of active channels that provide the amplification required to generate and propagate a nerve pulse. We noted that some types of neurons have no axon, and do most of their computation on analog "electrotonic" signals. In addition, many dendritic trees contain sites (hot spots) of voltage-gated channels; these trees thus contain multiple analog–digital interfaces involved in local integrative activity. In addition, there are many occasions when the nervous system needs to send signals over long distances; it uses action potentials (nerve pulses) to accomplish the task. There are known situations in which the nerve-pulse representation is an important part of the information-processing scheme. We will encounter such a case in the auditory system. If we are to be true to the biological metaphor, we can hardly escape building a credible circuit for the generation and propagation of action potentials.

An action-potential–generating neuron accumulates charge across its membrane. Nerve pulses originate in an area called the **axon hillock**, where the initial segment of the axon leaves the cell body. When the voltage across the membrane of the axon hillock reaches a certain value, nerve channels in the membrane engage in the positive-feedback cycle described by Hodgkin and Huxley, and discussed in Chapter 4. At this point, we note that the combination of positive feedback and delay that is responsible for the action potential is much like the one that caused the limit-cycle oscillation in the second-order section. A small increase in voltage causes nerve channels to open, which in turn allows a flow of current that causes an even faster increase in voltage. The positive feedback drives the voltage all the way to the rail, and a pulse is initiated. In this chapter, we will investigate an electronic circuit that generates pulses similar to those found in biological axons, and we will describe evolutions of that circuit that can be used to propagate action potentials in a manner analogous to the nodes of Ranvier.

Axons are very resistive; the salt water in the cytoplasm is such a poor conductor that repeaters are required at about 1-millimeter intervals. It is difficult to run an analog signal through a large number of repeaters without completely destroying the information in that signal. The pulse representation used by axons solved an important problem: How to transmit signal information over long distances without losing it in the process.

The nerve-pulse representation *encodes* the data, so that the signal level that was getting lost is restored, but still retains some of the analog properties of the data. Nerve pulses travel along the axon through many repeater stations, which reamplify and restore them, but leave them with the same duration. The signal arriving at the output synapses on the distal tips of the axonal arborization is much like the original signal generated at the axon hillock. It even retains some timing information—an attribute that is essential for processing temporal information for applications such as hearing or early vision. Pulses are started by *events*; the membrane in your inner ear wiggles a little bit and triggers one of the cells in the auditory nerve, or a feature of an image moves over a point in the visual field and your retina fires off a nerve pulse. The order of those occurrences can be preserved while the information about them is transported up toward the brain. Thus, it is not true that all the analog information is lost because a nerve-pulse representation is used. Once they had such a representation, biological systems started using it as a virtue. The evolution of biological systems has an insidious way of making virtues out of necessity. Many representations in the nervous system must have had their origins in the limitations of neural technology. The fact that biological systems have lousy wires we understand very well. Exactly what virtues have been developed from this flaw, however, we cannot tell with any certainty at the present time. Our approach will be to build a silicon circuit that generates and transmits nerve pulses, to use it in real applications, and thus to evolve our understanding to a higher degree.

THE AXON-HILLOCK CIRCUIT

In analogy with the behavior of a real nerve cell, we expect to inject a current into our electronic neuron. The circuit will integrate the current for some time, and then will fire off a nerve pulse. After the neuron fires, we keep putting in

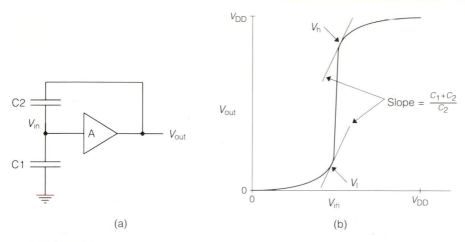

FIGURE 12.1 (a) Conceptual schematic of a circuit that generates an irreversible event due to positive feedback through the capacitor C2. (b) Transfer characteristic of the amplifier A. Due to the high gain near V_{in} approximately equal to $V_{DD}/2$, the gain will be much less than 1 for values of V_{in} very different from $V_{DD}/2$.

more current until we build up enough charge to fire off another nerve pulse. Many real neurons are *leaky*; it takes a *threshold current* just to break even. If we put in less than the threshold current, the cell just sits there, and it never generates any pulses.

To integrate the current that is coming in, we use a capacitor—call it C1. When the voltage on C1 increases to a certain value, V_l, the circuit will fire off a nerve pulse. Circuits that do something irreversible all have positive feedback. When a certain charge is built up, the circuit makes a decision and goes *bang!* It cannot stop halfway. Figure 12.1(a) is a circuit that exhibits this irreversible behavior. The amplifier has a gain A, and we put feedback around it with capacitor C2. Figure 12.1(b) shows the transfer characteristic of the amplifier—V_{out} as a function of V_{in}. This amplifier is noninverting and has high gain. There is some input voltage V_l at which the gain increases rapidly. If V_1 is less than V_l, the amplifier gain is less than 1, and the circuit cannot do anything exciting. We can charge the capacitor up to very nearly V_l, but if we stop supplying current, the voltage will sink back due to the leakage to ground. We can put enough charge in to bring V_1 up to $V_l - \epsilon$—but the voltage will still sink back. If V_1 ever increases above V_l, however, an irreversible sequence is initiated.

If the output voltage V_{out} changes, what will that change do to V_1? Initially, V_1 is equal to V_0, and then we change V_{out}. C1 and C2 form what is known as a **capacitive voltage divider**. Because capacitive voltage division is an important technique, we will take a brief excursion into the subject, and then return to our major topic.

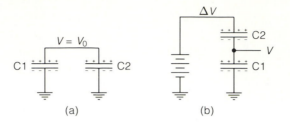

FIGURE 12.2 (a) Charge distribution on two capacitors with a common node initially at potential V_0. The second terminal of both capacitors is at ground. (b) Charge distribution on the two capacitors of (a) after the second terminal of C2 has been changed abruptly from ground to ΔV. The charge on the common node is the same as it was in (a).

Capacitive Voltage Divider

Figure 12.2(a) shows an example of an equivalent circuit of the two capacitors C1 and C2; it is an abstraction of the more complicated real circuit. To ascertain how capacitors act, we will not worry about the rest of the circuit in which the capacitors are embedded. Initially, capacitors C1 and C2 have voltage V_0 on the common node. There is some positive charge on both capacitors—we put it there as an initial condition. The total charge on the node is $(C_1 + C_2)V_0$; that is, it is the total capacitance times the voltage. This is just the definition of a (linear) capacitor: The charge is equal to the capacitance times the voltage. Now consider what happens when we change the voltage on the bottom of C2 from ground to ΔV. That situation is shown in Figure 12.2(b).

The charge on the common node in Figure 12.2(b) is the same as that in Figure 12.2(a); no charge got away. The charge in Figure 12.2(b) is $C_1 V - C_2(\Delta V - V)$, which is equal to the previous value of charge from Figure 12.2(a): $(C_1 + C_2)V_0$. So we can solve for V:

$$(C_1 + C_2)V = (C_1 + C_2)V_0 + C_2\Delta V$$

Dividing through by $C_1 + C_2$,

$$V = V_0 + \frac{C_2}{C_1 + C_2}\Delta V \tag{12.1}$$

This circuit is a straightforward exercise in conservation of charge. No matter how we derive it, the result is always the same. The change in the voltage between the capacitors is the change in the voltage at the end of C_2 multiplied by $C_2/(C_1 + C_2)$. That factor is called the **capacitive-voltage-divider fraction**, familiar to all electrical engineers; it is a straightforward reflection of the conservation of charge. Whenever there is no current flowing into a node, or whenever the current that is flowing causes the voltage to change slowly compared to the rate at which signals are switching, we can assume that, for short periods, the charge on that node is conserved, and we can find the initial conditions given by the conservation of charge. We write the conditions before and after a switching event, assuming that charge is the same, and we can find out what the voltage is afterward, in terms of what the voltage was before and of how much the ΔV node has changed.

Feedback Sequence

We are now in a position to analyze the way in which our axon hillock generates a nerve pulse (Figure 12.1 a). V_0 is the beginning voltage; it is the initial condition on the V_1 node before the feedback sequence takes place. Now, suppose we increase the input voltage a little. The output voltage starts to increase. As the output voltage increases, it pushes charge back through C2 and makes the input voltage increase, which makes the output voltage increase faster. Once the positive feedback starts to work, V_{out} goes *bang!* right up against the stop. What will voltage V_1 be after this irreversible sequence? Because the switching happens fast—much faster than any change due to the current we are feeding in—the charge on the V_1 node cannot change instantaneously. It would require an infinite current to make that happen. As long as the current we are feeding in changes the input voltage at a rate that is slow compared with the rate in which switching happens, we can predict the final value of V_1 from the capacitive-voltage-divider relation derived in the previous section.

The output voltage of the amplifier was shown as a function of the input voltage in Figure 12.1(b). There are two points at which the slope of this curve is $(C_1 + C_2)/C_2$; these are labeled V_l and V_h in the figure. As the output voltage starts to increase, only the fraction $C_2/(C_1 + C_2)$ of that change is reflected back in the input voltage. For input voltages between V_l and V_h, the gain of the amplifier is greater than the division through the capacitors, and the circuit is going to run away with itself. When we change the output voltage a little bit, that effect goes back to the input, gets amplified by the amplifier, and makes an even larger change in the output. If the gain around the loop is greater than 1, the voltage will increase exponentially. The gain around the loop will be greater than 1 when the slope of the transfer curve is greater than the division ratio going back through capacitors C1 and C2.

As we increase V_1 from low voltages, we reach a loop gain of unity at the lower voltage V_l. Coming down from high voltage, we reach the unity-gain point at the upper voltage V_h; V_h and V_l are slightly different, by perhaps 20 millivolts. In actual operation, V_1 is charging up because we are putting current into it. Eventually, V_1 reaches V_l. V_{out} then grows larger exponentially until it runs into the V_{DD} stop. *Bang!* The capacitive voltage divider prevents V_1 from being forced above V_{DD} or below ground.

The positive-feedback sequence in a biological axon hillock is achieved by voltage-dependent sodium channels, as described in Chapter 4. As the voltage inside the cell is increased, sodium channels open, driving the cytoplasm more positive, toward the sodium reversal potential. The neuron runs into the stop when the membrane is completely depolarized: The cytoplasmic voltage is very close to the sodium "power-supply" voltage (Figure 4.3 (p. 49)).

SELF-RESETTING NEURON

We have described a neuron that has a **prolonged depolarized state**, as biologists say. The neuron goes *bang!* and just stays on. Not many neurons have a prolonged depolarized period. A circuit with that behavior is good for making *one nerve pulse*. It is a fine system for controlling a proximity fuse to detonate something, when it does not matter whether the circuit ever resets itself. If we want to use the circuit again, as we do in a visual or auditory system, then we ought not to destroy the neuron by using it just once; we have to find a way to turn it off.

Resetting a neuron is not hard. One way to turn off a neuron is to leak some charge away to ground when the output is high; that is the purpose of transistors Q1 and Q2 in Figure 12.3. Q1 is a current-control transistor, just like the one at the bottom end of our differential amplifier of Chapter 5. We decide how long a pulse we want, and use Q1 as a **pulse-duration control**. Once the output is on, transistor Q2 is on, and we start to discharge the capacitance of the V_1 node through Q1 and Q2. If we bias Q1 on more, then we will leak charge away from C1 faster, and the circuit will turn itself off sooner. Once V_1 reaches V_h, the positive-feedback sequence is initiated once again. A small decrease in V_1 results in a large decrease in V_{out}, which results in an even further decrease in V_1. The output is slammed to ground, and the nerve pulse is terminated.

In a biological neuron, the role of the reset transistors $Q1$ and Q_2 is played by voltage-dependent potassium channels. These channels outnumber the sodium channels, but are slow to react to changes in membrane voltage. After the nerve

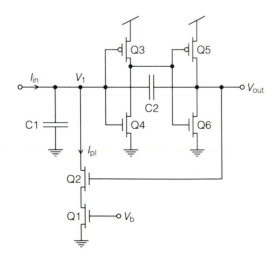

FIGURE 12.3 Schematic of the complete circuit for generating multiple action potentials. The current-control transistor Q1 limits the rate at which the circuit recovers when the output is high, and hence limits the pulse duration.

is fully depolarized, the population of open potassium channels gradually rises, and the population of open sodium channels decreases due to these channels' natural inactivation. When the open potassium channels outnumber the open sodium channels, the cytoplasm is driven negative, toward the potassium reversal potential. As the membrane is repolarized, the population of open sodium channels decreases even more rapidly, reducing the sodium current and causing an even faster decrease in cytoplasmic potential. The process terminates when the membrane is driven to the stop, very near the potassium reversal potential, where it is also near the resting potential. Finally, the potassium-channel population reverts to its closed state, and the membrane is once again ready for action.

Depolarization

If we put a steady current into the self-resetting neuron, the circuit will generate a train of pulses. To compute the pulse duration t_{high} and the time between pulses t_{low}, we need to be more precise about the upper curve in Figure 12.4. When a nerve pulse fires, V_{out} increases from ground to V_{DD}, and V_1 increases by $\Delta V_1 = V_{DD}C_2/(C_1 + C_2)$. So, V_1 does not go up all the way to the stop. If V_{DD} is 5 volts and $C_2/(C_1 + C_2)$ is 0.1, then V_1 will increase by 0.5 volt. When the nerve pulse ends, V_1 decreases by approximately the same amount. The time required to charge the V_1 node up by ΔV_1 is the time between pulses. As we change the voltage V_1, we charge both C1 and C2, so the total capacitance C is equal to $C_1 + C_2$, as long as the output terminal is at ground. The time between

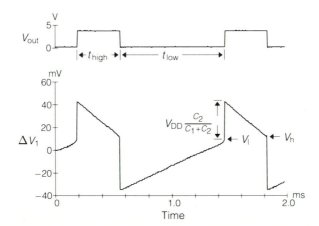

FIGURE 12.4 Waveforms of ΔV_1 (bottom trace) and V_{out} (top trace) measured on the circuit of Figure 12.3. Because the deviations are small, the bottom trace is shown as a deviation from its average value (approximately 2.5 volts). The difference between the amplitudes of the rising and falling edges of V_1 is due to the voltage dependence of the capacitor C1 used in this circuit.

pulses is just the time it takes I_{in} to charge V_1 by ΔV_1:

$$t_{low} = \frac{\Delta V_1}{dV_1/dt} = \frac{C\Delta V_1}{I_{in}}$$

The magnitude of ΔV_1 is a direct result of the capacitive voltage divider (Equation 12.1)—$\Delta V_1 = V_{DD}C_2/(C_1 + C_2)$. Hence,

$$t_{low} = \frac{C_2 V_{DD}}{I_{in}} \tag{12.2}$$

Repolarization

When the output voltage is high, Q1 is on, and a current I_{pl}, set by the saturation current of Q1, is leaking off the capacitor; that current decreases the voltage across C1 at a rate

$$\frac{dV_1}{dt} = -\frac{I_{pl}}{C_1 + C_2}$$

Once again, we must discharge both C1 and C2, so the capacitance is the sum of C_1 and C_2 as long as the output terminal is held at a constant voltage; for the duration of the pulse, it will be. The total current, however, is not just the current coming out; there is also a current coming in—the input current. So, the actual slope will be

$$\frac{dV_1}{dt} = \frac{I_{in} - I_{pl}}{C_1 + C_2}$$

Eventually, V_1 reaches V_h; when it gets to V_h, any change in V_1 will produce an even larger change in V_{out}, which in turn will produce an even larger change in V_1. We get an exponential runaway, except this time it is running *down* instead of up—the output will go *bang!*, and V_1 will be reduced again by $V_{DD}C_2/(C_1 + C_2)$. The decrement on the way down is approximately the same as the increment on the way up. The input current I_{in} then starts charging V_1 back up again:

$$t_{hi} = \frac{\Delta V_1}{dV_1/dt} = \frac{C\Delta V_1}{I_{pl} - I_{in}}$$

Once again, we note that $C = C_1 + C_2$ and $\Delta V_1 = V_{DD}C_2/(C_1 + C_2)$. Hence,

$$t_{hi} = \frac{C_2 V_{DD}}{I_{pl} - I_{in}} \tag{12.3}$$

These expressions assume that $V_h - V_l$ is much less than ΔV_1, as will be the case, normally. The pulse duration is determined by how long it takes I_{pl} to discharge V_1 by ΔV_1, in spite of its continued charging by I_{in}. From Equation 12.2, we can see that the time between pulses stays finite; if we terminate a pulse, a finite time always will elapse before we can generate a new one. This time lapse is what neurobiologists call the **refractory period**.

Saturation

If the input current is small (I_{in} is much smaller than I_{pl}), the pulse duration will be nearly independent of I_{in}. From Equation 12.3, however, we can see that the pulse *duration* does not have to stay finite at large values of I_{in}. I_{pl} can be equal to I_{in}. The difference between I_{pl} and I_{in} is the denominator of Equation 12.3; when the denominator goes to 0, the pulse duration goes to infinity, and the neuron stays turned on. No surprise. If we pump in more charge than the pulse-duration transistor Q1 can take away when the neuron is on, that neuron will just stay on. Most real neurons go to great lengths to prevent that kind of behavior. We also can choose to disallow unlimited pulse duration. The best way to limit the pulse duration is to turn off I_{in} when the neuron is turned on. If we disable the current coming in when the output is high, we guarantee that the pulse will terminate, and thus that the pulse duration will be independent of I_{in}.

There are times, however, when we might *want* the pulse to get wider as the input currents get bigger, until finally the output becomes a steady-state value. We can make wires that can transmit steady-state signal values around a chip. Such transmission cannot be done in a nervous system at any reasonable speed. There are situations where it is useful to go from a pulse representation to a steady-state one, which the neuron circuit does nicely. If we want the circuit to act like a real neuron, we just interrupt the flow of input current until the pulse is finished; then, we let the input current continue.

SILICON AXON

Many neurons in living systems generate nerve pulses that propagate throughout the cell, charging up the capacitance of the cell wall as they go. Because the capacitance of the cell wall is high and the conductivity of salt water inside the cell is low, propagation of pulses in this simple way is slow and energy consuming. As discussed in Chapter 4, larger and more complex animals have developed an insulating sheath that decreases the capacitance from the interior of the nerve fiber to the extracellular fluid. This sheath is made of a low-permittivity material, called **myelin**. A large **myelinated fiber** (wrapped with myelin), can conduct signals about 100 times faster than can an unmyelinated one. Even so, a nerve pulse will not travel more than a few millimeters unless it is periodically *restored* to its original shape. Myelinated fibers have a gap in their sheaths approximately every millimeter, where this restoration can take place. These repeater sites are called **nodes of Ranvier**.

Given that VLSI technology allows us to fabricate excellent wires with delay times six orders of magnitude shorter than neural delays are, it seems at first glance that an axon would be a useless appendage to one of our systems. As we have mentioned before, however, living systems take every opportunity to turn a limitation into a virtue. It turns out that slow wires with restored signals make excellent *delay lines*. Nerve pulses are a common representation for signals of different origins. The time coincidence of two nerve pulses can be computed

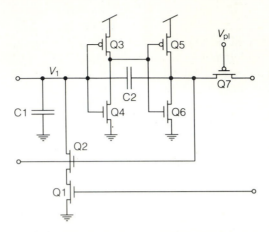

FIGURE 12.5   Schematic of an axon repeater circuit (node of Ranvier). A silicon axon is made up of a number of these sections connected in cascade. The output of any given stage is connected to the gate of Q1 on the previous stage. No current flows into the following stage until the output of the preceding stage is high. No current is allowed to leak off the V_1 node until the succeeding stage has fired. As a result, pulses from adjacent stages are spaced one pulse width apart.

much more simply than can the correlation between two analog signals. If we are to understand the nature of neural computation, we must certainly comprehend what can be done with nerve pulses. We will do so by building systems embodying these principles, and by characterizing their operation.

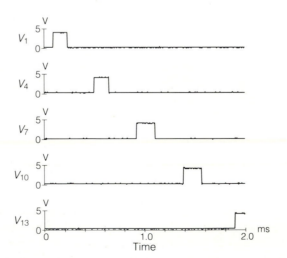

FIGURE 12.6   Waveforms measured at several taps of an axon formed by cascade connection of stages of the circuit shown in Figure 12.5. Taps were located at every third stage; thus, two outputs are not shown for each one that is.

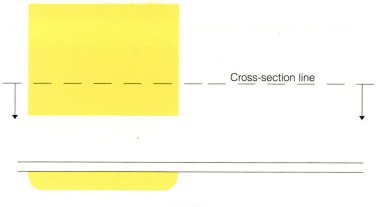

(a) Well.

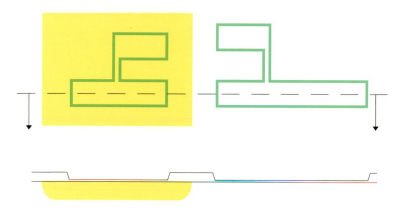

(b) Active.

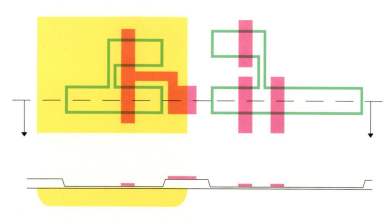

(c) Polysilicon.

PLATE 1 The CMOS process.

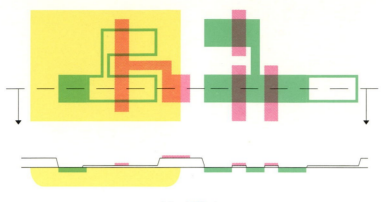

(d) *n*-Diffusion.

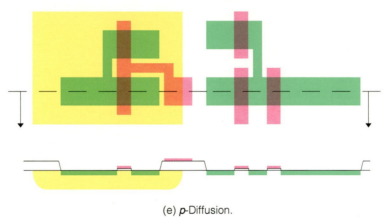

(e) *p*-Diffusion.

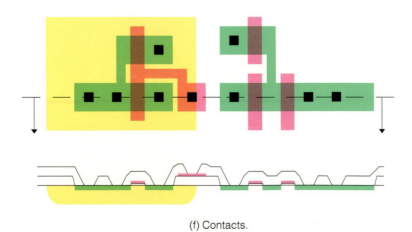

(f) Contacts.

PLATE 2 The CMOS process (continued).

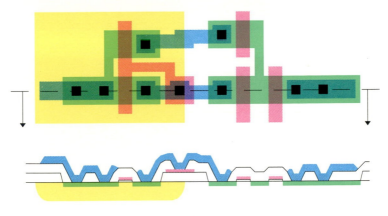

(g) Metal.

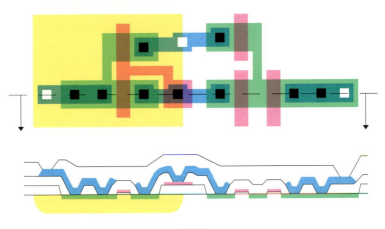

(h) Via.

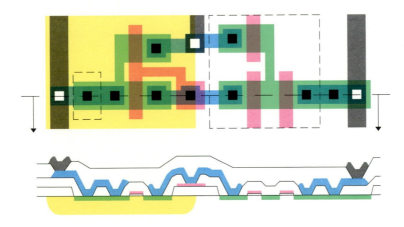

(i) Metal 2.

PLATE 3 The CMOS process (continued).

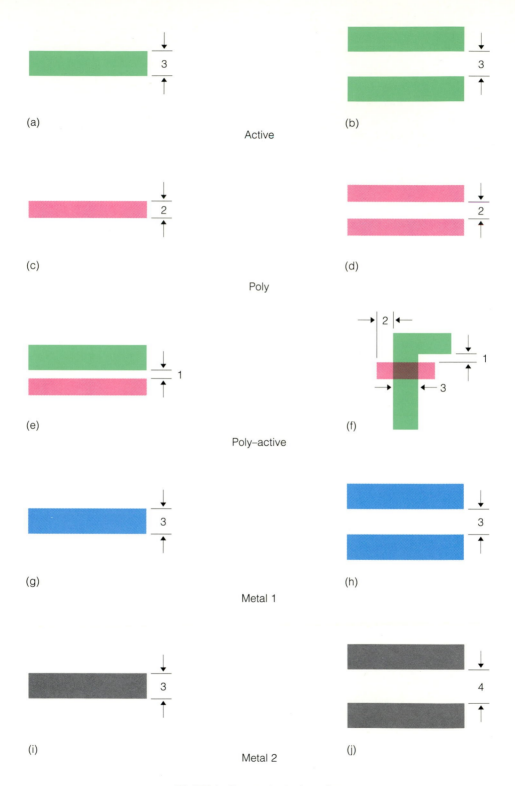

(a)

(b)

Active

(c)

(d)

Poly

(e)

(f)

Poly–active

(g)

(h)

Metal 1

(i)

(j)

Metal 2

PLATE 4 Geometric design rules.

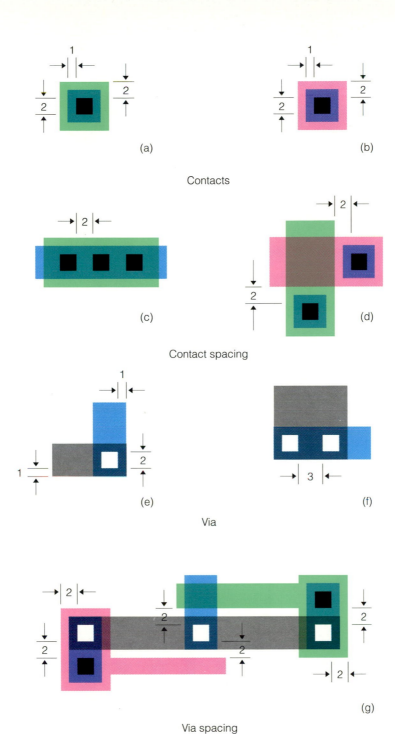

Contacts

Contact spacing

Via

Via spacing

PLATE 5 Contacts.

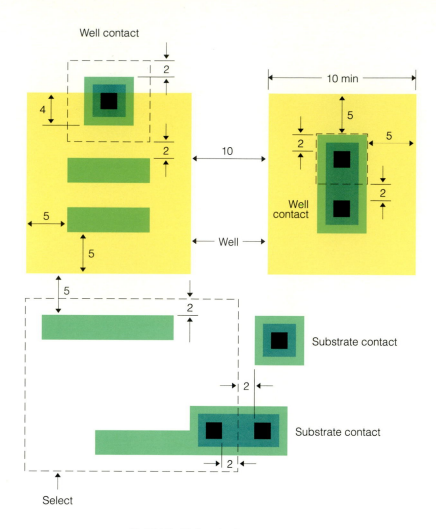

PLATE 6 Well and substrate contacts.

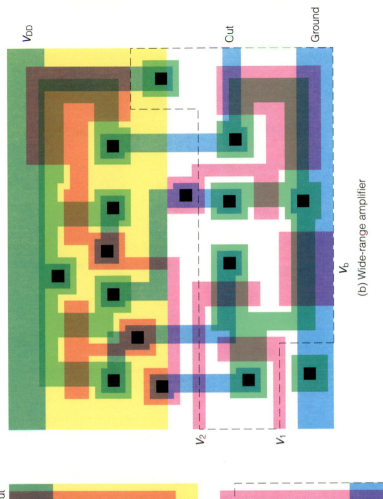

(a) Simple amplifier

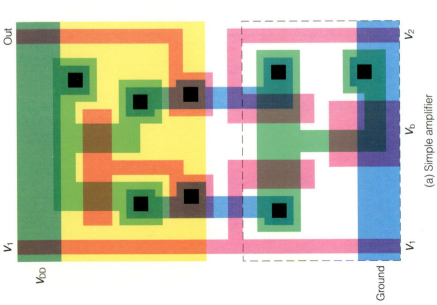

(b) Wide-range amplifier

PLATE 7 Transconductance amplifiers.

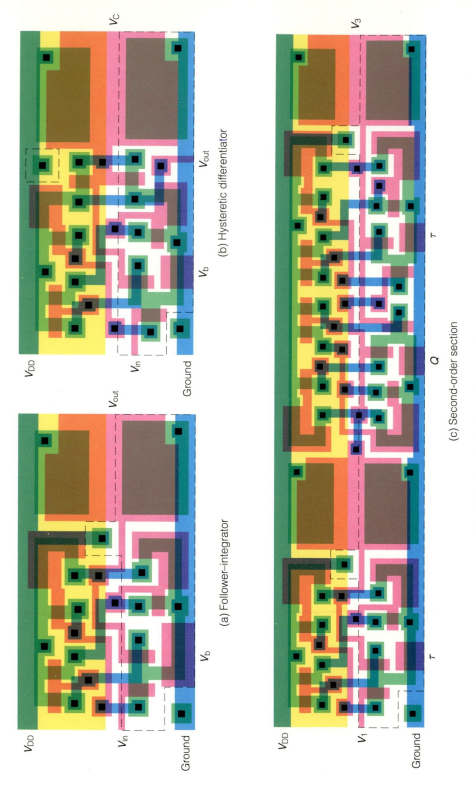

V_{DD}

V_C

V_{out}

V_{out}

V_b

(b) Hysteretic differentiator

V_{in}

Ground

V_{DD}

V_{out}

V_{in}

V_b

(a) Follower–integrator

Ground

V_{DD}

V_3

τ

Q

τ

V_1

(c) Second-order section

Ground

PLATE 8 Circuits implementing time-domain operations.

The design challenge in creating a silicon axon lies in coupling one restoring stage to its predecessor. The coupling must be strong enough to ensure that the pulse will not die out after a few stages, but it must not be so strong that the second stage will fire a few nanoseconds after the first one has fired. The circuit of Figure 12.3 can be extended to achieve this function, as shown in Figure 12.5.

The coupling between stages is provided by Q7, the gate of which acts as the pulse-duration control. When the output is low, the gate of the p-channel transistor Q7 is much more positive than is either its source or drain, and hence the transistor is off. When the output is at V_{DD}, Q7 can supply a current to the next stage; the magnitude of this current is set by the pulse-duration control. Instead of discharging C1 and C2 to determine the pulse duration, this current charges the capacitance of the next stage. When the next stage fires, Q1 is turned on, V_1 is discharged below V_h, and the output voltage returns to a low value. Hence, the pulse is high only slightly longer than is necessary to guarantee the firing of the succeeding stage. Waveforms illustrating the operation of the axon circuit are shown in Figure 12.6.

SUMMARY

The silicon axon, in addition to being a useful circuit, has exposed us to the technique of **piecewise-linear analysis**. We were able to analyze the circuit as though it was a time-independent linear circuit, until it went *bang!* Once it went *bang!*, we derived the condition after the discontinuity by assuming that any currents flowing in the circuit did not have a chance to transfer much charge *during the transient*, because the *bang!* happened so fast. So the *charge* just before the transient is nearly the same as that just after the transient. This method is very general; it allows us to analyze most circuits that have discontinuities in them, at least to a first approximation. As long as the switching time is short enough, no charge is lost during the discontinuity.

We can determine what the voltage is on the node after the *bang!* in terms of what it was before the *bang!* At first sight, circuits like this look impossible. But we can treat them as linear circuits—remembering that they are different linear circuits at one time than they are at another time. A switching power supply behaves in the same way. It is chugging along, and all of the sudden it switches, and then it is a whole new circuit. At first, there is an inductor there; after the discontinuity, the inductor is not there anymore. As long as we can tell *when* the circuit is going to make a transition, and *what it will be like* afterward, we can analyze it.

Computer scientists use this approach, because all computer programs have discontinuities. A program will go along, doing nice, gentle things. Then, all of the sudden, *bang!*—the program runs into an "if" statement. "If" statements are discontinuous. So the kind of thinking we use to analyze discontinuous circuits is similar to the reasoning computer scientists do when they analyze the behavior of a computer program. If we could not reason about circuits that have discontinuities, our domain would be like a computer language without an "if" statement—we could do toy problems but not anything real. So the piecewise-linear approach is a powerful extension to other methods we have for analyzing circuit behavior.

PART

IV

SYSTEM EXAMPLES

Once the limitation of standard parts with unique properties is introduced, it affects all higher levels as well. For it is a feature of our Universe that combinations of more elementary parts make systems with wholly new properties ... I would define these as emergent properties.

—C.F.A. Pantin   *The New Landscape* (1951)

C H A P T E R

13

SEEHEAR

Lars Nielsen   M.A. Mahowald   Carver Mead

The SeeHear is a system designed to help the blind to form a representation of their environment. The heart of the system is a single analog
chip onto which an image is projected by a lens. The function of the
system is to map visual signals from moving objects in the image into
auditory signals that can be projected through earphones to a listener.
A sensation is evoked similar to one that the listener would experience
if the moving objects were emitting sound. We hope that the auditory
signals provided by the SeeHear device, in addition to the sound cues
already present in the environment, will enable blind people to create an
internal model of their surroundings more detailed than one they could
extract from naturally occurring sound cues alone.

Information processing on the chip consists of

1. Encoding the intensity and position of a light source in a two-dimensional retinotopic projection
2. Processing the electrical signals representing the intensity information
   to emphasize temporal changes
3. Synthesizing a sound having the appropriate psychophysiologically
   determined cues for a sound source at that position

Adapted with permission from Nielson, L., Mahowald, M., and Mead, C., *SeeHear*.
1987, International Association for Pattern Recognition, 5th Scandinavian Conference on
Image Analysis.

Because of the microwatt power requirements of the subthreshold CMOS technology, the SeeHear device is small enough to be mounted on the head of the listener, and all source positions can be measured in the head-centered coordinate system natural to visual and auditory localization.

We have used biologically inspired representations of visual and auditory information in the inner processing of the chip. The optical processing done on the intensity information is based on signal processing in the vertebrate retina. This processing emphasizes motion information that, in the visual system, is capable of providing depth information when interpreted by higher centers of the brain. Auditory information is generated emphasizing transient events, which are known to provide optimal information for spatial localization.

BIOLOGICAL BASIS OF THE SEEHEAR SYSTEM

Information about sensory systems comes from a variety of sources, such as ethology, human psychology, and animal neurophysiology. Although each species of animal specialized to fill its own ecological niche, underlying structures of peripheral vision and hearing arose in response to fundamental environmental pressures common to all species. Humans and other vertebrates need to distinguish among myriad diverse stimuli to perceive objects in the physical world, to avoid obstacles and predators, to procure food, and to care for their young. Under these conditions, the evolutionary process has seen to it that the most primitive processing paradigm has been conserved across many species. By focusing on those characteristics that are common to many species of animals, we can understand the basic problems facing all higher animals, including humans.

Sensory systems enable animals to gather information about the environment; they transduce input from the environment into neural signals that are processed in the brain to create, in the animal, an internal model of the world. The animal bases all its actions on this model. Among other things, the internal model must contain information that will enable the animal to find food and to avoid danger. It is clear that the ability to sense objects from a distance and to maintain a sense of their locations in space is a great selective advantage; it is easier to find food if you do not have to run into it to realize that it is there, particularly if it is mobile. Furthermore, it is easier to delay becoming food if you can localize approaching predators and navigate through obstacles well enough to run in the opposite direction.

It is thus not surprising that the visual and auditory systems of widely diverse species are specialized, beginning at the earliest stages of neural processing, to localize visual and acoustic events. The mapping of light and sound inputs into neural representations appropriate for the localization of the sources of these inputs is performed by peripheral sensory systems. The mapping performed by the visual system differs from that done by the auditory system because the physics of light is different from the physics of sound.

Biological Visual Systems

Vertebrates have highly optimized methods for generating visual representations. The first steps of visual information processing are performed in the retina, onto which the visual scene is projected through a lens. There the light is sensed by a two-dimensional grid of photoreceptors, each of which generates an analog neural potential proportional to the logarithm of the intensity at that point in the image. The logarithm provides a large dynamic range of receptor response, and ensures that differences in receptor output will represent a contrast ratio that is independent of the absolute intensity with which the scene is illuminated. The light incident on a photoreceptor comes from a local region of space called the **receptive field** of that photoreceptor. The location of a photoreceptor on the retina encodes the direction to the light source in real space.

As the visual information is transmitted and processed through multiple layers of neurons, the location information is preserved through **retinotopic mapping**. The two-dimensional layers of neurons in the retina transmit their output through the optic nerve to two-dimensional sheets of neurons in the brain in a conformal mapping that maintains the relative spatial locations of the signals. Physiological investigations of the retina and of the various visual areas of primate brains have shown that the receptive fields of adjacent neurons correspond to adjacent regions of the visual field.

As the neural processing of the visual information proceeds, the representation becomes more complex. The transformation from simple intensity to more complex representations is begun in the retina itself; signals from the photoreceptors are transformed through several layers of neural processing before they are transmitted through the optic nerve to the brain. The output cells of the retina, called **retinal ganglion cells**, encode information about such things as local intensity gradients and time derivatives of intensity. On-center and off-center ganglion cells are sensitive to stationary edges, responding to spatial derivatives of intensity within their receptive fields, whereas on–off ganglion cells are motion sensitive, responding to only temporal derivatives of the intensity profile.

The visual centers of the brain must construct a model of three-dimensional space based on only the spatiotemporal pattern of signals they receive from the retina. In all animals, motion signals are an important part of the reconstruction process. A great number of vertebrates derive visual depth information exclusively from the relative motion of objects in the retinal image that results from the animal's own movements [Lorenz, 1981]. Although humans use binocular stereopsis for detailed information about depth at close range (less than 1 to 2 meters), parallax induced by head and body movements is an effective cue to depth even with one eye [Richards, 1975] and, at large distances, motion parallax is the only depth cue available.

Motion parallax is a simple geometric phenomenon; it is *not* dependent on binocular interaction. Different versions of the phenomenon occur dependent on how the eye and the line of sight are moving relative to the scene of interest [Carterette et al., 1975]. The simplest example can be demonstrated easily by introspection. If the eyes are fixated at infinity, and the head is moved, the apparent velocity of any object is a monotonic function of the distance to the object. The closest object moves fastest, whereas more distant objects move more slowly. Objects at infinity appear stationary.

In summary, three important points about visual processing in biological systems are

1. The first step in visual processing is performed by the photoreceptors; their output represents the logarithm of intensity. The logarithm expands the dynamic range of the photoreceptors and ensures that differences in receptor output represent a contrast ratio, which is independent of the illumination level of the scene.

2. The locations of light sources in a two-dimensional optical projection of real space are coded by the locations of neurons in retinotopic arrays.

3. The depth cues needed to reconstruct the third dimension of real space are provided by motion signals, which are generated early in visual processing, at the level of the retina. The basic motion cue reported by the retina is the time derivative of the intensity profile.

Auditory Psychophysiology

The SeeHear system depends on the ability to synthesize sounds that will appear to the listener to have come from a specified physical location. Fortunately, auditory psychophysiological research has led to an understanding of sound localization by humans that has made such a sound synthesis possible. Bloom and Kendall [Bloom, 1977a; Bloom, 1977b; Kendall et al., 1984] have succeeded in quantifying the acoustic cues that humans use for sound localization. Using these cues, they were able to synthesize sounds appearing to have come from arbitrarily specified directions. The cues used by Bloom and Kendall are a consequence of the interaction of sounds with the physical environment. The sound to be sensed by both ears must propagate through the air and around the head. The sound is then reflected by the pinna and tragus of the outer ear before entering the ear canal and arriving at the ear drum and the inner ear. The modifications of the sound in its journey to the right and left inner ears provide the cues to the location of the sound source.

There are two major horizontal-localization cues; these cues are both the result of binaural interactions, as illustrated in Figure 13.1. The first cue is due to the interaction of the sound with the head of the listener. Higher frequencies are attenuated when they travel around the head, as shown in Figure 13.1(a). The degree of the dispersion of the incoming sound wave depends on the details of the interaction with the listener's head, outer ear, and ear canal. In general, however, sound arriving at the right (contralateral) ear is more dispersed, having experienced greater high-frequency attenuation. We refer to the high-frequency attenuation as **acoustic headshadow**.

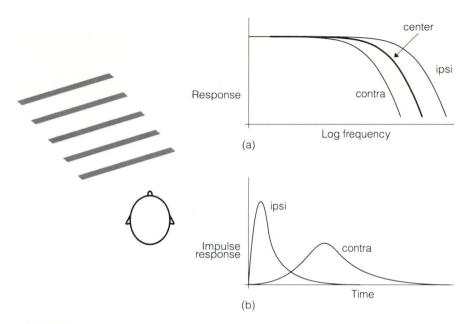

FIGURE 13.1 A model of the head, looking down from the top. A sound wave is impinging on the head from about 45 degrees left of center. Low frequencies present in the sound travel around the head with less attenuation than do high frequencies, creating the difference in frequency response of the left and right ears shown schematically in (a). In addition, the sound reaches the right ear later than it reaches the left ear. Both effects can be seen in the impulse response of the two ears sketched in (b). The response of the contralateral ear is delayed and broadened relative to that of the ipsilateral ear.

The second horizontal-localization cue is the difference in arrival time of a sound to the right and left ear, due to the difference in path length. A sound source directly in front of the listener is equidistant from the right and left ears, and therefore has no interaural time delay. Maximal delay occurs with a sound directly on the right or left of the listener; the length of the delay depends on the size of the binaural separation. For humans, typical values of the interaural time delay are between 350 and 650 microseconds.

The effects of both cues can be seen in the impulse response for the left and right ear canal, shown Figure 13.1(b). The response in the left ear is sharper and less delayed than is that in the right ear.

Localization of sound in the vertical direction is made possible by the pinna and tragus of the outer ear. Incoming sound can enter the ear canal via two paths, as shown in Figure 13.2. One path is as direct as possible, given the shape of the outer ear. The second path is longer; the incoming sound bounces from the pinna to the tragus and then into the ear canal. The signals traversing the two paths combine in the ear canal. The difference in path length between the two signals can be measured in psychoacoustic experiments as a notch in the spectral-sensitivity function, caused by destructive interference when the increase in path

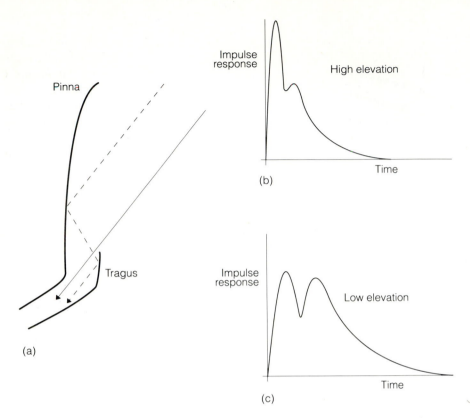

FIGURE 13.2   (a) Cross-section through the structures of the outer ear, where the primary cue for vertical localization is created. A sound wave traversing the indirect path (dashed line) bounces off the pinna to the tragus and thence into the ear canal. The delay in the indirect path is thus longer than that of the direct path (solid line). The difference in delay between the two paths is a monotonic function of elevation: It is short for higher elevations and longer for low elevations. The impulse response of a sound at high and low elevations is sketched in (b) and (c).

length due to pinna–tragus reflection is one-half the wavelength of the incoming sound. The time delay between the two paths is a function of elevation. The shape of the outer ear is unique in every individual, so the absolute values of the time delays vary. For all people, however, the length of the time delay is a monotonic function of elevation, with small delay at high elevations and large delay at low elevations. The impulse responses for sources at high and low elevations are shown in Figure 13.2. For humans, typical values of time delay are 35 to 80 microseconds.

In summary, the sufficient set of cues for sound localization is as follows:

1. Interaural time disparity—horizontal

2. Acoustic headshadow—horizontal

3. Pinna–tragus characteristics—vertical

Main Principles

We can now summarize basic effects and principles of vision and hearing. Visual processing at the retinal level detects motion mainly by taking time–space derivatives of the intensity profile of the visual scene. The transient nature of the time derivative localizes visual events in time. Motion of the observer causes neural events as edges in the visual scene move over receptors in the retina. The brain is able to construct a model of the three-dimensional world from these events by the use of motion parallax. Hearing also is mainly concerned with events; transients of sound are far easier to detect and localize than are repetitive sounds.

The basic difference between visual and auditory localization is the way position is represented in the peripheral sensory-processing stages. In vision, location of a pixel in a two-dimensional array of neurons in the retina corresponds to location of objects in a two-dimensional projection of the visual scene. The location information is preserved through parallel channels by retinotopic mapping. The auditory system, in contrast, has only two input channels; location information is encoded in the temporal patterns of signals in the two cochlea. These temporal patterns provide the cues that the higher auditory centers use to build a two-dimensional representation of the acoustic environment, similar to the visual one, in which the position of a neuron corresponds to the location of the stimulus that it detects.

THE SEEHEAR DESIGN

At this point, we are in a position to formulate the needed *function* of the SeeHear system. Signals representing visual events must be transformed into acoustic events. The *location* of each visual event must be encoded, and that encoding must be used to synthesize an acoustic signal that will provide the hearing cues appropriate for an acoustic event at that location. Events occurring simultaneously in a two-dimensional projection of a visual scene must be transformed into an acoustic signal coded in only two channels. Information that would allow the reconstruction of depth (motion-parallax cues, for example) must be preserved. If the SeeHear system successfully performs the overall function, users can create an internal model of the visual world using their auditory systems.

Designing a chip that will perform the function needed is an interesting architectural challenge. Processing elements and their interconnections must be designed and spatially arranged on the chip. The key problem is to find an arrangement of specific subsystems that, in aggregate, will perform the overall function. Each subsystem is built up out of circuits described in earlier chapters.

Vision

The SeeHear visual system is similar to the vertebrate eye. A lens maps the scene onto a two-dimensional array of pixels. Each pixel contains a photosen-

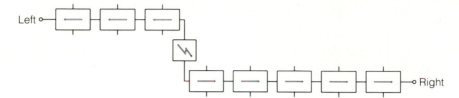

FIGURE 13.3   An electronic circuit that creates the illusion of horizontal localization of a sound. A sound source feeds the inputs of two delay lines, one leading to the right ear and the other to the left ear. Each delay line delays and broadens the sound increasingly with length. With the arrangement shown, the sound appears to come from left of center, and has the horizontal cues shown in Figure 13.1.

sor and associated local processing. The light falling on one pixel in the array comes from a specific direction in real space. The location of a pixel in the array corresponds to the location of a particular feature in a two-dimensional projection of the visual scene. As in biology, the visual system first takes an analog logarithm of the intensity, and then takes an analog time derivative. This computation is done locally on the chip, thereby maintaining directional information. The visual processing in the SeeHear system thus incorporates two main biologically relevant features: The location of light sources is encoded in the retinotopic array of pixels, and motion information in the visual processing is emphasized by computation of the analog time derivative of an unsampled time-varying signal. This signal, when used as input to the sound-synthesis machinery, generates appropriate sound signals for the auditory system.

Sound Synthesis

The SeeHear sound-synthesis system is capable of generating the hearing cues shown in Figures 13.1 and 13.2 for events at any specified location. Consistent with the continuous nature of the visual part of the SeeHear design, we use continuous sound-synthesis methods that conserve the analog nature of the signal from the pixels, and take advantage of the place information in the retinotopic visual array.

One auditory source   We start with the simplest sound-synthesis problem: We wish to generate only one auditory event from a single horizontal location. The design of such a horizontal auditory-cue generator for one source is illustrated in Figure 13.3. An event-generating signal source is connected to two delay lines one leading to the left of the source, and the other to the right. Each line delays an input signal by an amount per unit length specified by a variable control. This system is capable of giving the auditory direction cues shown in Figure 13.1. The input device generates a pulse input signal for both delay lines. If the left delay line is shorter than the right one is, the signal will reach the left output first.

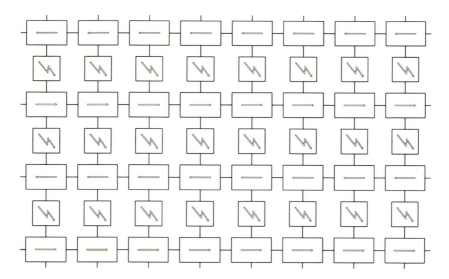

FIGURE 13.4 An arrangement for generating horizontal-localization cues for a number of sources at different apparent angles. The principle of superposition is used to share the left- and right-directed delay lines. Each delay stage adds the local sound-source output to the delayed version of its input, and passes on the composite signal to its successor.

The output of the device can be used directly to produce sound that can be presented through earphones or loudspeakers. In addition to providing a delay, the analog processing in the delay lines filters the higher frequencies from the signal. The farther the signal travels, the more dispersed it becomes. We thus generate both the binaural time-disparity cue and the acoustic-headshadow cue from the delay lines. The horizontal direction is determined by the difference in length of the left and right delay lines. We therefore call the delay lines a **binaural-headshadow model**.

Multiple auditory sources   An auditory-cue generator for multiple sources is illustrated in Figure 13.4. The system has a two-dimensional set of input devices. Each row of input devices provides signals coupled into its two adjacent delay lines, one leading to the left, the other to the right. In any given row, each input device represents a different horizontal location. The extended system shown in Figure 13.4 is able to synthesize sounds appearing to have come from multiple sound sources simultaneously. Each pair of delay lines can be shared by input devices in two rows. This sharing is possible because, at the signal values we are using, the analog processing in the delay lines is linear. We can have more than one input device, and the signal from each device will be superimposed on the signal already present in the delay lines at that position. The different inputs are added linearly in the delay lines, just as sound pressure waves at moderate levels are combined in air.

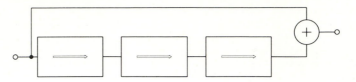

FIGURE 13.5   Electronic model of the pinna–tragus cue. The output of a headshadow-model delay line such as that shown in Figure 13.4 is added to a delayed version of itself. The apparent elevation of the sound is set by adjustment of the delay of the sections.

The vertical position of a signal source is encoded in the position of the delay line to which its outputs are coupled. We control the size of the auditory field by setting the total delay of the delay lines. The maximal total delay of one delay line (corresponding to an auditory field of 180 degrees) is the time required for sound to travel the distance between the ears. The relative simplicity of the implementation is a result of the analog processing of the delay lines emulating the superposition of sound pressure waves in air.

Pinna–tragus model   The pinna–tragus vertical cue shown in Figure 13.2 is the result of two paths by which sound can reach a single ear canal. The reflected path is delayed slightly relative to the direct path. We can synthesize this cue by adding a delay–add section to the end of each delay line in Figure 13.4. The structure of the analog delay–add section is shown in Figure 13.5. The output of the section is the sum of the signal, and a delayed version of the signal, just as the sound pressure in the ear canal is the sum of the sound from the direct path and that from the reflected path. The size of the delay determines the length of the longer path relative to that of the direct path, and hence the apparent elevation angle of the sound source. Setting the delay in the delay–add section generates the elevation cue. For this reason, we call the delay–add sections a **pinna–tragus model**.

We have now synthesized exactly the signals present in the ear canals, as shown in Figures 13.1 and 13.2. Sounds generated from these signals, presented through earphones inserted in a user's ear canals, give the illusion of a sound source localized in space.

THE SEEHEAR CHIP

The principle concept of the SeeHear chip is shown in Figure 13.6. The pixel array is oriented such that the delay lines run in the horizontal direction. The processing in each pixel strongly emphasizes time derivatives, so edges in the visual scene moving over the photoreceptors generate large, pulselike transient signals. The pixel outputs in each row act as input devices for a hearing-cue generator, like the one in Figure 13.4. Each pixel provides input to both delay lines of the hearing-cue generator at the point physically adjacent to the pixel.

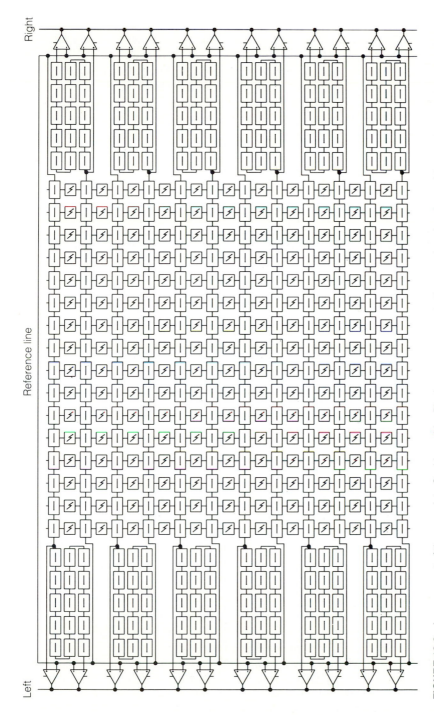

FIGURE 13.6 Arrangement of the complete SeeHear chip. Pixel processors create time-varying signals as objects move over the chip's field of view. These signals are coupled into the headshadow-model delay lines, in which the horizontal cues appropriate for their position are computed. A pinna–tragus delay at the end of each headshadow-model delay computes the vertical cue appropriate for the elevation of that particular row. The outputs of all channels are summed into the left and right auditory outputs. A fabrication layout of a small version of this chip is presented on the inside of the back cover.

The signals from the pixels along the row are delayed and filtered by an amount that is a function of the horizontal position of the pixel. This delay and filtering generates the horizontal hearing cues. For the vertical cues, we observe that all the pixels in one row of the array correspond to the same elevation angle in real space. The pinna–tragus model (delay–add section) at the end of each row therefore is tuned to have a delay corresponding to its elevation. This delay generates the vertical hearing cue. To form the output to the earphones, we represent the outputs from the pinna–tragus models by currents. The outputs for the left and right ears are summed separately: Kirchhoff's law automatically provides linear superposition of information in each output channel.

The analog nature of the processing in the SeeHear system leads to a remarkable simplicity of design, and to an economy of computational elements. The superposition of signals in the auditory-cue generator allows the parallel computation of sound cues for events occurring simultaneously in the visual scene, and encodes the information in only two output channels. A multiple-channel visual representation is thus transformed into a time-varying acoustic representation appropriate for perception by the auditory system. Thus, not only are computational elements of the auditory-cue generator shared by several pixels, but also no additional computational machinery is introduced to provide clocking or sampling; time is its own representation and memory is spatially encoded.

Implementation

The basic building blocks of the SeeHear system are all formed of primitive circuit elements described in earlier chapters. These building blocks are composed to generate the final chip layout, which follows precisely the plan shown in Figure 13.6. A row includes a row of pixels, a single delay line, and a pinna section at the output of the delay line. Alternate rows are mirrored to generate a roughly hexagonal array of photoreceptors, and alternating rightward- and leftward-propagating delay lines. The chip generates the signals for the right and left channels by summing the current outputs of the pinna–tragus models onto output wires running vertically along the right and left sides, respectively. The actual chip contained 32 rows of 36 pixels each.

The three building blocks that constitute the system are the retina model (pixel), the binaural-headshadow model (analog delay lines), and the pinna–tragus model (delay–add sections).

Retina model The pixel circuit is composed of a receptor (the light-transducing element) and a differentiator that emphasizes the temporal derivative of the intensity at that receptor. Each photoreceptor provides an output voltage that is logarithmic in the light intensity over four to five orders of magnitude. The intensity range covered is comparable to that covered by the *cones* in human visual systems. The logarithmic characteristic provides an output voltage-difference proportional to the *contrast ratio*, independent of the absolute illumination of the scene.

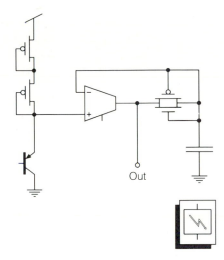

FIGURE 13.7 Schematic of the pixel processor. The photoreceptor output on the left computes the logarithm of the incident intensity. The time-derivative of the signal is computed by a hysteretic-differentiator described in Figure 10.11 (p. 174). The output of the differentiator is capacitively coupled to the adjacent delay lines. The symbol for the circuit is shown in the inset.

The schematic of the pixel is shown in Figure 13.7; a detailed discussion of the operation of the bipolar phototransistor is given in Chapter 15. Bipolar transistor structures are a natural byproduct of the bulk CMOS process used to implement the SeeHear system. They usually are considered to be a parasitic device, and can lead to certain problems in standard logic circuits. They are, however, excellent photodetectors, giving between 100 and 1000 electrons out per absorbed photon in. We use a large-area bipolar phototransistor of this type as our primary receptor. Two diode-connected MOS transistors operating in subthreshold are used to create an output voltage that is a logarithmic function of the photocurrent, as described in Chapter 6. This output voltage changes about 275 millivolts for each decade change in light intensity. The range of the output voltage is 1 volt to 2.5 volts below V_{DD}, where direct coupling to subsequent stages is accomplished readily.

The differentiator used in the pixel is the hysteretic differentiator described in Chapter 10. The circuit generates sharp transitions in its output voltage when the time derivative of its input voltage changes sign. Maximum outputs will therefore occur when high-contrast features move over the retina. This emphasis on derivatives provides maximum opportunity for users to generate information by body movement, as sighted people do with normal visual processing.

Binaural-headshadow model   All auditory processing is accomplished by way of analog delay lines, each of which is simply a long string of follower–integrator sections, as described in Chapter 9. Each section delays the incoming signal and broadens it slightly. The time required for a signal to reach the output of the line, and the degree of attenuation of high frequencies in the signal, are both monotonic functions of the number of sections through which that signal must propagate. The delay of the line from one end to the other (which determines the range of interaural time disparities that the SeeHear system can

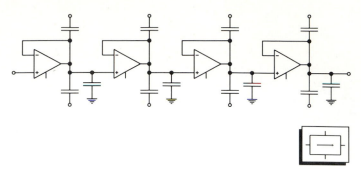

FIGURE 13.8 Delay line used in the headshadow model. Each stage is capacitively coupled to two pixels, one above and one below. The total delay is set by the transconductance of the amplifiers. The symbol for a single stage is shown in the inset.

encode) is controlled by the number of sections, and by the time constant of each section.

Coupling from an individual pixel output is accomplished by means of a capacitor connected from the differentiator output to a node in the delay line, as shown in Figure 13.8. The capacitive voltage-divider ratio is chosen to inject about 200 millivolts into the line for a 1.5-volt excursion of the pixel-differentiator output signal. The inputs to all delay lines are supplied with a DC reference level V_{ref} from offchip.

Pinna–tragus model The combined, processed outputs of two adjacent rows of pixels appear at the output of each headshadow-model delay line. Each such output is equipped with its own pinna–tragus model. Each pinna–tragus model consists of 18 delay sections that act as a final section of the analog delay line. The delay of the pinna–tragus model, which must vary as a function of elevation, is set by the time constant of the sections, which is controlled separately from that of the headshadow delay line.

Because the inputs of all delay lines are connected to V_{ref}, the total of all signals coupled into a particular delay line is represented by the difference between the output voltage of the line and V_{ref}. This difference is converted to a current by one transconductance amplifier at the output of the headshadow-model delay line, representing the direct signal into the ear canal, and by an additional amplifier at the output of the pinna–tragus delay line representing the reflected path. These currents are summed directly onto the appropriate output wire. The output amplifiers are operated well above threshold, where their linear range is sufficient to represent the full range of signal excursions encountered.

To realize the decrease in pinna–tragus delay with elevation, the transconductance controls of the amplifiers in the delay–add sections are connected to a polysilicon line that runs vertically along the edge of the chip. Each end of the line is brought out to an offchip pad. By application of different voltages to the two ends of the line, we can achieve any desired gradient in pinna–tragus delay.

PERFORMANCE

We can test the generation of horizontal cues by observing the chip outputs with the pinna–tragus delay disabled. Figure 13.9 shows the output of a single headshadow delay line for one pixel excited by a small step in light intensity. In Figure 13.9(a), the light was focused on a pixel near the left side of the chip. In Figure 13.9(b), the light was focused on a pixel near the right side of the chip. Note that the qualitative features required by the binaural-headshadow model are nicely embodied in the delay-line implementation.

By enabling the pinna–tragus delays, we can observe the vertical cues generated by the system. Under these conditions, the SeeHear output signals to the two ears, in response to a flashing stimulus, are as shown in Figure 13.10. For this set of measurements, the interaural time delay of the headshadow delay lines was adjusted to slightly under 4 milliseconds, corresponding to an interaural spacing of about 4.5 feet—an appropriate spacing for demonstrating the operation of the system on a set of loudspeakers. The pinna tragus delays were set to 3 milliseconds for the bottom row, and to about 1.5 milliseconds for the top row. These values correspond reasonably well to the hearing system of a large elephant, and have therefore become known as our "Jumbo" configuration. The direct and reflected signals are clearly resolved in both the left and right channels at lower elevations. Even for the contralateral ear channel, the pinna reflection is lost in the headshadow at only the highest elevation. In listening tests, the system provides an astoundingly realistic sense of horizontal localization, and a mildly convincing vertical cue that is easily learned by most listeners.

An instructive alternative view of the operation of the SeeHear chip is shown in Figure 13.11. Here the response of each ear is shown as a function of frequency.

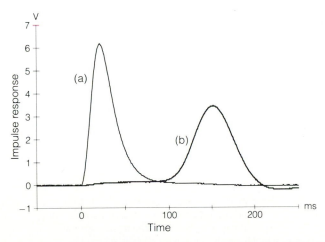

FIGURE 13.9 Measured output of a headshadow-model delay-line channel excited by a light source emitting an impulse of light at $t = 0$. (a) The source was focused near the output of the line. (b) The source was focused near the input of the line. The horizontal cues shown correspond to those of Figure 13.1.

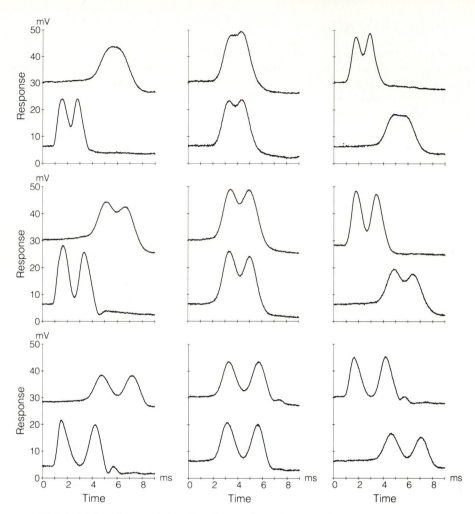

FIGURE 13.10 Measured time-domain response of the two SeeHear outputs to the onset of illumination of a small-area light source. The response was measured with the source located at nine positions in the field of view of the chip. In each plot, the lower trace is the output for the left ear, and the upper trace, which has been displaced for clarity, is the output for the right ear. The position of each plot on the page corresponds to the position of the source in the field of view. All plots have the same *x* and *y* scales, which have been labeled on only the left and bottom plots. The delay settings were appropriate for demonstrating the system with a pair of loudspeakers.

The peaked nature of the response is due to the differentiation associated with the capacitive coupling between the pixel output and the head-model delay lines. Two distinct peaks are visible in all but two of the traces. The first peak is the direct output of the head model, and the second peak is the delayed output from the pinna–tragus model. The pinna–tragus delay was set to decrease with elevation, thus generating a vertical-position cue that is easily learned by most listeners.

The relative delay between the left and right traces in each plot is due to the head-model delay lines. As expected, this horizontal cue is directly correlated with the horizontal location of the source.

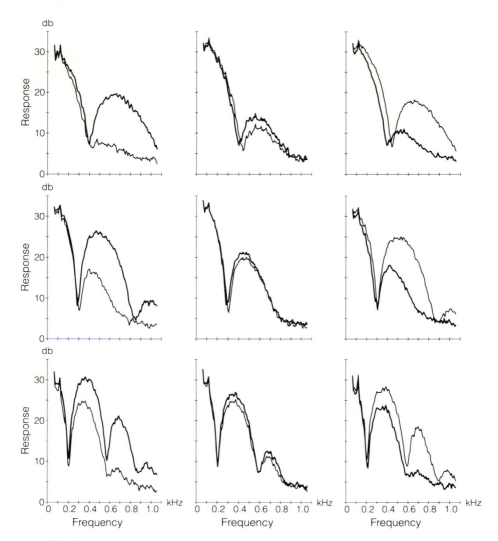

FIGURE 13.11 Measured frequency response of the two SeeHear outputs for the same delay settings as those used in Figure 13.10. We measured the response by modulating the illumination of a small-area light source with white noise, and integrating the resulting output over a long period on a commercial spectrum analyzer. Spectra were recorded with the source located at nine positions in the field of view of the chip. In each plot, the solid trace is the output for the left ear, and the shaded trace is the output for the right ear. The position of each plot on the page corresponds to the position of the source in the field of view. All plots have the same *x* and *y* scales, which have been labeled on only the left and bottom plots.

The general decrease in response at higher frequencies is due to the head-model delay lines. As expected, the effect is much more pronounced for the contralateral ear than it is for the ipsilateral ear, giving a strong impression of horizontal localization.

The effect of the pinna–tragus model is evident as a sharp notch in the frequency response. This notch occurs at higher frequencies as the source is moved to higher elevations, thus generating the vertical position cue.

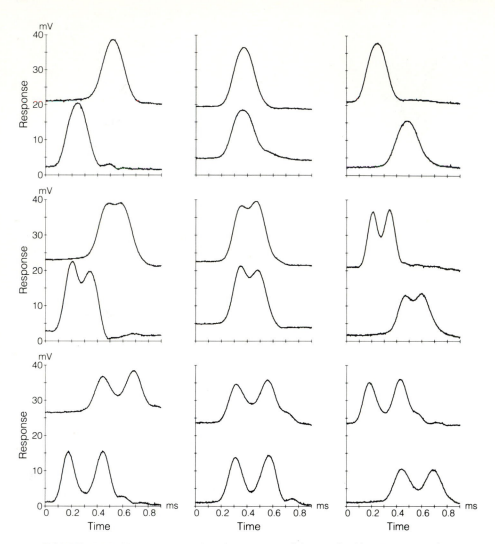

FIGURE 13.12 Measured time-domain response of the two SeeHear outputs to the onset of illumination of a small-area light source. The response was measured with the source located at nine positions in the field of view of the chip. In each plot, the lower trace is the output for the left ear, and the upper trace, which has been displaced for clarity, is the output for the right ear. The position of each plot on the page corresponds to the position of the source in the field of view. All plots have the same x and y scales, which have been labeled on only the left and bottom plots. The interaural time-delay setting is appropriate for a human listener, but the pinna–tragus delay corresponds to a much larger outer ear, such as that of a deer.

Two distinct peaks are visible at lower elevations, but are smeared out at higher elevations. This failure of the system response to scale to shorter times is a result of our running the follower–integrator circuits in the pinna–tragus model somewhat above threshold to achieve the short delays, and can be overcome by use of smaller capacitors in these delay stages. Even though much of the information is lost by the filtering action of the pinna–tragus delay lines, the vertical position is still discernible by many listeners.

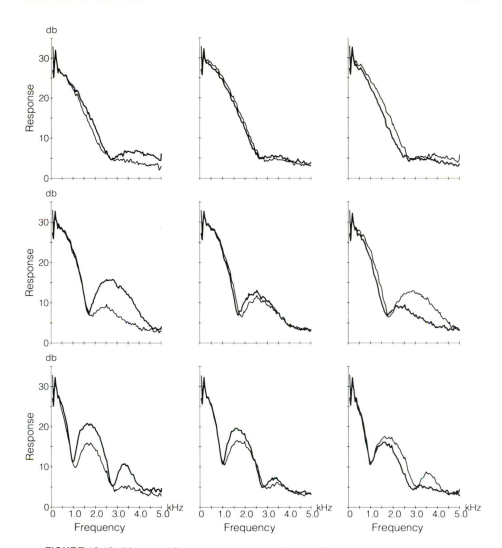

FIGURE 13.13 Measured frequency response of the two SeeHear outputs for the same delay settings as those used in Figure 13.12. We measured the response by modulating the illumination of a small-area light source with white noise, and integrating the resulting output over a long period on a commercial spectrum analyzer. Spectra were recorded with the source located at nine positions in the field of view of the chip. In each plot, the solid trace is the output for the left ear, and the shaded trace is the output for the right ear. The position of each plot on the page corresponds to the position of the source in the field of view. All plots have the same x and y scales, which have been labeled on only the left and bottom plots.

The general decrease in response at higher frequencies is due to the head-model delay lines. As expected, the effect is much more pronounced for the contralateral ear than it is for the ipsilateral ear, giving a strong impression of horizontal localization.

The spectral notch due to the pinna–tragus model is evident at low elevations, but is much less pronounced at high elevations. For this reason, the vertical position cue is not as striking with this setting as it was with longer delays.

The general rolloff of the curves at high frequency is due to the headshadow effect. The sharp notches in the spectra are due to the pinna–tragus reflection; they are the result of the cancellation in amplitude that occurs at frequencies where the indirect path is delayed just 180 degrees in phase from the direct path. The vertical cue can be seen clearly in the shift of the spectral notches to higher frequencies with elevation.

When the delays are adjusted to values more suited to the separation of human ears, the results are somewhat less convincing. The data shown in Figure 13.12 correspond to a maximum interaural delay of about 600 microseconds. The minimum pinna–tragus delay that could be achieved with the amplifiers operating in their subthreshold range was about 300 microseconds. This value corresponds to an outer ear considerably larger than that of a human—more like that of a deer. For this reason, these settings have become known as our "Bambi" configuration. At low elevations, the system performs nearly as well as Jumbo. At high elevations, the pinna–tragus delay is short enough that the indirect signal is lost in the width of the direct signal. The frequency response of the configuration is shown in Figure 13.13. Even at the highest elevations, there is still a distinct notch in the spectrum corresponding to the pinna–tragus delay.

The SeeHear chip thus is capable of generating the three principle auditory-localization cues in response to visual signals anywhere in its field of view. We have performed a number of listening tests to evaluate the realism of the localization cues generated by the device. The SeeHear chip creates a remarkably realistic auditory image of a flashing stimulus when the delays are set to correspond to the distance between two loudspeakers. Due to the headshadow cue, the illusion of horizontal localization is much more convincing than is that obtainable with time disparity alone. When the delays are set for operation with headphones, equally convincing horizontal localization is obtained. The pinna–tragus vertical cue, although not as vivid as the horizontal cues, allows most listeners to achieve a sense of the elevation of a light source, especially if that source is moving.

SUMMARY

In this chapter, we have described a complete system, the organizing principles of which were inspired by those found in biological systems. The system has been implemented in the neural paradigm described in the first three parts of this book. The result is a vast amount of both auditory and visual computation performed by a system measuring only a few square millimeters, using only a few milliwatts of power. The mapping of sensory input into an appropriate internal representation has been the key to achieving a compact and efficient implementation of what might otherwise have been a much more complex system.

The natural mapping of space and time in an analog VLSI system parallels the kind of processing found in the brain, because both VLSI and neural systems use the properties of physical devices as computational primitives, and both technologies are limited by the interconnections rather than by the computations themselves.

As we evolve our VLSI system, any improvement in either the visual or the auditory subsystems should be immediately noticeable by a user. For that reason, the chip should be a valuable proving ground within which to develop a deeper understanding of both sensory modalities. We can learn a great deal about both modes of perception by studying the visual and auditory systems in animals. Chapters 15 and 16 describe the syntheses of systems that mimic, as closely as we can manage, the corresponding function found in living animals.

REFERENCES

Bloom, P.J. Determination of monaural sensitivity changes due to the pinna by use of minimum-audible-field measurements in the lateral vertical plane. *Journal of the Acoustical Society of America,* 61:820, 1977a.

Bloom, P.J. Creating source elevation illusions by spectral manipulation. *Journal of the Audio Engineering Society,* 25:560, 1977b.

Carterette, E.C. and Friedman, M.P. *Handbook of Perception,* vol 5. New York: Academic Press, 1975.

Kendall, G.S. and Martens, W.L. Simulating the Cues of Spatial Hearing in Natural Environments. In Buxston, W. (ed), *Proceedings of the 1984 International Computer Music Conference.* Paris: IRCAM, 1984.

Lorenz, K.Z. *The Foundations of Ethology.* New York: Springer-Verlag, 1981.

Richards, W. Visual Space Perception. In Carterette, E.C. and Friedman, M.P. (eds), *Handbook of Perception,* vol 5. New York: Academic Press, 1975, p. 351.

14

OPTICAL MOTION SENSOR

John Tanner   Carver Mead

Future machines that interact flexibly with their environment must process raw sensory data and extract meaningful information from them. Vision is a valuable means of gathering a variety of information about the external environment. The extraction of motion in the visual field, although only a small part of vision processing, provides signals useful in tracking moving objects and gives clues about an object's extent and distance away.

This chapter describes the theory and implementation of an integrated system that reports the uniform velocity of an image focused directly on it. The chip contains an integrated photoreceptor array to sense the image, and has closely coupled custom circuits to perform computation and data extraction.

The integrated optical motion detector was designed to use local analog image-intensity information as much as possible to extract image motion. The logarithmic photoreceptor described in Chapter 15 and analog computation elements are combined in a novel approach to extracting velocity information from a uniformly moving image. The new motion detector has a number of features that overcome the shortcomings of previous designs [Lyon, 1981; Tanner et al., 1984].

Portions reprinted with permission from *VLSI Signal Processing*, Kung, Owen, and Nash, eds., IEEE Press, pp. 59–76. © 1987 IEEE.

- The continuous, nonclocked analog photoreceptor has been demonstrated to operate over more than four orders of magnitude of light intensity [Mead, 1985]; this range is much greater than that video-camera–based vision systems have.

- The system analyzes information contained in the analog light-intensity variations in the image. Sharp edges can be used but are not required. The image-contrast requirements are small.

- Local image gradients rather than global patterns are used; global notions such as object boundaries are not needed.

- The analog circuitry prevents the information loss inherent in thresholding or digitization.

- Temporal aliasing is avoided by continuous computation; there is no clocking or temporal sampling (there is spatial sampling).

A TWO-DIMENSIONAL ANALOG MOTION DETECTOR

An algorithm for two-dimensional velocity detection must address the problem that arises from an inherent ambiguity between motions along the two axes. This ambiguity occurs when the field of view is limited, as is the view through an aperture. The **aperture problem** is well known for binary-valued images. Figure 14.1 shows the view through a square aperture. A black-and-white image containing a single straight edge is moving at some velocity; the position of the edge at a later time is shown by the dashed line. The velocity cannot be uniquely determined from these two snapshots. There is an infinite family of possible velocities, as illustrated by the arrows. The image velocity components v_x and v_y can be viewed as the x and y coordinates in a **velocity plane**. In this plane, the actual velocity of the image defines a point. The family of possible image velocities defines a **constraint line** in velocity space that has the same orientation

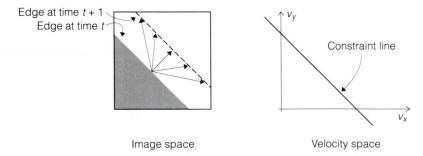

FIGURE 14.1 The aperture problem: Local information is not sufficient to determine two-dimensional velocity uniquely. The family of possible velocities, denoted by the arrows in image space, define the constraint line in velocity space. The constraint line has the same orientation as does the edge in physical space.

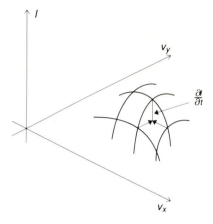

FIGURE 14.2 The intensity surface of a two-dimensional image. The change in intensity from a present high value to a future lower one, $\partial I/\partial t$, could be the result of many possible motions of the intensity surface. The arrows represent two possible motions.

as does the edge in physical space. To be consistent with the visual information from the local aperture, the actual velocity point is constrained to lie on the line in velocity space.

Note that Figure 14.1 illustrates the ambiguity problem but does *not* depict the operation of our system. The velocity detector described in this chapter represents intensity values continuously (the images considered are *not* just black and white) and represents time continuously (there is *no* notion of snapshots of the image or of clocking in this system).

Using analog values for intensities and gradients does not eliminate the ambiguity problem. Figure 14.2 shows the intensity plot of an image that contains gray-scale information and varies smoothly in intensity throughout. Intensity is plotted as height above the image plane for each point in the x, y image plane, and is a function of the objects in view. As the image moves, the shape of the intensity surface stays the same but translates in the image plane. A stationary sensor will detect changes in intensity due to the movement of the image. The change in intensity with time, $\partial I/\partial t$, is a change in height of the intensity surface at a fixed point. The local sensor cannot tell whether its upward or downward movement is due to motion of the intensity surface along only the x axis, only the y axis, or both axes. Two of these possibilities are shown as arrows in Figure 14.2. The inherent ambiguity cannot be resolved by strictly local information.

Following Horn and Schunk [Horn et al., 1981], the expression that relates the intensity derivatives to the velocity is

$$\frac{\partial I}{\partial t} = -\frac{\partial I}{\partial x}v_x - \frac{\partial I}{\partial y}v_y \tag{14.1}$$

The intensity of Figure 14.2, a function of the two spatial variables x and y, has spatial derivatives $\partial I/\partial x$ and $\partial I/\partial y$. The x and y components of velocity are v_x and v_y, and $\partial I/\partial t$ is the change in intensity with respect to time at a stationary observation point. This equation shows that the values of three local

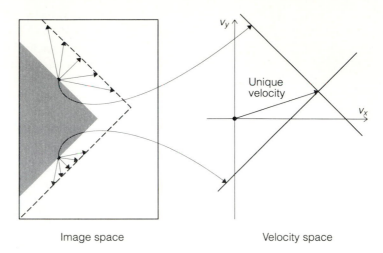

Image space   Velocity space

FIGURE 14.3   Uniquely determining velocity by the intersection of constraint lines.

derivatives of the intensity do not allow velocity to be determined uniquely; there is an inherent ambiguity.

The local intensity derivatives do provide useful information—they constrain the possible values of the x and y components of velocity, just as the black-and-white images in the aperture problem constrained the velocity components. Writing Equation 14.1 in the form of the line equation

$$Ax + By + C = 0$$

yields

$$\frac{\partial I}{\partial x}v_x + \frac{\partial I}{\partial y}v_y + \frac{\partial I}{\partial t} = 0$$

Each local set of three derivatives defines a line in the velocity plane along which the actual velocity must lie. The slope of this constraint line is $-(\partial I/\partial x)/(\partial I/\partial y)$. If the gray-scale image is viewed as having a fuzzy edge with orientation perpendicular to the intensity gradient, the constraint line has the same orientation in velocity space as the edge has in physical space. This orientation is the same as the constraint line of the black-and-white image.

The aperture problem for binary-valued images is just a special case of the general two-dimensional velocity ambiguity. Local images—gray scale or black and white—can provide only a family of possible velocities. This set of velocities can be represented by the coefficients of the equation for the constraint line.

It is much easier to determine the constraint line if the analog information is retained. For gray-scale images, the coefficients of the constraint-line equation are just the three partial derivatives that can be measured locally— $\partial I/\partial x$, $\partial I/\partial y$, and $\partial I/\partial t$. We can use thresholding to transform an image with continuous intensity values into a black-and-white image. Determining the orientation of the edge of the binary-valued image (and so its constraint line) is a more global problem of determining the boundary between black regions and white regions and of fitting a line to the boundary. To determine the velocity constraint line, we find it much easier to measure the coefficients locally than to throw away the information and then to try to reconstruct it with a global process.

We can resolve the ambiguity of a single local set of measurements by using another set of local values from a nearby location. These values define another line in the velocity plane. The intersection of these two lines uniquely determines the actual velocity (Figure 14.3).

Solution of Simultaneous Constraints

In practice, to find the actual velocity, we must ensure that all sites on the sensor array contribute constraints. Using only a small number of sites that are close together relative to an object size results in a few constraint lines in the velocity plane that are nearly parallel. A small error in any of the derivatives or in the constraint solver can then result in a large error in the computed velocity. Errors are kept to a minimum when two lines in the velocity plane cross at right angles. This intersection occurs when there are contributions from two sites on edges that are perpendicular. An *edge* in this case is loosely a line perpendicular to the direction of greatest intensity change. Taking contributions from a large number of sites will then ensure the existence of orthogonal constraints for any reasonable image.

The barber pole is a well-known example of an illusion that occurs because the orthogonality of constraint lines cannot be ensured. In this illusion, the rotating cylinder produces a purely horizontal velocity. Our vision system erroneously reports "seeing" a vertical velocity. Images such as gratings and stripe patterns with intensity variations along only one axis cause this mistake. All constraint lines are coincident, so their intersection is not unique. It is not possible for human, computer, or chip to disambiguate the motion of such a pattern.

In practice, there is no such thing as a perfect stripe pattern. The ability to disambiguate velocity correctly is thus a matter of degree. Our chip should reliably report the actual velocity unless the signals resulting from intensity variation along one axis lie below the noise level.

Constraint-Solving Circuits

Our constraint-solving circuit contains a set of global wires that distributes a best guess of velocity to all the individual constraint-generating sites (Figure 14.4). Each locale performs a computation to check whether the global velocity satisfies its constraint. If there is an error, circuitry within the local site then supplies a *force* that tends to move the global velocity toward satisfying the local constraint. The global velocity components are represented as analog voltages on the set of global wires. The correcting forces are currents that charge or discharge the global wires.

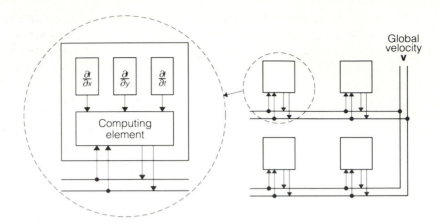

FIGURE 14.4   Block diagram of the constraint-solver cell and array. The three locally derived derivatives, $\partial I/\partial x$, $\partial I/\partial y$, and $\partial I/\partial t$, along with the present value of the globally distributed velocity components, are inputs to a circuit that continuously computes a correction to the global velocities.

Finding the intersection of many lines is an overconstrained problem. Any errors will result in a region of intersection in which the real desired point is most likely to lie. To compute a most probable intersection point (velocity), we must know what types of errors to expect, define "most probable," and select on the basis of that definition a forcing function that varies with detected error. In the absence of rigor, we can make reasonable guesses for the forcing function. It should be monotonic—the greater the error, the harder the chip should push in the right direction. Because a forcing function linear in error distance is easiest to implement, we have selected it. The constraint solver minimizes the error by finding the least-squares fit of the velocity point to all the constraint lines.

The direction of the correction force should be perpendicular to the constraint line (Figure 14.5). Based on local information alone, each motion-detector cell knows that the global velocity should lie on its locally defined constraint line, but it knows nothing about where along the line the global velocity lies. If a nonorthogonal component in the correction force were generated by the cell, an undue preference for the position of the global velocity on the constraint line would be expressed.

We ensure orthogonality by using a direct perpendicular construction for the correction force. If we rearrange the constraint-line equation

$$\frac{\partial I}{\partial x}v_x + \frac{\partial I}{\partial y}v_y + \frac{\partial I}{\partial t} = 0$$

from the implicit form $Ax + By + C = 0$ to the slope-intercept form $y = mx + b$ we get

$$v_y = -\frac{\partial I/\partial x}{\partial I/\partial y}v_x - \frac{\partial I/\partial t}{\partial I/\partial y}$$

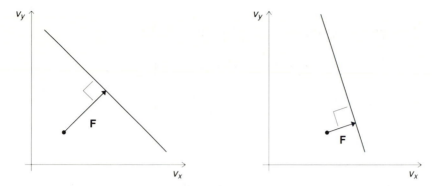

FIGURE 14.5 The correction force should be perpendicular to the constraint line in order to express only information obtained from the image.

The slope of the constraint line, where defined, is

$$m = -\frac{\partial I/\partial x}{\partial I/\partial y}$$

so the slope of the desired perpendicular correction force is then the negative reciprocal,

$$-\frac{1}{m} = \frac{\partial I/\partial y}{\partial I/\partial x}$$

A unit vector in this direction is

$$\frac{\nabla \mathbf{I}}{|\nabla \mathbf{I}|} = \left\langle \frac{\partial I/\partial x}{\sqrt{(\partial I/\partial x)^2 + (\partial I/\partial y)^2}}, \frac{\partial I/\partial y}{\sqrt{(\partial I/\partial x)^2 + (\partial I/\partial y)^2}} \right\rangle$$

The magnitude of the correction force should be greater if the present point in velocity space is farther away from the constraint line. The force should be zero for points lying on the constraint line. The direction of the force always should be perpendicular to the constraint line, and should have a sign such that the global velocity point will move toward the constraint line. A forcing function that is linear with error distance fulfills all these requirements and can be easily computed as

$$D = -\frac{(\partial I/\partial x)v_x + (\partial I/\partial y)v_y + \partial I/\partial t}{\sqrt{(\partial I/\partial x)^2 + (\partial I/\partial y)^2}}$$

If we just substitute the values for the velocity components into the line equation and normalize by the quantity under the radical, we get D, a signed distance. The magnitude of D is the distance from the present velocity point $\langle v_x, v_y \rangle$ to the constraint line. The sign of D indicates on which side of the line the point is and therefore the direction of the correcting force. The error vector, $\mathbf{e}$, from the current velocity to the point on the constraint line is then

$$\mathbf{e} = D \cdot \frac{\nabla \mathbf{I}}{|\nabla \mathbf{I}|}$$

$$= \left\langle D \frac{\partial I/\partial x}{\sqrt{(\partial I/\partial x)^2 + (\partial I/\partial y)^2}}, D \frac{\partial I/\partial y}{\sqrt{(\partial I/\partial x)^2 + (\partial I/\partial y)^2}} \right\rangle$$

$$= \left\langle -\frac{(\partial I/\partial x)v_x + (\partial I/\partial y)v_y + \partial I/\partial t}{(\partial I/\partial x)^2 + (\partial I/\partial y)^2} \frac{\partial I}{\partial x}, -\frac{(\partial I/\partial x)v_x + (\partial I/\partial y)v_y + \partial I/\partial t}{(\partial I/\partial x)^2 + (\partial I/\partial y)^2} \frac{\partial I}{\partial y} \right\rangle$$

Each cell should produce a force (electrical current), $\mathbf{F}$, that will tend to move the global velocity proportional to the detected error, $\mathbf{\Delta v}$. We also would like to scale this correcting force according to our confidence in the local data, C:

$$\mathbf{F} = C \cdot \mathbf{e}$$

There is more information in a higher-contrast edge, or at least there is a higher signal-to-noise ratio. A greater weight should be afforded to the correcting forces in those higher-contrast areas. Our measure of contrast in the image is the intensity gradient, a vector quantity:

$$\nabla \mathbf{I} = \left\langle \frac{\partial I}{\partial x}, \frac{\partial I}{\partial y} \right\rangle$$

Confidence is related to the magnitude of the gradient,

$$|\nabla \mathbf{I}| = \sqrt{\left(\frac{\partial I}{\partial x}\right)^2 + \left(\frac{\partial I}{\partial y}\right)^2}$$

If we choose our confidence, C, to be the square of the magnitude of the intensity gradient, we have

$$C = |\nabla \mathbf{I}|^2 = \left(\frac{\partial I}{\partial x}\right)^2 + \left(\frac{\partial I}{\partial y}\right)^2$$

This choice greatly simplifies the correcting-force calculation by canceling out the denominator. Our force equation becomes

$$\mathbf{F} = \left\langle -\left(\frac{\partial I}{\partial x}v_x + \frac{\partial I}{\partial y}v_y + \frac{\partial I}{\partial t}\right)\frac{\partial I}{\partial x}, -\left(\frac{\partial I}{\partial x}v_x + \frac{\partial I}{\partial y}v_y + \frac{\partial I}{\partial t}\right)\frac{\partial I}{\partial y} \right\rangle$$

Writing the two components of this vector equation separately, we have

$$F_x = -\left(\frac{\partial I}{\partial x}v_x + \frac{\partial I}{\partial y}v_y + \frac{\partial I}{\partial t}\right)\frac{\partial I}{\partial x}$$

$$F_y = -\left(\frac{\partial I}{\partial x}v_x + \frac{\partial I}{\partial y}v_y + \frac{\partial I}{\partial t}\right)\frac{\partial I}{\partial y} \tag{14.2}$$

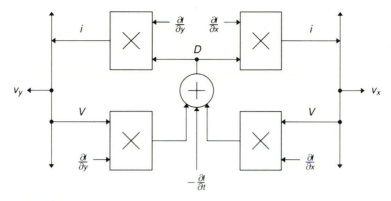

FIGURE 14.6 Block diagram for each cell's motion-detection circuitry.

Analog computational elements within each cell of a two-dimensional array implement the calculations described by Equation 14.2. The block diagram of an implementation of the orthogonal two-dimensional formulation is shown in Figure 14.6.

The two-dimensional constraint solver can be viewed in terms of feedback. Each cell computes an error, the signed scalar quantity D, which is the distance in velocity space from the global average velocity to the locally known constraint line. This distance error is used as feedback to correct the system. It is multiplied by the appropriate two-dimensional vector perpendicular to the constraint line, to generate a correction force in the same direction and thus to correct the global velocity vector.

The constraint-solving system for two-dimensional motion detection is collective in nature. Local information, weighted by confidence, is aggregated to compute a global result. Each cell performs a simple calculation based on moving the global velocity state into closer agreement with its locally measured information. The collective behavior that emerges is the tracking of the intersection of constraint lines to solve the two-dimensional ambiguity, when possible, and to report accurately the two-dimensional analog velocity of the image.

Our motion-detector chip consists of a two-dimensional array of cells. Each cell contains a photoreceptor and computational circuitry. The outputs of the photoreceptors are routed to adjacent cells, so that the computational elements of each cell can monitor the light intensity at the nearest neighbor in each dimension, as well as the cell's own intensity. The x and y components of velocity are distributed on wires globally to each cell. These values represent the present best guess for the global velocity. The voltages on these velocity wires are inputs to each cell. From the global velocity inputs and the local light-intensity inputs, each cell calculates a correction to the global velocity and expresses this correction in terms of currents that it applies to the same global velocity wires with an appropriate magnitude and sign. The global velocity wires perform a current sum of the correction contributions from all cells. The velocity voltages change according to the net correction from all the cells.

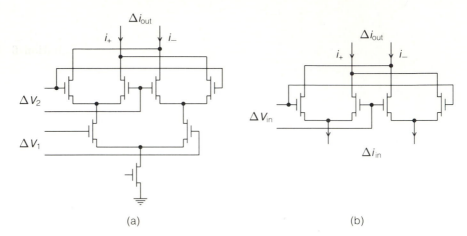

FIGURE 14.7 Two variations of the four-quadrant multiplier with differential-current outputs. (a) Both inputs are differential voltages. (b) One input is a differential voltage, the other is a differential current.

The inputs to the chip consist of the optical image focused on the die (the motion of which the chip measures) and several analog wires to control the gain of each component of the cells' circuitry. The outputs of the chip are the analog voltages on the global velocity wires.

Each cell contains four analog multipliers, a differential amplifier, and current-summing nodes to implement the correction computation of Equation 14.2, as shown in the block diagram of Figure 14.6. In addition, each cell contains a photoreceptor circuit and a differentiator.

The analog multipliers are variations of the Gilbert transconductance multiplier described in Chapter 6. The first variation is shown in Figure 14.7(a). Here we dispense with the top current mirror that was used to subtract the two currents, i_+ and i_-. Instead, we use the difference between these two currents, carried on two separate wires, as the output of the multiplier. Even though the two currents are not subtracted by hardware, Equation 6.10 (p. 93) still holds, and for small voltages becomes

$$\Delta i_{\text{out}} \propto \Delta V_{\text{in1}} \Delta V_{\text{in2}}$$

We see that the output current is proportional to the product of the two voltage inputs.

Carrying a signal on two wires, either as a current or voltage difference, is natural for CMOS analog design. We have already seen that the basic transconductance amplifier and many of its variations use differential inputs to solve the signal-reference problem. Circuits such as the topless multiplier produce outputs on two wires. This dual-rail signaling scheme is used throughout the design of the motion-detector chip.

A second multiplier variation, shown in Figure 14.7(b), leaves off the bottom differential pair and requires two currents as inputs in place of the two voltages. This circuit is identical to the one shown in Figure 6.7 (p. 91). Equation 6.9 (p. 93) describes the behavior of this circuit. For small voltages, this equation reduces to

$$\Delta i_{\text{out}} \propto \Delta i_{\text{in}} \Delta V_{\text{in}}$$

This variation is a four-quadrant multiplier with one voltage-input and one current-input pair, and with a current output.

Figure 14.8 shows a detailed schematic for the circuitry in one cell. A transconductance amplifier and capacitor integrate the output of the logarithmic photoreceptor with a time constant set with the external analog current control labeled τ. A choice in the range of 0.3 to 0.4 volt for the τ control knob allows operation for velocities typically encountered by a mouse pointing device. The difference between the intensity signal and its integrated value is amplified by a transconductance amplifier and is summed onto the pair of nodes labeled D (for distance in velocity space of the current global velocity point from this cell's constraint line). The amplifier gain is set externally by the TS (for time-derivative scaling) analog control.

We estimate the spatial derivatives by taking the difference in the intensity values of adjacent sensors. The two spatial derivatives are multiplied by the corresponding velocity components and the two results are summed onto the D nodes as differential currents. The gain of the multipliers is controlled by the external analog control labeled GS (for gradient scaling) that sets the multiplier bias current i_b. The scaling of the gradient relative to the time derivative by the two respective analog controls determines the scaling of the global velocity output. In practice, the GS and TS controls usually are the same and are operated between 0.5 and 0.7 volt.

The differential current summed onto the D nodes represents the distance term, which is the common term in the two parts of Equation 14.2. This D current pair is passed through two double current mirrors. The mirrors allow the current pair to be duplicated and to be used in two places in the next stage of computation. Each copy of the D currents is used as input to another four-quadrant multiplier of the variety with one set of current inputs. These multipliers multiply the D currents by the appropriate spatial derivative and sum the resulting current back onto the global velocity wires.

In the present version of the chip, the global velocity wires are brought out to pads, so that the pull-down resistors can be varied to set the operating point, and enough capacitance can be added to ensure one dominant time constant and thus to prevent oscillation. In practice, the stray capacitance is sufficient to prevent oscillation. Appropriate values for external pull-down resistors are in the range of 100 to 1000 megaohms due to the small subthreshold currents. These unusually large resistors can be obtained, and can be used as loads. A better way to provide pulldowns is to use the two pairs of onchip n-type transistors as high-resistance current sources. The current through these transistors is set by

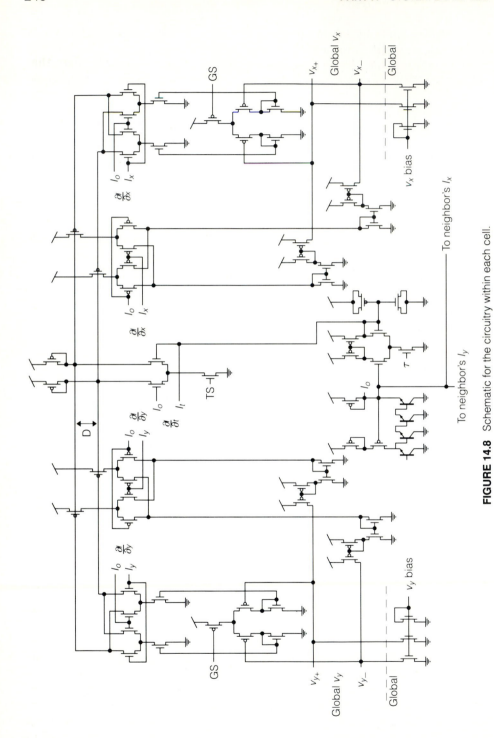

FIGURE 14.8 Schematic for the circuitry within each cell.

the analog v bias controls and is chosen to keep the common-mode voltage of the v_+ and v_- lines at an appropriate operating point.

Early versions of the chip used the simple four-quadrant multipliers that have constraints between the common-mode operating point of the two inputs and between the inputs and the outputs. Recent versions of the chip use wide-range multipliers. We ease the operating-point restrictions by inserting current mirrors between the two stages of a multiplier and between multiplier stages, as shown in Figure 14.8. The settings of the analog v bias controls are less critical.

The output currents of the inner two multipliers tend to charge the global velocity lines. Current is taken from the velocity lines by matched pairs of n-type pull-down transistors. The gate voltage is the same for both transistors in the pair and is chosen such that the common-mode voltage of the pair of velocity lines is within operating range—about 2.5 volts. The nonideality of the current sources connected to the velocity lines—both the pulldowns and the multipliers—tends to keep the velocity voltages near each other. Although not a strong effect, this tendency becomes important for low-contrast images. We discuss this effect in the next section, and present experimental data there. The pull-down transistors in their saturation region provide a much greater dynamic resistance and therefore a smaller nonideality than do the external pull-down resistors.

The high dynamic resistance of the pull-down transistors makes the transistors act as good current sources but makes the common-mode voltage of the global velocity lines highly dependent on the controlling gate voltages, v_x bias and v_y bias. For any given image and any setting of the GS and TS control knobs, there is a setting for the bias voltage that will keep the common-mode velocity voltage near 2.5 volts. As the image intensity varies, the optimum setting of the bias changes as well. To make full use of the wide dynamic range of the photoreceptors, we need a mechanism for adjusting the bias voltages automatically. The present prototype chip is augmented with an external operational amplifier to provide this automatic bias. The common-mode voltage is compared to a fixed voltage of 2.5 volts, and the error is fed back to the gate of the n-type transistor pulldowns. There are two circuits, one for the x component and one for the y component. Future versions of the motion detector will include a similar circuit onchip.

The circuitry in each cell forms two interconnected loops. These loops must be constructed to have negative feedback, both differential mode and common mode. We can alter the sign of the differential-mode feedback by swapping the connection of the dual-rail lines at any of several places in the circuit. The common-mode gain of the multiplier circuits is due to the nonideality of these circuits' current sources. An incorrectly constructed loop has common-mode positive feedback around the loop, which effectively forms a bistable latch. In this case, the operating point tends to migrate out of the desired range toward one of the rails. Attempting to correct the operating point with the bias voltage on the pulldowns causes the operating point to snap to the other state, out of range in the other direction. The automatic correction circuitry causes a continuous oscillation of the common-mode operating point. An extra pair of current mirrors is included in the present design between the output of the multipliers and the global velocity lines to keep the sign of the common-mode feedback negative.

An eight by eight array of motion-detector cells was fabricated on a standard MOSIS CMOS-bulk fabrication run. A λ of 1.5 microns yielded a die size of about 4500 by 3500 microns.

PERFORMANCE

We have tested the eight by eight array chip extensively by simulating motion electronically and by projecting actual moving images. In the first set of experiments, we used an electronically controlled light source to apply to the chip an intensity field that varied spatially across the chip and also varied with time. The space and time derivatives of intensity were controlled to simulate a moving intensity pattern while the velocity outputs from the chip were monitored. In the second set of experiments, we focused actual images on the chip and measured the chip's response. We verified the constraint-line behavior and mapped the correction force for different images.

Characterization of the Motion Output

The setup for the motion-simulation test is shown in Figure 14.9. Any changes in the light intensity were assumed to be due only to motion of the image, not to changes in the illumination level. Rapidly changing the illumination level under experimental control allowed us to simulate the motion of a spatial intensity gradient.

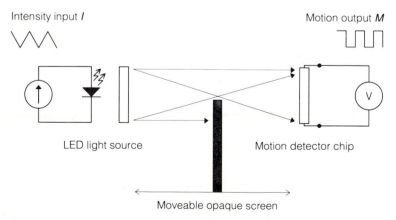

FIGURE 14.9 The test setup to simulate motion electronically. An array of LEDs casts light directly onto the motion-detector chip. Varying the LED current produced a controlled $\partial I/\partial t$. An opaque screen made a shadow edge on the chip. The distance from the chip to the screen controlled the sharpness of the edge, $\partial I/\partial x$.

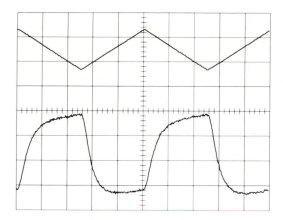

FIGURE 14.10 Oscilloscope traces of LED current (top) and reported velocity from the chip (bottom) for frequency of 20 hertz.

We generated a time derivative by changing the current through the LED light source. A triangle-wave intensity, used in these experiments, made a $\partial I/\partial t$ that was a square wave. The magnitude of the $\partial I/\partial t$ square wave was the slope of the triangle wave, which was dependent on the amplitude and frequency of the triangle wave. Frequency was used to vary $\partial I/\partial t$.

An opaque screen between the LED and the chip partially occluded the light and caused a spatial derivative of intensity (an edge) to fall on the chip. Moving the screen closer to the chip made a greater $\partial I/\partial x$ (a sharper edge). We adjusted the position of the screen until the measured spatial gradient was the desired value.

When we applied to the motion-detector chip a spatial intensity gradient that varied in time as a triangle wave, the differential voltage on the chip's velocity outputs was a square wave. Figure 14.10 shows an oscilloscope trace of the LED input current and of the velocity output of the chip. For these experiments, the screen producing the spatial gradient was aligned with the y axis of the chip. As the intensities varied with time, the y component of velocity reported by the chip was nearly zero.

With experimental control of $\partial I/\partial x$ and $\partial I/\partial t$, we tested the velocity output of the chip to verify that the reciprocal relationship for velocity held:

$$v_x = -\frac{\partial I/\partial t}{\partial I/\partial x}$$

This relationship comes from Equation 14.1, with v_y set to zero. We took two sets of measurements. First, we plotted reported velocity as a function of $\partial I/\partial t$ for fixed values of $\partial I/\partial x$; we expected a straight-line graph. Second, we held constant the triangle-wave frequency generating $\partial I/\partial t$ and varied the spatial gradient; the expected curve was a hyperbola. For all plots, the reported velocity was the amplitude of the square wave of the x component of the velocity output from the chip.

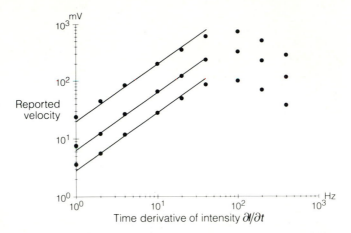

FIGURE 14.11 Measured motion response of the chip as a function of $\partial I/\partial t$ for three different values of $\partial I/\partial x$. The straight lines represent an ideal linear response.

Figure 14.11 shows plots of reported velocity versus $\partial I/\partial t$ (frequency) for three fixed values of $\partial I/\partial x$. The straight lines represent the theoretical proportional behavior, as shown on the log–log plot. The experimental results matched the predicted ones in the range from 1 to 40 hertz. Beyond that frequency, the amplitude of the output rolled off. One pole of the rolloff is accounted for by the capacitance of the sensor itself. The corner frequency is a function of absolute light level, as shown in [Mead, 1985]. The other pole is set by the output current driving the capacitive output node. We can increase this corner frequency by increasing the operating-current level of the entire chip.

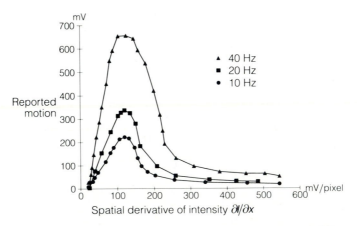

FIGURE 14.12 Measured motion response of the chip as a function of $\partial I/\partial x$ for three values of $\partial I/\partial t$. The response approximates a hyperbola over most of its range, as expected for velocity. Near zero, the response is linear with $\partial I/\partial x$.

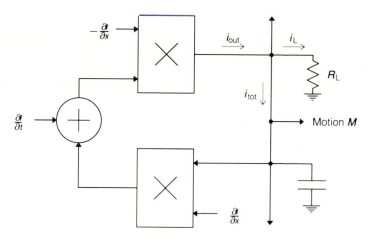

FIGURE 14.13   Schematic of the motion-cell circuitry with the finite load resistance, R_L.

Figure 14.12 shows a plot of reported velocity on the vertical axis versus applied $\partial I/\partial x$ on the horizontal axis for three fixed values of $\partial I/\partial t$. The curves approximate a hyperbola over most of their range. The experimental curve to the left of the peaks deviates significantly from a hyperbola.

As $\partial I/\partial x$ decreases, the reported velocity should increase; the resistance of the circuitry will increase, however, causing it to have less effect on the reported velocity. When $\partial I/\partial x$ is equal to 0, the reported velocity can take on any value because it is not affected at all by the local cells. The current source loads on the v_x and v_y lines in our implementation have large but finite resistance, so, in the absence of any information from the visual field, the reported velocity will tend toward zero. The schematic representing this effect is shown in Figure 14.13. For simplicity, we consider only the one-dimensional case, which we can derive from the two-dimensional case by setting $\partial I/\partial y$ to zero. For large $\partial I/\partial x$ (contrast ratios), the resistance of the local circuits is much smaller than that of the loads, so the loads' effect on reported velocity is negligible. As the contrast ratio is reduced, the load resistance must be taken into account.

So far, we have referred to the output of the chip as the velocity v. We have now shown, however, that under some circumstances the values on these global output lines may not be the actual velocity, so we will distinguish the chip's output by calling it the reported motion, M.

The output voltage on the global velocity lines is determined by the total charge on the node given by

$$M \propto \int i_{\text{tot}} \, dt$$

The condition for the system to be in steady state is therefore $i_{\text{tot}} = 0$. Before the load resistance is considered, i_{tot} is equal to i_{out}. When the load resistance is included, i_{tot} is equal to $i_{\text{out}} - i_{\text{L}}$; so, for steady state

$$i_{\text{out}} = i_{\text{L}} = M \frac{1}{R_{\text{L}}}$$

The output current, i_{out}, produced by the top multiplier is

$$i_{\text{out}} = -\left(M \frac{\partial I}{\partial x} + \frac{\partial I}{\partial t} \right) \frac{\partial I}{\partial x}$$

Thus, the steady state solution becomes

$$M \frac{1}{R_{\text{L}}} = -\left(M \frac{\partial I}{\partial x} + \frac{\partial I}{\partial t} \right) \frac{\partial I}{\partial x}$$

Solving for M, we get

$$M = -\frac{\partial I/\partial x}{(\partial I/\partial x)^2 + 1/R_{\text{L}}} \frac{\partial I}{\partial t} \tag{14.3}$$

A plot of this mathematical function is shown in Figure 14.14. For sufficiently large $\partial I/\partial x$, $(\partial I/\partial x)^2$ is much greater than $1/R_{\text{L}}$, so Equation 14.3 reduces to

$$M = -\frac{\partial I/\partial t}{\partial I/\partial x} = v \tag{14.4}$$

As $\partial I/\partial x$ approaches zero, $(\partial I/\partial x)^2$ becomes much smaller than $1/R_{\text{L}}$, and the equation becomes

$$M = -\frac{\partial I}{\partial t} \frac{\partial I}{\partial x} R_{\text{L}} \tag{14.5}$$

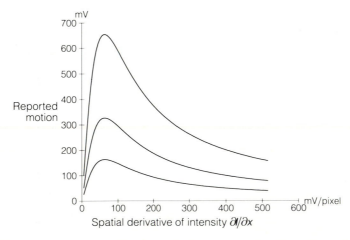

FIGURE 14.14   Plot of the theoretical motion-response curve as a function of $\partial I/\partial x$ according to Equation 14.3. This curve approximates a hyperbolic response to the right and a linear response near zero.

This analysis allows us to determine the chip's behavior for images that have different contrast ratios. When there is sufficient difference between light and dark areas, the motion-detector chip will report velocity accurately. As contrast in the image is reduced, the motion output M will change smoothly to become a function proportional to both $\partial I/\partial t$ and $\partial I/\partial x$. This change in behavior seems a particularly graceful way for a system to fail as the contrast ratio in its field of view is reduced to the point at which velocity no longer can be extracted. For a strict velocity detector, the zero-contrast case is undefined, so a device that reported "true velocity" could take on any value in the absence of information. Our motion detector has the virtue that it reports zero motion when it can detect no spatial-intensity variation.

Note that, if we want the multiplicative definition of motion over the entire operating range, we can easily make the motion-detector chip do this calculation. Setting the control current to zero on the feedback multiplier makes i_{out} equal to $(\partial I/\partial t)(\partial I/\partial x)$. This current can be turned into a voltage by the load resistor or by a higher-performance current-sensing arrangement offchip.

Over the complete range of $\partial I/\partial x$s, and in particular in both the hyperbolic and linear regimes of operation, Equations 14.4 and 14.5 show that the magnitude of the motion response should be proportional to $\partial I/\partial t$. The three curves of Figure 14.12—taken at frequencies of 10, 20, and 40 hertz—are scaled versions of the same curve and so bear out this proportionality over the range of $\partial I/\partial x$. Figure 14.11 shows a plot of reported motion as a function of $\partial I/\partial t$. The three curves are for fixed $\partial I/\partial x$s, one chosen from the right of the peak of the Figure 14.12 plot (the hyperbolic regime), one chosen from the left of the peak (the linear regime), and one chosen at the peak (midway in the transition region between the hyperbolic and linear regimes).

Verification of Constraint-Line Behavior

The collection of circuits in each cell (see Figure 14.6), working in concert, tries to satisfy the constraint between the x and y components of velocity according to the line equation

$$\frac{\partial I}{\partial x}v_x + \frac{\partial I}{\partial y}v_y + \frac{\partial I}{\partial t} = 0$$

This constraint is defined by the three inputs, the locally measured intensity derivatives, $\partial I/\partial x$, $\partial I/\partial y$, and $\partial I/\partial t$. If we force the voltage representing one of the components of velocity to a particular value, the circuit will drive the other component of velocity until the latter's value satisfies the constraint. For a given image input, we can determine the entire constraint line by sweeping the forced velocity value. Figure 14.15 plots three constraint lines from the measured response of the motion-detector chip. A single edge was projected onto the chip so that all the constraint lines of each cell in the array would coincide. The x component of velocity was driven to a sequence of values. For each value, the chip determined the y component, and the resulting point in velocity space was

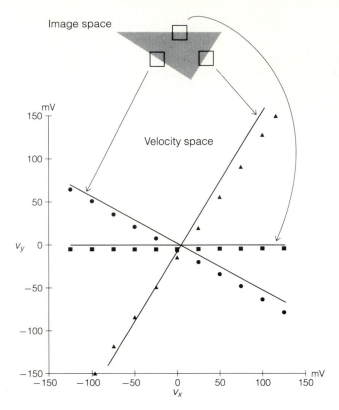

FIGURE 14.15 Demonstration of the constraint-line behavior of the motion-detector chip. The x component of velocity was swept while v_x versus v_y was plotted. The three trials were for the edge in the image oriented at 0, 60, and 30 degrees. The lines are the ideal constraint lines.

plotted. The image was not moving relative to the chip, so we predicted that the constraint line would pass through the origin. A constraint line was plotted for three different orientations of the edge. To ensure the relative angles of the three orientations, we used a single triangle as the image for each trial. Between trials, the part of the image falling on the chip was adjusted by translations only. Although the data deviated from the ideal slightly, this experiment clearly demonstrated the constraint-line behavior of the motion-detector chip.

Velocity-Space Maps

To demonstrate the two-dimensional collective operation of the motion-detector chip, we focused an image of a single high-contrast edge onto the chip. Because the image was stationary, the chip should have reported zero motion. The global output lines were driven externally to take on a sequence of values chosen to scan the velocity space in a regular grid. For each x, y pair of voltages driven onto the chip, the chip responded with a current intended to move the global point in velocity space into agreement with the velocity of its image input; namely, zero velocity. These resulting x, y pairs of currents were measured for each point and were displayed as a small vector originating at the forced point in velocity space. The resulting maps of these vectors (Figures 14.16 through 14.18) show the direction and magnitude of the force exerted by the chip on the global velocity lines. The point of stability—the **attractor point**—is near zero, as it should be. The amount by which the chip pulls as the global line moves far-ther away from the attractor depends on the structure of the applied image. An image containing a single edge was used in the experiment that produced Figures 14.16 and 14.17. A one-dimensional image, such as a single edge, pro-vides information about the velocity only perpendicular to the edge. Thus, the chip should pull harder when the velocity lines are forced away from the real ve-locity in a direction perpendicular to the one-dimensional image stimulus. The image contains less information about the velocity parallel to the applied edge, so forced displacements of velocity away from zero in that direction result in much smaller restoring forces. A more complex image was used in the experi-ment that produced Figure 14.18. Presented with an unambiguous image, the chip pulls evenly toward a unique velocity when displaced from that velocity in any direction.

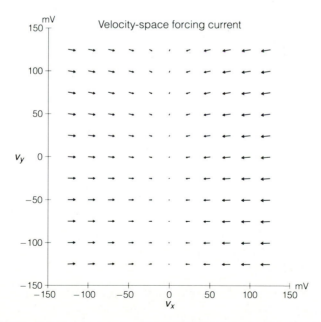

FIGURE 14.16   Velocity-space map of the restoring forces generated by the motion-detector chip in response to an edge at 90 degrees.

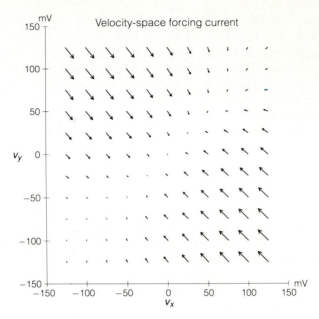

FIGURE 14.17   Velocity-space map of the restoring forces generated by the motion-detector chip in response to an edge at 45 degrees.

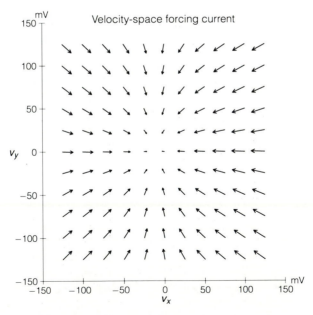

FIGURE 14.18   Velocity-space map of restoring force for a bright circle on a dark background. Edges of all orientations are represented.

LEAST-SQUARES METHODS AND GRADIENT-DESCENT SOLUTIONS

John Wyatt

In this section, we show how the optical motion sensor implements a gradient-descent solution to a general least-squares problem. We shift our emphasis from the *underspecified* nature of a single measurement for estimating the velocity (the aperture problem) to the *overspecified* nature of a system of many such measurements.

Notation

We number the cells of the array in any order from 1 to N ($N = 64$ for this particular chip), and let $\partial I/\partial x\,|_k$, $\partial I/\partial y\,|_k$ and $\partial I/\partial t\,|_k$ denote the results of the three local image measurements performed by cell number k. The motion sensor attempts to solve the following equations for v_x and v_y:

$$\left.\frac{\partial I}{\partial x}\right|_1 v_x + \left.\frac{\partial I}{\partial y}\right|_1 v_y = -\left.\frac{\partial I}{\partial t}\right|_1$$

$$\left.\frac{\partial I}{\partial x}\right|_2 v_x + \left.\frac{\partial I}{\partial y}\right|_2 v_y = -\left.\frac{\partial I}{\partial t}\right|_2$$

$$\vdots$$

$$\left.\frac{\partial I}{\partial x}\right|_N v_x + \left.\frac{\partial I}{\partial y}\right|_N v_y = -\left.\frac{\partial I}{\partial t}\right|_N \tag{14.6}$$

To focus attention on the general problem, we change notation to the generic form

$$a_{11}(t)v_x + a_{12}(t)v_y = b_1(t)$$

$$\vdots$$

$$a_{N1}(t)v_x + a_{N2}(t)v_y = b_N(t) \tag{14.7}$$

or, in matrix notation

$$\mathbf{A}(t)(\mathbf{v}) = \mathbf{b}(t)$$

where $\mathbf{A}(t)$ is an $N \times 2$ matrix, and $\mathbf{v} = (v_x, v_y)^T$ is a column vector (the superscript T denotes the transpose operation). Since there are more equations than there are unknowns, there generally will be no solution when the coefficients are obtained from necessarily imperfect image measurements. Thus, we concede at the outset that there must be errors; we try to establish control of the situation by giving these errors names! Let $e_k(\mathbf{v}, t)$ be the amount by which a candidate solution $\mathbf{v}$ fails to satisfy the kth equation in the system Equation 14.7;

that is,

$$e_k(\mathbf{v}, t) = a_{k1}(t)v_1 + a_{k2}(t)v_2 - b_k(t) \tag{14.8}$$

A reasonable goal is to minimize the sum of the squares of these errors; that is, to minimize

$$E(\mathbf{v}, t) = \tfrac{1}{2} \sum_{k=1}^{N} e_k^2(\mathbf{v}, t) = \tfrac{1}{2} \big(\mathbf{A}(t)\mathbf{v} - \mathbf{b}\big)^T \big(\mathbf{A}(t)\mathbf{v} - \mathbf{b}\big) \tag{14.9}$$

The Static Least-Squares Problem

Since E is quadratic in $\mathbf{v}$ and nonnegative, we look for a minimum at the point or points where its gradient vanishes. A straightforward calculation based on Equation 14.9 shows that

$$\nabla E(\mathbf{v}, t) = \mathbf{A}^T(t)\big(\mathbf{A}(t)\mathbf{v} - \mathbf{b}(t)\big) \tag{14.10}$$

where $\nabla E = (\partial E/\partial v_x, \partial E/\partial v_y)^T$. The arrows in Figures 14.16 through 14.18 show the gradient of this error function as calculated by the actual chip for three simple stationary images. Equating the right side of Equation 14.10 to zero yields the well-known *normal equations* [Strang, 1980] for the solution to the least-squares problem. The best way to relate this result to the motion sensor is to substitute the terms of Equation 14.6 into Equation 14.8 and to note that

$$\frac{\partial}{\partial v_x}\left(\tfrac{1}{2}e_k^2\right) = \left(\frac{\partial I}{\partial x}\bigg|_k v_x + \frac{\partial I}{\partial y}\bigg|_k v_y + \frac{\partial I}{\partial t}\bigg|_k\right)\frac{\partial I}{\partial x}\bigg|_k = -F_{x,k}$$

$$\frac{\partial}{\partial v_y}\left(\tfrac{1}{2}e_k^2\right) = \left(\frac{\partial I}{\partial x}\bigg|_k v_x + \frac{\partial I}{\partial y}\bigg|_k v_y + \frac{\partial I}{\partial t}\bigg|_k\right)\frac{\partial I}{\partial y}\bigg|_k = -F_{y,k}$$

where $F_{x,k}$ and $F_{y,k}$ represent the "forces" calculated by cell number k, as in Equation 14.2. Thus, the normal equations for the system Equation 14.6 take the form

$$\frac{\partial E}{\partial v_x} = -\sum_{k=1}^{N} F_{x,k} = 0$$

$$\frac{\partial E}{\partial v_y} = -\sum_{k=1}^{N} F_{y,k} = 0$$

and their solution is achieved as a balance of forces when the chip is at equilibrium. In the steady state, the chip calculates a velocity estimate that minimizes the sum of the squares of the errors.

The Dynamic Least-Squares Problem

A dynamic analysis shows that, when the image velocity changes too rapidly for the circuits to follow precisely, the motion sensor responds appropriately by forcing the velocity estimate (v_x, v_y) to move *straight down the gradient* of the error landscape as rapidly as the circuit time constants permit.[1] Stated more abstractly, the system implements the coupled first-order gradient system of differential equations

$$\frac{d\mathbf{v}}{dt} = -\lambda \nabla E(\mathbf{v}, t) \tag{14.11}$$

where λ is a nonnegative constant to be determined.

To verify that the chip implements this desirable gradient-descent behavior, we recall that each cell injects differential currents into two pairs of global signal lines. These currents are, by design, proportional to the forces in Equation 14.2; that is,

$$i_{x,k} = GF_{x,k}$$

$$i_{y,k} = GF_{y,k}$$

where the constant G is determined by the bias currents on the multipliers. The two pairs of signal lines sum the injected currents. The differential voltage on each pair evolves in time according to $dv/dt = i/C$, where C is the total distributed capacitance per pair. We ignore scaling issues for the moment and equate the estimated velocities v_x and v_y to the differential voltages. The result is

$$\frac{dv_x}{dt} = \frac{G}{C} \sum_{k=1}^{N} F_{x,k} = -\frac{G}{C} \frac{\partial E}{\partial v_x}$$

$$\frac{dv_y}{dt} = \frac{G}{C} \sum_{k=1}^{N} F_{y,k} = -\frac{G}{C} \frac{\partial E}{\partial v_y} \tag{14.12}$$

which has the form of Equation 14.11 with $\lambda = G/C$.

The global wires are doing a lot of computation and communication in this design. Each wire sums the error signals from $N = 64$ processors by Kirchhoff's current law, integrates the differential equation (Equation 14.12) using $dv/dt = i/C$, and instantaneously communicates the result, encoded as a voltage, back to the processors. This technique is a strikingly efficient use of the physics of the medium to perform a computation. The net result—gradient descent down an

---

[1] The phrase "straight down the gradient" can be misleading. In the first place, the path of the velocity estimate $\mathbf{v}(t)$ need not be a straight line, any more than is the path of a skier who goes straight down the fall line of a complicated mountain terrain. Furthermore, the error landscape can vary in time, so the error could, in principle, *increase* even while the solution is evolving straight down its gradient. Thus a more accurate analogy might be the path of a skier going straight down the fall line during an avalanche!

error or "energy" landscape—is somewhat similar to that of other neural network algorithms typically implemented on digital computers [Hopfield, 1982; Ackley et al., 1985; Rumelhart et al., 1986]. The major differences are that the motion-sensor energy landscape (1) can be time-dependent; (2) is always convex—that is, it *cannot* have multiple, isolated local minima; and (3) becomes flat when the image contrast goes to zero.

SUMMARY

We have designed and built the first integrated motion detector using analog circuit elements and collective computation. We formulated the algorithm and designed the architecture to exhibit collective behavior through the aggregation of locally derived quantities. We used closely coupled analog photoreceptors and small analog computational elements, making feasible the parallel operation of large arrays of sensors and computing elements. The system makes extensive use of local intensity information and therefore operates in the presence of global intensity gradients. This local computing also eliminates the need for any prior higher-level processing, such as edge detection or object recognition.

The motion-detector architecture, along with local analog computational elements, provides a dense, reliable means of processing high-bandwidth visual data. The motion-detector chip demonstrates the suitability of analog VLSI circuits to process sensory data.

The motion-detector chip is one of the first of a growing class of systems that employ collective computation. As we gain experience with this type of system, we may expand the range of application beyond that of processing sensory data. The motion-detector chip proved to be a good first example. Although it has a crisp, solid mathematical foundation, the motion-detector chip exhibits the collective behavior that is so necessary for processing sensory data from the fuzzy real world.

REFERENCES

Ackley, D.H., Hinton, G.E., and Sejnowski, T.J. A learning algorithm for Boltzmann machines. *Cognitive Science,* 9:147, 1985.

Hopfield, J.J. Neural networks and physical systems with emergent collective computational abilities. *Proceedings of the National Academy of Science,* 79:2554, 1982.

Horn, B.K.P. and Schunck, B.G. Determining optical flow. *Artificial Intelligence,* 17:185, 1981.

Lyon, R.F. The optical mouse, and an architectural methodology for smart digital sensors. *Carnegie-Mellon University Conference on VLSI Systems and Computations, Pittsburg, PA.* Rockville, MD: Computer Science Press, 1981, p. 1.

Mead, C. A sensitive electronic photoreceptor. In Fuchs, H. (ed), *1985 Chapel Hill Conference on Very Large Scale Integration.* Chapel Hill, NC: Computer Science Press, 1985, p. 463.

Rumelhart, D.E., McClelland, J.L., and the PDP Research Group. *Parallel Distributed Processing: Explorations in the Microstructure of Cognition.* vol 1. Cambridge, MA: MIT Press, 1986.

Strang, G. *Linear Algebra and Its Applications.* 2nd ed., New York: Academic Press, 1980.

Tanner, J.E. and Mead, C. A correlating optical motion detector. In Penfield, P. (ed), *Proceedings, Conference on Advanced Research in VLSI: January 23–25 1984, MIT, Cambridge, MA.* Dedham, MA: Artech House, 1984, p. 57.

SILICON RETINA

M. A. Mahowald   Carver Mead

The retina is a thin sheet of neural tissue that partially lines the orb of the eye. This tiny outpost of the central nervous system is responsible for collecting all the visual information that reaches the brain. Signals from the retina must carry reliable information about properties of objects in the world over many orders of magnitude of illumination.

The high degree to which a perceived image is independent of the absolute illumination level is, in large part, a result of the initial analog stages of retinal processing, from the photoreceptors through the outer-plexiform layer. This processing relies on lateral inhibition to adapt the system to a wide range of viewing conditions, and to produce an output that is independent of the absolute illumination level. A byproduct of the mechanism of lateral inhibition is the enhancement of spatial edges in the image; in signal-processing terms, the operation performed by the chip resembles a Laplacian filter.

We have built a silicon retina that is modeled on the distal portion of the vertebrate retina. This chip generates, in real time, outputs that correspond directly to signals observed in the corresponding levels of biological retinas. The chip design uses the principles of signal aggregation discussed in Chapter 7. It demonstrates a tolerance for device imperfections that is characteristic of a collective system.

Portions reprinted with permission from *Neural Networks*, Vol. 1. Mead, C. and Mahowald, M.A. A Silicon Model of Early Visual Processing. © 1988, Pergamon Press.

RETINAL STRUCTURE

A thorough review of the biological literature up to 1973 is given in *The Vertebrate Retina* [Rodieck, 1973], and one of more recent work is presented in *The Retina: An Approachable Part of the Brain* [Dowling, 1987]. Although the details of each animal's anatomy are unique, the gross structure of the retina has been conserved throughout the vertebrates.

The major divisions of the retina are shown in cross-section in Figure 15.1. Light is transduced into an electrical potential by the photoreceptors at the top. The primary signal pathway proceeds from the photoreceptors through the **triad synapses** to the **bipolar cells**, and thence to the **retinal ganglion cells**, the output cells of the retina. This pathway penetrates two dense layers of neural processes and associated synapses. The **horizontal cells** are located just below the photoreceptors, in the **outer-plexiform layer**. The **inner-plexiform layer**, just above the ganglion cell bodies, contains amacrine cells. The horizontal and **amacrine cells** spread across a large area of the retina, in layers transverse to the primary signal flow.

Each cell type in the retina has unique characteristics. The horizontal cells, along with the photoreceptors and bipolar cells, represent information with smoothly-varying analog signals. The amacrine cells, which are concerned with extracting motion events, have active channels in their processes that propagate temporally sharp signals in response to broad inputs. The amacrine and hori-

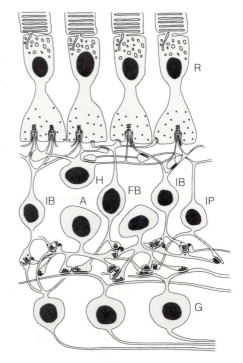

FIGURE 15.1   Artist's conception of a cross-section of a primate retina, indicating the primary cell types and signal pathways. The outer-plexiform layer is beneath the foot of the photoreceptors. The invagination into the foot of the photoreceptor is the site of the triad synapse. In the center of the invagination is a bipolar-cell process, flanked by two horizontal cell processes. R: photoreceptor, H: horizontal cell, IB: invaginating bipolar cell, FB: flat bipolar cell, A: amacrine cell, IP: interplexiform cell, G: ganglion cell. (*Source:* Adapted from [Dowling, 1987, p. 18].)

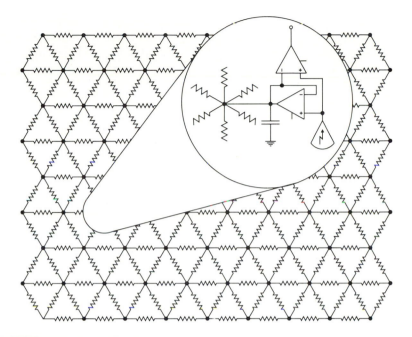

FIGURE 15.2   Diagram of the silicon retina showing the resistive network; a single pixel element is illustrated in the circular window. The silicon model of the triad synapse consists of a follower-connected transconductance amplifier by which the photoreceptor drives the resistive network, and an amplifier that takes the difference between the photoreceptor output and the voltage stored on the capacitance of the resistive network. These pixels are tiled in a hexagonal array. The resistive network results from a hexagonal tiling of pixels.

zontal cells are examples of *axonless* neurons. They receive inputs and generate outputs along the same neuronal processes. In contrast, the retinal ganglion cell possesses distinct dendrites and an axon that produces action potentials that are quasidigital (digital in amplitude but analog in time). The two-dimensional sheet of the retina is a marvelous canvas painted with the rich palate of biophysics. The diversity of cell types and computations demonstrates the power of combining a small number of physical elements in a hierarchical structure. Modeling the retina in silicon, we hope to develop a repertoire of computations based on the physics of the medium.

We begin with a simple model of the analog processing that occurs in the distal portion of the retina. Because our model of retinal processing is implemented on a physical substrate, it has a straightforward structural relationship to the vertebrate retina. A simplified plan of the silicon retina is shown in Figure 15.2. This view emphasizes the lateral spread of the resistive network, corresponding to the horizontal cell layer. The primary signal pathway proceeds through the photoreceptor and the circuitry representing the bipolar cell shown in the inset. The image signal is processed in parallel at each node of the network.

The key processing element in the outer-plexiform layer is the *triad synapse*, which is found in the base of the photoreceptor. The triad synapse is the point of contact among the photoreceptor, the horizontal cells, and the bipolar cells. We can describe our model of the computation performed at the triad synapse in terms of the synapse's three elements:

1. The photoreceptor takes the logarithm of the intensity

2. The horizontal cells form a resistive network that spatially and temporally averages the photoreceptor output

3. The bipolar cell's output is proportional to the difference between the photoreceptor signal and the horizontal cell signal

We will describe these elements in detail in the following sections.

Photoreceptor Circuit

The primary function of the **photoreceptor** is to transduce light into an electrical signal. For intermediate levels of illumination, this signal is proportional to the logarithm of the incoming light intensity. The logarithmic nature of the output of the biological photoreceptor is supported by psychophysical and electrophysiological evidence. Psychophysical investigations of human visual-sensitivity thresholds show that the threshold increment of illumination for detection of a stimulus is proportional to the background illumination over several orders of magnitude [Shapley et al., 1984]. Physiological recordings show that the photoreceptors' electrical response is logarithmic in light intensity over the central part of the photoreceptors' range, as are the responses of other cells in the distal retina [Rodieck, 1973]. The logarithmic nature of the response has two important system-level consequences:

1. An intensity range of many orders of magnitude is compressed into a manageable excursion in signal level.

2. The voltage difference between two points is proportional to the **contrast ratio** between the two corresponding points in the image. In a natural image, the contrast ratio is the ratio between the reflectances of two adjacent objects, reflectances which are independent of the illumination level.

The silicon photoreceptor circuit consists of a **photodetector**, which transduces light falling onto the retina into an electrical photocurrent, and a logarithmic element, which converts the photocurrent into an electrical potential proportional to the logarithm of the local light intensity. Our photodetector is a **vertical bipolar transistor**, which occurs as a natural byproduct in the CMOS process described in Appendix A. The base of the transistor is an isolated section of well, the emitter is a diffused area in the well, and the collector is the substrate. Photons with energies greater than the band gap of silicon create electron–hole pairs as they are absorbed. Electrons are collected by the n-type base of the *pnp* phototransistor, thereby lowering the energy barrier from emitter to base, and

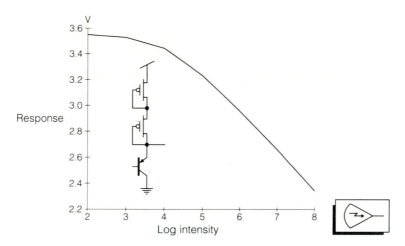

FIGURE 15.3   Measured response of a logarithmic photoreceptor. Photocurrent is proportional to incident-light intensity. Response is logarithmic over more than four orders of magnitude in intensity. Direct exposure of the chip to room illumination resulted in an output voltage of 2.1 volts. The symbol for the photoreceptor circuit is shown in the inset.

increasing the flow of holes from emitter to collector. The gain of this process is determined by the number of holes that can cross the base before one hole recombines with an electron in the base. The photodetector in our silicon photoreceptor produces several hundred electrons for every photon absorbed by the structure.

The current from the photodetector is fed into two diode-connected MOS transistors in series. The photocurrent biases these transistors in the subthreshold region. This arrangement was described in Chapter 6; it produces a voltage proportional to the logarithm of the current, and therefore to the logarithm of the incoming intensity. We use two transistors to ensure that, under normal illumination conditions, the output voltage will be within the limited allowable voltage range of the resistive network. Even so, at very low light levels, the output voltage of the photoreceptor may be close enough to V_{DD} that the resistor bias circuit described in Chapter 7 cannot adequately bias the horizontal resistive connections.

The voltage out of this photoreceptor circuit is logarithmic over four to five orders of magnitude of incoming light intensity, as shown in Figure 15.3. The lowest photocurrent is about 10^{-14} amps, which translates to a light level of 10^5 photons per second. This level corresponds approximately to a moonlit scene focused on the chip through a standard camera lens, which is about the lowest illumination level visible to the cones in a vertebrate retina.

Horizontal Resistive Layer

The retina provides an excellent example of the computation that can be performed using a resistive network. The horizontal cells in most species are connected to one another by gap junctions to form an electrically continuous network in which signals propagate by electrotonic spread [Dowling, 1987]. The lateral spread of information at the outer-plexiform layer is thus mediated by the resistive network formed by the horizontal cells. The voltage at every point in the network represents a spatially weighted average of the photoreceptor inputs. The farther away an input is from a point in the network, the less weight it is given. The horizontal cells usually are modeled as passive cables, in which the weighting function decreases exponentially with distance.

The properties of passive resistive networks were described in Chapter 7; additional details are given in Appendix C. Our silicon retina includes one such network, patterned after the horizontal cells of the retina. Each photoreceptor in the network is linked to its six neighbors with resistive elements, to form the hexagonal array shown in Figure 15.2. Each node of the array has a single bias circuit to control the strength of the six associated resistive connections. The photoreceptors act as voltage inputs that drive the horizontal network through conductances. This method of providing input to a resistive network is shown in Figure 7.12 (p. 120). By using a wide-range amplifier in place of a bidirectional conductance, we have turned the photoreceptor into an effective voltage source. No current can be drawn from the output node of the photoreceptor, because the amplifier input is connected to only the gate of a transistor.

The horizontal network computes a spatially weighted average of photoreceptor inputs. The spatial scale of the weighting function is determined by the product of the lateral resistance and the conductance coupling the photoreceptors into the network. Varying the conductance of the wide-range amplifier or the strength of the resistors changes the space constant of the network, and thus changes the effective area over which signals are averaged.

Both biological and silicon resistive networks have associated parasitic capacitances. The fine unmyelinated processes of the horizontal cells have a large surface-to-volume ratio, so their membrane capacitance to the extracellular fluid will average input signals over time as well as over space. Our integrated resistive elements have an unavoidable capacitance to the silicon substrate, so they provide the same kind of time integration as do their biological counterparts. The effects of delays due to electrotonic propagation in the network are most apparent when the input image changes suddenly.

Triad Synapse Computation

The receptive field of the bipolar cell shows an antagonistic center-surround response [Werblin, 1974]. The center of the bipolar cell receptive field is excited by the photoreceptors, whereas the antagonistic surround is due to the horizontal cells. The triad synapse is thus the obvious anatomical substrate for this computation. In our model, the center-surround computation is a result of the interaction of the photoreceptors, the horizontal cells, and the bipolar cells in the triad synapse.

The output of our silicon retina is analogous to the output of a bipolar cell in a vertebrate retina. Our triad synapse consists of two elements (Figure 15.2):

1. A wide-range amplifier provides a conductance through which the resistive network is driven toward the photoreceptor output potential

2. A second amplifier senses the voltage difference across the conductance, and generates an output proportional to the difference between the photoreceptor output and the network potential at that location

The output of our bipolar cell thus represents the difference between a center intensity and a weighted average of the intensities of surrounding points in the image.

IMPLEMENTATION

The floorplan for the retina is shown in Figure 15.4. The chip consists of an array of pixels, and a scanning arrangement for reading the results of retinal processing. The output of any pixel can be accessed through the scanner, which is made up of a vertical scan register along the left side of the chip and a horizontal scan register along the bottom of the chip. Each scan-register stage has 1-bit of

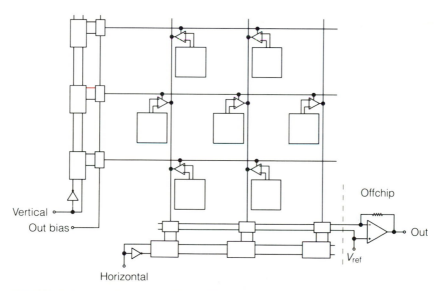

FIGURE 15.4 Layout of the retina chip. The main pixel array is made up of alternating rows of rectangular tiles, arranged to form a hexagonal array. The scanner along the left side allows any row of pixels to be selected. The scanner along the bottom allows the output current of any selected pixel to be gated onto the output line, where it is sensed by the offchip current-sensing amplifier. A schematic illustration of the shift-register cell used in the scanners is shown in Figure 15.6. The horizontal and vertical switching circuits are shown in Figure 15.7. The complete schematic of the pixel is shown in Figure 15.5. In the completed chip, the array was 48 by 48 pixels in extent. A fabrication layout of a small version of this chip is presented on the inside of the front cover.

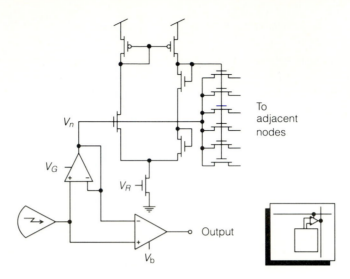

To
adjacent
nodes

Output

FIGURE 15.5 Detailed schematic illustration of all circuitry within an individual pixel
of the silicon retina. The logarithmic photoreceptor circuit is shown in the lower-left
corner. The follower-connected transconductance amplifier forms the G conductance
for that node of the resistive network. The six pass transistors form this end of the
resistive connections to the six neighboring pixels. The single bias circuit, described in
Figure 7.10 (p. 118), is shared among all six pass transistors. The output amplifier does
not need to have a wide-range design, because the output line can be run at a constant
potential, near V_{DD}. In the design described in this chapter, each pixel was 109 λ wide
by 97 λ high. The symbol for the pixel circuit is shown in the inset.

shift register, with the associated signal-selection circuits. Each register normally
is operated with a binary 1 in the selected stage, and binary 0s in all other stages.
The selected stage of the vertical register connects the *out-bias* voltage to the
horizontal scan line running through all pixels in the corresponding row of the
array. The deselected stages force the voltage on their horizontal scan lines to
ground. Each horizontal scan line is connected to the bias control (V_b) of the
output amplifiers of all pixels in the row. The output of each pixel in a selected
row is represented by a current; that current is enabled onto the vertical scan
line by the V_b bias on the horizontal scan line. The current scale for all outputs is
set by the out-bias voltage, which is supplied from offchip. A schematic diagram
of all circuits in the pixel is shown in Figure 15.5.

The shift-register stage is made with complementary set–reset logic (CSRL)
[Mead et al., 1985], and is shown in Figure 15.6. Signals are two-rail; the data
value is represented on the top rail, and its complement is represented on the
bottom rail. As ϕ_2 rises, the power supply to the second pair of cross-coupled
inverters is limited by the upper p-channel power-down transistor. By the time
ϕ_2 reaches the threshold of the two pass transistors, the current to the second
pair of cross-coupled inverters is limited to about one-half of the maximum that
can be supplied when the clock is low. For this reason, the first stage, which is

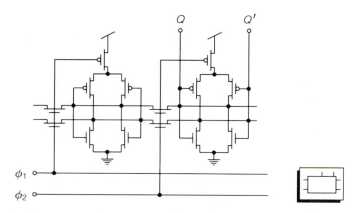

FIGURE 15.6 Shift-register stage used in the horizontal and vertical scanner. Each stage consists of a pair of cross-coupled inverters, which have a p-channel transistor in series with their common power supply. Because the output of each inverter feeds the input of the other, the cross-coupled stage has two stable states: (1) a binary 1 is stored on the top rail and a 0 on the bottom rail; or (2) a binary 0 is stored on the top rail and a 1 on the bottom rail.

On the rising edge of ϕ_2, the power to the second cross-coupled stage is cut off, and the data from the previous stage are able to pass through the pass transistors. When ϕ_2 falls, power is restored, and the data are held statically. A similar transfer occurs to the following stage during ϕ_1.

fully powered up, can force its state through the pass transistors into the second stage on the rising edge of ϕ_2. Similarly, the second stage can transfer its contents into the following stage on the rising edge of ϕ_1. Unidirectionality of the transfer is guaranteed because the clock signals are used both for the pass transistors and for the power-down transistor of the receiving stage. The clocks must be nonoverlapping.

We can envision the dynamics of a transfer by considering the interesting case, when the new datum is a 0 (upper rail low) and the previously stored datum is a 1 (upper rail high). While ϕ_2 is high, the upper rail discharges toward ground and the lower rail charges toward V_{DD}. The clock rates are limited by the capacitances of the nodes and the resistances of the pass transistors. After some time, the two voltages cross over. The clock ϕ_2 may return to zero any time after the crossover occurs, and a successful transfer will result. There is no need to wait for the two signal rails to pass any absolute threshold. Each cross-coupled stage can be viewed as a sense amplifier with very high differential gain. The positive-feedback action will fully restore both datum and complement, as long as the *relative* values of these two signals are of correct sign when the clock falls. If we attempt to bring the clock low before the crossover time at which the two signals become equal, the signals return to their previous values, and the transfer fails. The crossover time thus represents the minimum time during which the clock must be high, and thereby limits the maximum frequency of operation. At all times, at least one clock is low, so the CSRL shift register is fully static.

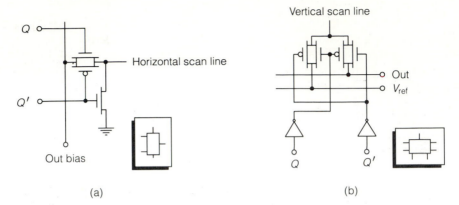

(a)   (b)

FIGURE 15.7   (a) Schematic diagram of the driver for a horizontal scan line. (b) Multi-plexor for a vertical scan line. A binary 1 in the vertical scan register gates the *out-bias* voltage onto the selected row, while the scan lines to the other rows are held at ground. A 1 in the horizontal scan register gates the output of the corresponding column onto the output line; all other output lines are connected to the reference line.

The circuits associated with driving a horizontal scan line and selecting data from a vertical scan line are shown in Figure 15.7. The current in a vertical scan line is connected to one of two output lines through a pair of complementary pass-transistor analog switches. If a binary 1 is stored in the corresponding stage of the horizontal shift-register, the vertical scan line is connected to the line labeled *out*. If a binary 0 is stored in the stage, the vertical scan line is connected to the line labeled V_{ref}. The current from the selected column thus flows in the *out* line, and the current from all unselected columns flows in the V_{ref} line. The chip is designed to be used with the off-chip current-sense amplifier shown to the right of the broken line in Figure 15.4. The *out* line is held at the V_{ref} potential by negative feedback from the amplifier output through the resistor. The principal advantage of this arrangement is that all vertical scan lines—selected and unselected—are held at the same potential. Thus, no transient is introduced as the vertical scan line is selected. In addition, capacitive transients due to the charge in the pass-transistor channels are minimized by the complementary nature of the analog switches [Sivilotti et al., 1987].

The scanners can be operated in one of two modes: static probe or serial access. In static-probe mode, a single row and column are selected, and the output of a single pixel is observed as a function of time, as the stimulus incident on the chip is changed. In serial-access mode, both vertical and horizontal shift registers are clocked at regular intervals to provide a sequential scan of the processed image for display on a television monitor. A binary 1 is applied at *horizontal*, and is clocked through the horizontal shift register in the time required by a single scan line in the television display. A binary 1 is applied at *vertical*, and is clocked through the vertical shift register in the time required by one frame of the television display. The vertical scan lines are accessed in sequential order via a single binary 1 being clocked through the horizontal shift register. After all pixels in a given row have been accessed, the single binary 1 in the vertical shift register is advanced to the next position, and the horizontal scan is repeated. The horizontal scan can be fast because it involves current steering and does not require voltage changes on the capacitance of a long scan wire. The vertical selection, which involves the settling of the output bias on the selected amplifiers, has the entire horizontal flyback time of the television display to settle, before it must be stable for the next horizontal scan.

The core of the chip is made up of rectangular tiles with height-to-width ratios of $\sqrt{3}$ to 2. Each tile contains the circuitry for a single pixel, as shown in Figure 15.5, with the wiring necessary to connect the pixel to its nearest neighbors. Each tile also contains the sections of global wiring necessary to form signal nets for V_{DD}, the bias controls for the resistive network, and the horizontal and vertical scan lines. The photoreceptors are located near the vertical scan line, such that alternating rows of left- and right-facing cells form a hexagonal array. This arrangement allows the vertical scan wire to be shared between adjacent rows, being accessed from the left by the odd rows, and from the right by even rows. To protect the processing circuitry from the effects of stray minority carriers, we have covered the entire chip with a solid sheet of second-layer metal, with openings directly over the photoreceptors; this layer is used for distributing ground to the pixels. We designed several versions of this chip over 3 years. A small section of the array of the most recent version is shown on the front endpaper of this book.

PERFORMANCE

Neurophysiologists have undertaken a tremendous variety of experiments in an attempt to understand how the retina performs computations, and they have come up with many explanations for retinal operation. Different investigators emphasize different aspects of retinal function, such as spatial-frequency filtering, adaptation and gain control, edge enhancement, and statistical optimization [Srinivasan et al., 1982]. It is entirely in the nature of biological systems that the results of several experiments designed to demonstrate one or another of these points of view can be explained by the properties of the single underlying structure. A highly evolved mechanism is able to subserve a multitude of purposes simultaneously.

Our experiments on the silicon retina have yielded results remarkably similar to those obtained from biological systems. From an engineering point of view, the primary function of the computation performed by silicon retina is to provide an automatic gain control that extends the useful operating range of the system. It is essential that a sensory system be sensitive to changes in its input, no matter what the viewing conditions. The structure executing this gain-control operation can perform many other functions as well, such as computing the contrast ratio or enhancing edges in the image. Thus, the mechanisms responsible for keeping the system operating over an enormous range of image intensity and contrast have important consequences with regard to the representation of data.

Sensitivity Curves

The computation performed in the distal portion of the retina prevents the output from saturating over an incredible range of illumination levels. By logarithmically compressing the input signal, the photoreceptor takes the first step toward increasing the retina's dynamic range. The next step is a level normalization, implemented by means of the resistive network. The horizontal cells of the retina provide a spatially averaged version of the photoreceptor outputs, with which the local photoreceptor potential can be compared. The triad synapse senses the difference between the photoreceptor output and the potential of the horizontal cells, and generates a bipolar-cell output from this difference. The maximum response occurs when the photoreceptor potential is different from the space–time averaged outputs of many photoreceptors in the local neighborhood. This situation occurs when the image is changing rapidly in either space or time.

Figure 15.8 shows the shift in operating point of the bipolar-cell output of both a biological and a silicon retina, as a function of surround illumination. At a fixed surround illumination level, the output of the bipolar cell has a familiar tanh characteristic; it saturates to produce a constant output at very low or very

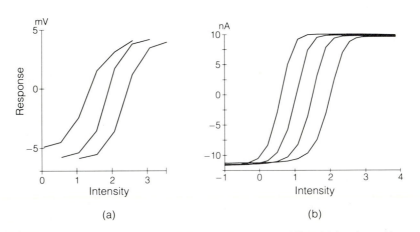

(a)   (b)

FIGURE 15.8 Curve shifting. Intensity-response curves shift to higher intensities at higher background illuminations. (a) Intensity-response curves for a depolarizing bipolar cell elicited by full-field flashes. The test flashes were substituted for constant background illuminations. These curves are plotted from the peaks of bipolar response to substituted test flashes. Peak responses are plotted, measured from the membrane potential just prior to response. (*Source:* Data from [Werblin, 1974]) (b) Intensity-response curves for a single pixel of the silicon retina. Curves are plotted for four different background intensities. The stimulus was a small disk centered on the receptive field of the pixel. The steady-state response is plotted.

high center intensities, and it is sensitive to changes in input over the middle of its range. Using the potential of the resistive network as a reference centers the range over which the output responds on the signal level averaged over the local surround. The full gain of the triad synapse can thus be used to report features of the image without fear that the output will be driven into saturation in the absence of local image information.

The action of the horizontal cell layer is an example of lateral inhibition, a ubiquitous feature of peripheral sensory systems [von Békésy, 1967]. Lateral inhibition is used to provide a reference value with which to compare the signal. This reference value is the operating point of the system. In the retina, the operating point of the system is the local average of intensity as computed by the horizontal cells. Because it uses a local rather than a global average, the eye is able to see detail in both the light and dark areas of high-contrast scenes, a task that would overwhelm a television camera, which uses only global adaptation.

Time Response

Time is an intrinsic part of an analog computation. In analog perception systems, the time scale of the computation must be matched to the time scale of external events, and to other real-time parts of the system. Biological vision systems use an inherently dynamic processing strategy. As emphasized in Chapter 13, body and eye movements are an important part of the computation.

Figure 15.9 shows the response of a single output to a sudden increase in incident illumination. Output from a bipolar cell in a biological retina is provided for comparison. The initial peak represents the difference between the voltage at the photoreceptor caused by the step input and the old averaged voltage stored on the capacitance of the resistive network. As the resistive network equilibrates to the new input level, the output of the amplifier diminishes. The final plateau value is a function of the size of the stimulus, which changes the average value of the intensity of the image as computed by the resistive network. Having computed a new average value of intensity, the resistive network causes the output of the amplifier to overshoot when the stimulus is turned off. As the network decays to its former value, the output returns to the baseline.

The temporal response of the silicon retina depends on the properties of the horizontal network. The voltage stored on the capacitance of the resistive network is the temporally as well as spatially averaged output of the photoreceptors. The horizontal network is like the follower–integrator circuit discussed in Chapter 9, which weights its input by an amount that decreases exponentially into the past. The time constant of integration is set by the bias voltages of the wide-range amplifier and of the resistors. The time constant can be varied independently of the space constant, which depends on only the difference between these bias voltages, rather than on their absolute magnitude.

The form of time response of the system varies with the space constant of the network. When the resistance value is low, γ approaches one, and the network

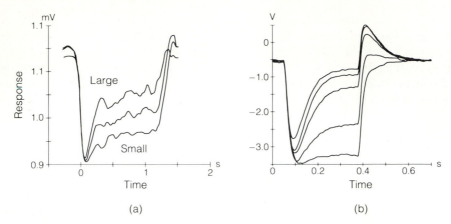

FIGURE 15.9 Temporal response to different-sized test flashes. (a) Response of
a bipolar cell of the mud puppy, *Necturus maculosus*. (*Source:* Data from [Werblin,
1974]) (b) Output of a pixel in the silicon retina. Test flashes of the same intensity but of
different diameters were centered on the receptive field of the unit. The space constant
of the network was $\gamma = 0.3$. Larger flashes increased the excitation of the surround.
The surround response was delayed due to the capacitance of the resistive network.
Because the surround level is subtracted from the center response, the output shows
a decrease for long times. This decrease is larger for larger flashes. The overshoot at
stimulus offset decays as the surround returns to its resting level.

is computing the global average. A test flash of any limited size will produce a
sustained output. Conversely, when the resistance value is high, γ approaches
zero, and the triad synapse is just a diff1 circuit (Figure 10.5 (p. 167)), which
has no sustained output. Because the rise time of the photoreceptor is finite, the
space constant also can affect the initial peak of the time response. The dynamics
of a small test flash are dominated by a pixel charging the capacitance of the
surrounding area through the resistive network. In contrast, a pixel in the middle
of a large test flash is charging mainly its own capacitance, because adjacent
nodes of the network are being charged by their associated photoreceptors. The
peak value of the output is thus larger for a small test flash than it is for larger
test flashes.

Edge Response

We can view the suppression of spatially and temporally smooth image information as a filtering operation designed to enhance edges in the image. The
outputs of the bipolar cells directly drive the sustained X-type retinal-ganglion
cells of the mud puppy, *Necturus maculosus*. Consequently, the receptive-field
properties of this type of ganglion cell can be traced to those of the bipolar cells
[Werblin et al., 1969]. Although the formation of the receptive field of the X-type
ganglion cells of the cat is somewhat more complex [Dowling, 1987], the end result is qualitatively similar. The receptive fields of these cells are described as

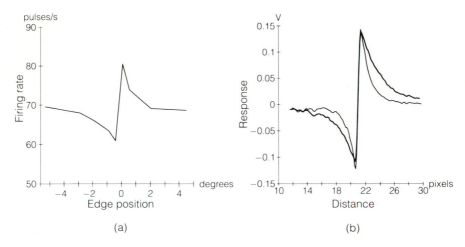

FIGURE 15.10   Spatial-derivative response of a retinal ganglion cell and of a pixel to a contrast edge. The vertical edge was held stationary at different distances from the receptive-field center. Contrast of the edge was 0.2 in both experiments. (a) On-center X-type ganglion cell of the cat. The contrast edge was turned alternately on and off. The average pulse density over the period 10 to 20 seconds after the introduction of the edge was measured for each edge position (*Source:* [Enroth-Cugell et al., 1966]). (b) Pixel output measured at steady state as the edge was moved in increments of 0.01 centimeters at the image plane. Interpixel spacing corresponded to 0.11 centimeters at the image plane. Response is shown for two different space constants. The rate of decay of the response is determined by the space constant of the resistive network.

antagonistic center-surround fields. Activation of the center of the receptive field stimulates the cell's response, and activation of the surround produces inhibition. Cells with this organization are strongly affected by discontinuities in intensity. The response of a sustained X-type ganglion cell to a contrast edge placed at different positions relative to its receptive field is shown in Figure 15.10(a). The spatial pattern of activity found in the cat is similar to the response of our silicon retina to a spatial-intensity step, as shown in Figure 15.10(b). The way the second spatial derivative is computed is illustrated in Figure 15.11. The surround value computed by the resistive network reflects the average intensity over a restricted region of the image. As the sharp edge passes over the receptive-field center, the output undergoes a sharp transition from lower than the average to above the average. Sharp edges thus generate large output, whereas smooth areas of the image produce no output, because the local center intensity matches the average intensity.

The center-surround computation sometimes is referred to as *a difference of Gaussians.* Laplacian filters, which have been used widely in computer vision systems, can be approximated by a difference of Gaussians [Marr, 1982]. These filters have been used to help computers localize objects; they work because discontinuities in intensity frequently correspond to object edges. Both of these mathematical forms express, in an analytically tractable way, the computation

FIGURE 15.11 Model illustrating the mechanism of the generation of pixel response to spatial edge in intensity. The solid line, labeled *receptors*, represents the voltage outputs of the photoreceptors along a cross-section perpendicular to the edge. The resistive network computes a weighted local average of the photoreceptor intensity, shown by the dashed line. The average intensity differs from the actual intensity at the stimulus edge, because the photoreceptors on one side of the edge pull the network on the other side toward their potential. The difference between the photoreceptor output and the resistive network is the predicted pixel output, shown in the trace labeled *difference*. This mechanism results in increased output at places in the image where the first derivative of the intensity is changing.

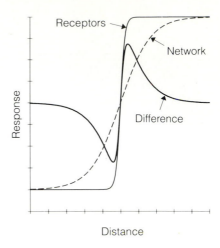

that occurs as a natural result of an efficient physical implementation of local level normalization.

Space Constant of the Resistive Network

The resistive net is an economical way to generate a center-surround type of receptive field because the wiring is shared among many elements. Furthermore, we can vary the extent of the surround by changing the space constant of the network. In several species, the space constant of the horizontal-cell network is modulated by the release of dopamine [Dowling, 1987].

Figure 15.12 shows the exponential nature of the spatial decay of the response on one side of an edge for different space constants. The edge stimulus, being uniform in one dimension, generates current flow in only the transverse direction. The one-dimensional network therefore is a good approximation to the response of the two-dimensional network to an edge. As we noted in Chapter 7, the continuum approximation to the solution for a one-dimensional network is

$$V = V_0 e^{-\frac{1}{L}|x|} \tag{7.1}$$

where

$$\frac{1}{L} = \sqrt{RG} \tag{7.2}$$

As discussed in Appendix C, when we choose the unit of length to be $\sqrt{3}/2$ times the spacing of points in the horizontal lattice, the continuum approximation is very good, even for values of L as low as 1. The value of L is determined by the product of the conductance G and the resistance R. Both G and R are exponential functions of their respective bias controls:

$$G \propto e^{V_G} \quad \text{and} \quad R \propto e^{-V_R} \tag{15.1}$$

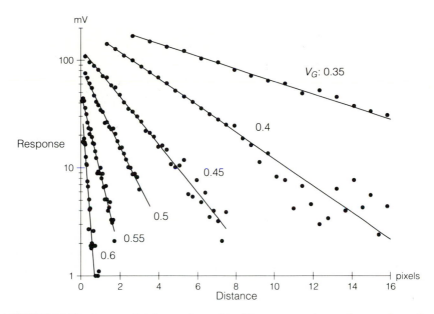

FIGURE 15.12   Exponential decay of one side of the response to an edge, as shown in Figure 15.10(b). Each curve was taken with the setting of the V_G control shown. For all curves, V_R was 0.55 volt. The slope of the decay corresponds to the space constant of the network.

Substituting Equation 15.1 into Equation 7.1 (p. 108), we obtain

$$\frac{1}{L} = \sqrt{RG} \propto e^{(V_G - V_R)/2} \tag{15.2}$$

The space constant thus should be a function of $V_G - V_R$, and should not be dependent on the absolute voltage level. The constant of proportionality in Equation 15.2 contains the width-to-length ratios for transistors in the horizontal resistor and in the resistor bias circuit, and those for transistors in the transconductance amplifier. Figure 15.13 shows the edge response of the silicon retina measured for several values of bias voltages, with a fixed difference between V_G and V_R, and thus a fixed ratio between the transconductance bias current and the resistor bias current. The form of the static response of the system is unchanged, as expected.

If we assume the continuum form of the decay, Equation 7.2 (p. 108) applies to the horizontal network over the range of L values involved, and we can compare the slopes of the decay curves in Figure 15.12 with the theoretical expression given in Equation 15.2, where all voltages are expressed in terms of $kT/(q\kappa)$. The comparison is shown in Figure 15.14; the voltage dependence of the decay constant is in excellent agreement with the theoretical prediction. The absolute value of the curve in Figure 15.14 was adjusted for the best fit to the data, and is higher, by a factor of about two, than the value deduced from the device geometries in

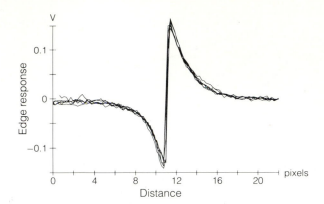

FIGURE 15.13 The response of a pixel to a 0.2 contrast edge measured for a fixed difference between the conductance bias voltage and the resistor bias voltage. (DC offsets in the response were subtracted out.) The space constant of the network depends on only the ratio of conductance bias current to resistor bias current. Resistor bias voltages were 100 millivolts greater than were the conductance bias voltages. The form of the response stayed essentially unchanged as bias voltages were swept over a 250-millivolt range, thereby changing the bias current by more than three orders of magnitude.

the resistive connections and in the transconductance amplifiers. A number of factors may be responsible for this discrepancy, including inaccurate calibration of the interpixel spacing, partial saturation of resistive connections due to voltage offsets, uncertainties in the channel lengths of short-channel devices, and so on. None of these factors should have a large effect on the voltage dependence of the decay, in keeping with our observations.

The space constant determines the peak amplitude of the response as well as the decay constant of the exponential. The decay length L is small when the conductance feeding the local input to the network is large relative to the

FIGURE 15.14 Space constant of the response data of Figure 15.12, plotted as a function of $V_G - V_R$. The straight line is the theoretical expression taken from Equation 15.2, using the measured value of $\kappa = 0.73$. The magnitude of the curve was adjusted for best fit to the data, and is about a factor of two higher than expected from the width-to-length ratios of transistors in the transconductance amplifier and in the resistor bias circuit.

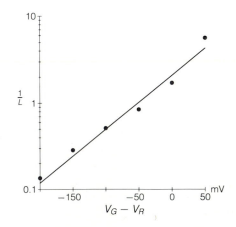

lateral conductance. Under these conditions, the difference between the local photoreceptor and the network also is small, because the average is dominated by the local input. The decay length L is large when the conductance feeding the local input to the network is small relative to the lateral conductance. Under these conditions, the difference between the local photoreceptor and the network approaches the full difference between the local photoreceptor and the average over many photoreceptors, because the average is affected very little by the local input. This dependence of peak amplitude on space constant can be seen in the curves in Figure 15.12. The precise nature of this dependence cannot be determined from the continuum limit, because the input conductance is inherently tied to the discrete nature of the network. Feinstein discusses these matters in more detail [Feinstein, 1988].

Mach Bands

Retinal processing has important consequences for higher-level vision. Many of the most striking phenomena known from perceptual psychology are a result of the first levels of neural processing. In the visual systems of higher animals, the center-surround response to local stimuli is responsible for some of the strongest visual illusions. For example, Mach bands, the Hermann–Hering grid illusion, and the Craik–O'Brian–Cornsweet illusion may all be traced to simple inhibitory interactions among elements of the retina [Ratliff, 1965; Julesz, 1971].

The response of a pixel to a ramp stimulus is plotted in Figure 15.15. Because the retina performs a second-order filtering of the image, changes in the first derivative of intensity are enhanced. **Mach bands** are illusory bright and dark bands that appear at the edges of an intensity ramp. The positions of the illusory bands correspond to the positions where the retinal output is enhanced due to changes in the first derivative of the intensity.

The retina, as the first stage in the visual system, provides gain control and image enhancement, as well as transduction of light into electrical signals. The evolutionary advantage of this kind of preprocessing is evidenced by the ubiquitous occurrence of retina structures in the vertebrates, and even in invertebrates such as the octopus. From an engineering viewpoint, the retina greatly reduces the signal bandwidth required to transmit visual information to the brain, thereby greatly reducing the size of the optic nerve and allowing more effective computation at the next level. Thus, the retina is a prime example of a system that performs information processing by *selectively rejecting irrelevant information*. Any operation that discards information will, of necessity, create **ambiguities**, in which several distinct input images create an output that is indistinguishable by the next level of processing. To the visual researcher, these *optical illusions* provide valuable insight into the nature of information processing at various stages in the visual system. The fact that our retinal model generates an illusory output when exposed to the same stimulus that evokes a Mach-band illusion in humans gives us additional confidence that we have correctly interpreted the principles on which the biological system operates.

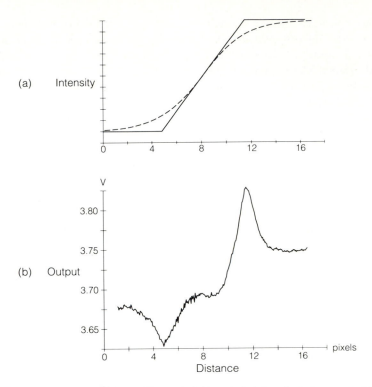

(a)   Intensity

(b)   Output

FIGURE 15.15   Mach bands are illusory bright and dark bands that appear at the edges of a ramp of intensity. The interaction between retinal output and higher-level neural processing is believed to explain the perception of Mach bands.

(a) Ramp stimulus illustrates the function of a second-order filter. The solid line indicates the intensity profile of an ideal Mach-band stimulus. The dashed line is the weighted local average of the intensity. The difference between the local average and the point intensity is the output of the retina. The magnitude of the difference is large at the point in the image where the first derivative is changing.

(b) Response of a pixel to ramp stimulus. This stimulus is a shadow cast by an opaque sheet between an extended light source and the image plane. The stimulus is moved over the retina in 50-micron steps. The enhanced response at the edges of the ramp is due to the second-order behavior of the retinal response. The shift in DC value across the response is due to intensity variation as the light source approaches the pixel.

SUMMARY

We have taken the first step in simulating the computations done by the brain to process a visual image. We have used a medium that has a structure in many ways similar to neurobiological structures. Following the biological metaphor has led us to develop a system that is nearly optimal from many points of view. The constraints on our silicon system are similar to those on neurobiological systems. As in the biological retina, density is limited by the total amount of wire required to accomplish the computation. The retina, like many other areas of the brain, minimizes wire by arranging the signal representation such that as much wire as possible can be shared. The resistive network is the ultimate example of shared wiring. By including a pixel's own input in the average, we can compute the weighted average over a neighborhood for every position in the image, using the same shared structure.

The principle of shared wire is found, in less extreme forms, throughout the brain. Computation is always done in the context of neighboring information. For a neighborhood to be meaningful, nearby areas in the neural structure must represent information that is more closely related than is that represented by areas farther away. Visual areas in the cortex that begin the processing sequence are mapped retinotopically. Higher-level areas represent more abstract information, but areas that are close together still represent similar information. It is this *map* property that organizes the cortex such that most wires can be short and highly shared; it is perhaps the single most important architectural principle in the brain.

REFERENCES

Dowling, J.E. *The Retina: An Approachable Part of the Brain.* Cambridge, MA: Belknap Press of Harvard University Press, 1987.

Enroth-Cugell, C. and Robson, J.G. The contrast sensitivity of retinal ganglion cells of the cat. *Journal of Physiology,* 187:517, 1966.

Feinstein, D. The hexagonal resistive network and the circular approximation. *Caltech Computer Science Technical Report,* Caltech-CS-TR-88-7, California Institute of Technology, Pasadena, CA, 1988.

Julesz, B. *Foundations of Cyclopean Perception.* Chicago, IL: The University of Chicago Press, 1971.

Marr, D. *Vision.* San Francisco, CA: W.H. Freeman, 1982.

Mead, C. and Wawrzynek, J. A new discipline for CMOS design. In Fuchs, H. (ed), *1985 Chapel Hill Conference on Very Large Scale Integration.* Chapel Hill, NC: Computer Science Press, 1985, p. 87.

Ratliff, F. *Mach Bands: Quantitative Studies on Neural Networks in the Retina.* San Francisco: Holden-Day, 1965.

Rodieck, R.W. *The Vertebrate Retina.* San Francisco, CA: W.H. Freeman, 1973.

Shapley, R. and Enroth-Cugell, C. Visual adaptation and retinal gain controls. In Osborne, N.N. and Chader, G.J. (eds), *Progress in Retinal Research,* vol 3. Oxford, England: Pergamon Press, 1984, p. 263.

Sivilotti, M.A., Mahowald, M.A., and Mead, C.A. Real-time visual computations using analog CMOS processing arrays. In Losleben, P. (ed), *Stanford Conference on Very Large Scale Integration.* Cambridge, MA: MIT Press, 1987, p. 295.

Srinivasan, M.V., Laughlin, S.B., and Dubs, A. Predictive coding: A fresh view of inhibition in the retina. *Proceedings of the Royal Society of London,* Series B, 216:427, 1982.

von Békésy, G. *Sensory Inhibition*. Princeton, NJ: Princeton University Press, 1967.

Werblin, F.S. and Dowling, J.E. Organization of the retina of the mudpuppy, *Necturus maculosus*. II. Intracellular recording. *Journal of Neurophysiology*, 32:339, 1969.

Werblin, F.S. Control of retinal sensitivity, II. Lateral interactions at the outer plexiform layer. *Journal of General Physiology*, 63:62, 1974.

ELECTRONIC COCHLEA

Richard F. Lyon   Carver Mead

When we understand how hearing works, we will be able to build amazing machines with brainlike abilities to interpret the world through sounds—that is, to *hear*. As part of our endeavor to decipher the auditory nervous system, we can use models that incorporate current ideas of how that system works to engineer simple *electronic* systems that hear in simple ways. The relative success of these *engineered* systems then helps us to evaluate our knowledge about hearing, and helps to motivate further research.

As a first step in building machines that hear, we have implemented an analog electronic cochlea that incorporates much of the current state of knowledge about cochlear structure and function. The biological **cochlea** (inner ear) is a complex three-dimensional fluid-dynamic system, illustrated schematically in Figure 16.1. In the process of designing, building, and testing the electronic cochlea, we have had to put together a coherent view of the function of the biological cochlea from the diverse ideas in the literature. This view and the resulting design are the subjects of this chapter.

We hear through the sound-analyzing action of the cochlea and of the auditory centers of the brain. As does vision, hearing provides a representation of events and objects in the world that are relevant to survival.

Portions reprinted with permission from *IEEE Transactions on Acoustics, Speech, and Signal Processing*, Vol. 36, No. 7, July 1988. © IEEE 1988.

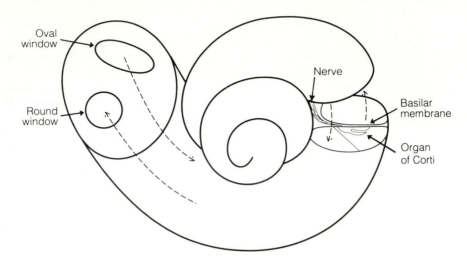

FIGURE 16.1　Artist's conception of the cochlea, with cutaway showing a cross section of a cochlear duct. The bending of the cochlear partition causes a shearing between it and the tectorial membrane, which can be both sensed and amplified by hair cells in the organ of Corti. The dashed lines indicate fluid paths from the input at the oval window and back to the round window for pressure relief.

Just as the natural environment of light rays is cluttered, so is that of sound waves. Hearing systems therefore have evolved to exploit many cues to separate out complex sounds. The same systems that have evolved to help cats to catch mice and to warn rabbits of wolves also serve to let humans speak with other humans. Except for the highest level of the brain (the auditory cortex), the hearing systems of these animals are essentially identical.

BASIC MECHANISMS OF HEARING

The cochlea consists of a coiled fluid-filled tube (see Figure 16.1) with a stiff **cochlear partition** (the **basilar membrane** and associated structures) separating the tube lengthwise into two chambers (called ducts, or **scalae**). At one end of the tube, called the **basal end** or simply the **base**, a pair of flexible membranes called **windows** connect the cochlea acoustically to the middle-ear cavity. A trio of small bones called **middle-ear ossicles** couple sound from the **tympanic membrane** (eardrum) into one of the windows, called the **oval window**. When the oval window is pushed in by a sound wave, the fluid in the cochlea moves, the partition between the ducts distorts, and the fluid bulges back out through the **round window**. Transducers called **hair cells** sit along the edge of the partition in a structure known as the **organ of Corti**, and are arranged to couple with the partition motion and the fluid flow that goes with that motion.

The distortion of the cochlear partition by sounds takes the form of a traveling wave, starting at the base and propagating toward the far end of the cochlear ducts, known as the **apical end**, or **apex**. As the wave propagates, a filtering action occurs in which high frequencies are strongly attenuated; the cutoff frequency gradually lowers with distance from base to apex. The **inner hair cells**, of which there are several thousand, detect the fluid velocity of the wave as it passes. At low sound levels, some frequencies are amplified as they propagate, due to the energy added by the **outer hair cells**, of which there are about three times as many as inner hair cells. As the sound level changes, the effective gain provided by the outer hair cells is adjusted to keep the mechanical response within a more limited range of amplitude.

The propagation of sound energy as hydrodynamic waves in the fluid and partition system is essentially a distributed low-pass filter. The membrane velocity detected at each hair cell is essentially a bandpass-filtered version of the original sound. Analyzing and modeling the function of these lowpass and bandpass mechanisms is the key to understanding the first stage of hearing. Because analog circuits cannot easily be made precise, they must be made self-adjusting; if the circuits must adjust for their own long-term offsets and drifts, they might as well also adjust to the signal. The use of adaptation to optimize the system response seems to be a pervasive principle in perception systems, which are built from sensitive but imprecise components. **Lateral inhibition** is one term often applied to physiological systems that self-adjust [von Békésy, 1967].

Traveling Waves

As sounds push on the oval window, a pressure wave is initiated between the ducts. The fluid is incompressible, and the bone around the cochlea is incompressible, so as the pressure wave moves, it displaces the basilar membrane. When the eardrum is tapped, the middle-ear ossicles tap on the oval window, and a pressure pulse travels down the length of the cochlea. In propagating, the pressure pulse deforms the basilar membrane upward; if we could watch, we would see a little bump traveling along the basilar membrane. There is a well-defined velocity at which a signal will travel on such a structure, depending on the physical parameters of the membrane.

If the basilar membrane is thick and stiff, the wave will travel very quickly along the cochlea; if it is thin and flexible, the wave will travel very slowly. The changing properties of the basilar membrane control the velocity of propagation of a wave. Hearing starts by spreading out the sound along this continuous traveling-wave structure. The velocity of propagation is a nearly exponential function of the distance along the membrane. The signal starts near the oval window with very *high* velocity of propagation, because the basilar membrane is very thick and stiff at the basal end. As the signal travels away from the oval window, toward the apical end, the basilar membrane becomes thinner, wider, and more flexible, so the velocity of propagation *decreases*—it changes by a factor of about 100 along the length of the cochlea.

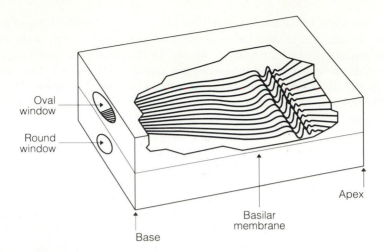

FIGURE 16.2 A sinusoidal traveling wave on the basilar membrane, in a simplified rectangular-box model. The basilar membrane (the flexible part of the cochlear partition between the bony shelves) starts out stiff and narrow at the base and becomes more compliant and wider toward the apex. Thus, a wave's propagation velocity and wavelength decrease—the wavenumber, or spatial frequency, increases—as the wave travels from base to apex.

Sine-Wave Response

When the sound is a sine wave of a given frequency, it vibrates the basilar membrane sinusoidally. The wave travels very quickly at the basal end, so it has a long wavelength. A constant energy per unit time is being put in, but, as the wave slows down and the wavelength gets shorter, the energy per unit length builds up, so the basilar membrane gets more and more stretched by the wave. For any given frequency, there is a region beyond which the wave can no longer propagate efficiently. The energy is dissipated in the membrane and its associated detection machinery. Past this region, the wave amplitude decreases rapidly (faster than exponentially). Figure 16.2 is an artist's conception of what the membrane deflection might look like for a given sine wave.

Neural Machinery

The auditory-nerve signal comes out of the machinery in the organ of Corti, along one side of the basilar membrane. A protrusion called the **tectorial membrane** is located just above the basilar membrane. We can think about the tectorial membrane's relation to the organ of Corti this way: As the pressure wave travels along the cochlea, it bends the basilar membrane up and down; when the basilar membrane is pushed up, the tectorial membrane moves to the right relative to the basilar membrane. This linkage arrangement is a way of converting up-and-down motion on the basilar membrane to shearing motion between it and the tectorial membrane.

Mounted on the top of the basilar membrane is a row of inner hair cells. The single row of 3500 (in humans) inner hair cells that runs along the length of the membrane is the only source of the nerve pulses that travel to the cochlear nucleus and on up into the brain. All the auditory information is carried by about 28,000 (in humans) nerve fibers. Everything we hear is dependent on that set of hair cells and nerve cells. Fine hairs, called **stereocilia**, protrude from the end of the inner hair cells; they detect the shearing motion of the membranes and act as the *transducers* that convert deflection to an ion current.

Let us consider the behavior of the auditory system for loud signals, in which situation the outer hair cells are not needed. Signals are propagating down the cochlea, so there are bumps traveling along the basilar membrane. The bumps travel quickly at first, and then they slow down. For any given frequency, there is a point at which the displacement is maximum; this is the point of maximum velocity of the vibration of hair cells with respect to the tectorial membrane.

On the scale of a hair cell's stereocilia—a small fraction of a micron—the viscosity of the fluid is high. The fans of cilia sticking out of the hair cells have enough resistance to the motion of the fluid that they bend. When the cilia are bent one way, the hair cells stimulate the primary auditory neurons to fire. When the cilia are bent the other way, no pulses are generated. When the cilia are bent to some position at which the neurons fire, and then are left undisturbed for some time, the neurons stop firing. From then on, bending the cilia in the preferred direction away from that new position causes firings. So the inner hair cells act as auto-zeroing half-wave rectifiers for the velocity of the motion of the fluid.

Outer Hair Cells

The large structure of the organ of Corti on top of the membrane absorbs energy from the traveling wave. In the absence of intervention from the outer hair cells, the membrane response is reasonably damped. The ear was designed to hear transients, and therefore the basilar membrane itself is not a highly resonant structure.

What then is the purpose of the outer hair cells? There are only a few slow afferent (*to* the brain) nerve fibers coming into the auditory nerve from the outer hair cells. On the other hand, there are a large number of slow fibers coming *down* from higher places in the brain into the cochlea, that synapse onto these outer hair cells. The outer hair cells are *not* used primarily as receptors—they are used as *muscles*. If they are not inhibited by the efferent (*from* the brain) fibers, they provide *positive* feedback into the membrane. If they are bent, they push even harder in the same direction. They can put enough energy back into the basilar membrane that it will actually oscillate under some conditions; the resulting ringing in the ears is called **tinnitus**.

Tinnitus is not caused by an out-of-control sensory neuron as one might suppose. It is a *mechanical oscillation* in the cochlea that is driven by the outer hair cells. The cells pump energy back into the oscillations of the basilar membrane, and they can pump enough energy to make the traveling-wave structure unstable, so it creates an oscillatory wave that propagates back out through the eardrum into the air. In 1981, Zurek and Clark [Zurek et al., 1981] reported spontaneous acoustic emission from a chinchilla that made such a squeal that it could be heard from several meters away by a human's unaided ear. An excellent and insightful overview of the role of outer hair cells for active gain control in the auditory system is given by Kim. In a classic monument of understatement, he comments on the chinchilla results, "It is highly implausible that such an intense and sustained acoustic signal could emanate from a passive mechanical system" [Kim, 1984, p. 251].

So, the outer hair cells are used as muscles and their function is to reduce the damping of the basilar membrane when the sound input would be otherwise too weak to hear. This arrangement provides not just gain, but also control of the gain, it controls gain by a factor of 100 in amplitude (10,000 in energy). When the signal is small, the outer hair cells are not inhibited and they feedback energy. This system of *automatic gain control* (AGC) works for sound power levels within a few decades of the bottom end of our hearing range by making the structure slightly more resonant and thereby much higher gain—by reducing the damping until it is negative in some regions. We will discuss the details of gain control after we have developed the basilar membrane model.

Based on the threshold of hearing and linear extrapolations from observations on loud signals, researchers once estimated that a displacement of the cilia by less than one-thousandth of an angstrom (10^{-3} angstrom or 10^{-13} meter) would be large enough to give a reasonable probability of evoking a nerve pulse. Because the detectability of sounds near the threshold of hearing involves active mechanical amplification, the actual motion sensed probably is on the order of 1 angstrom of basilar-membrane displacement or hair-cell bending.

WAVE PROPAGATION

As we have discussed, sounds entering the cochlea initiate traveling waves of fluid pressure and cochlear-partition motion that propagate from the base toward the apex. The fluid-mechanical system of ducts separated by a flexible partition is like a waveguide, in which wavelength and propagation velocity depend on the frequency of a wave and on the physical properties of the waveguide. In the cochlea, the physical properties of the partition are not constant with x, but instead change radically from base to apex. The changing parameters lead to the desirable behavior of sorting out sounds by their frequencies or time scales; unfortunately, the parameter variation makes the wave analysis a bit more complex. In this section, we will discuss the mathematics of waves in uniform and nonuniform media, including the cochlea.

The instantaneous value W of the pressure or displacement of a wave propagating in a one-dimensional uniform medium due to a sine-wave input can be expressed as

$$W(x,t) = A(x)\cos(kx - \omega t)$$

If frequency ω and wavenumber k (spatial frequency) are positive and real and A is constant, W is a wave propagating to the right (toward $+x$) at a phase velocity $c = \omega/k$ with no change in amplitude. If the wavenumber k is complex, the wave will either grow or die out exponentially with distance, depending on the sign of the imaginary part of k.

Differential equations for W can be derived from some approximation to the physics of the system. We can then convert the differential equations to algebraic equations involving ω, k, and parameters of the system by a generalization of the technique described in Chapter 8, noting that W can be factored out of its derivatives when $A(x)$ is constant (or if A is assumed constant when it is nearly so). These algebraic equations relating ω and k are referred to as **dispersion relations**. Pairs of ω and k that satisfy the dispersion relations represent waves compatible with the physical system.

From the dispersion relations, we can calculate the velocity of the wave. If the velocity is independent of ω, all frequencies travel at the same speed and the medium is said to be **nondispersive**. In the cochlea, higher frequencies are known to propagate more slowly than do lower frequencies, and the basilar membrane is therefore **dispersive**. In a dispersive medium, we distinguish two different velocities. The **phase velocity** $c = \omega/k$ is the velocity at which any given crest or valley of the wave propagates. The **group velocity** $U = d\omega/dk$ is the speed at which the wave envelope and energy propagate.

Dispersion relations generally have symmetric solutions, such that any wave traveling in one direction has a corresponding solution, of the same frequency, traveling with the same speed in the opposite direction. If, for a given real value of ω, the solution for k is complex, then the equations imply a wave amplitude that is growing or diminishing exponentially with distance x. If the imaginary part k_i of $k = k_r + jk_i$ is positive (for the complex exponential wave conventions we have adopted), the wave diminishes toward the right $(+x)$; in any dissipative system, a wave diminishes in the direction that it travels. The wave may thus be written as the damped sinusoid

$$W(x,t) = A \cos\left(k_r x - \omega t\right)e^{-k_i x}$$

Fluid Mechanics of the Cochlea

In the cochlea, finding the relations between ω and k is more complex than is determining them for a one-dimensional wave system, such as a vibrating string. We must first work out the fluid-flow problem in two or three dimensions; ultimately, we can represent displacement, velocity, and pressure waves on the cochlear partition in one dimension as the relation between k and ω changes with x (conventionally referred to as the cochlear **place** dimension).

It is highly likely that the lowest-order loss mechanism in the cochlea is the viscous drag of fluid moving in a boundary layer near the basilar membrane and through the small spaces of the organ of Corti. The sensitive cilia of the inner hair cells that detect motion are moved by viscous drag. The outer hair cells also interact with the fluid and membranes in the organ of Corti, and are known to be a source of energy, rather than a sink. At low sound levels, the outer hair cells can supply more than enough energy to make up for the energy lost to viscous drag. We therefore model the effects of the outer hair cells as a negative damping.

The analysis of the hydrodynamic system of the cochlea yields a relation among frequency, place, and complex wavenumber. The analyses we used are based on three approximations commonly employed to make the hydrodynamics problem relatively simple:

1. We assume that the cochlear fluids have essentially zero viscosity, so the sound energy is not dissipated in the bulk of the fluid, but rather is transferred into motion of the organ of Corti

2. We assume that the fluid is incompressible, or equivalently that the velocity of sound in the fluid is large compared to the velocities of the waves on the cochlear partition

3. We assume the fluid motions to be small, so we can neglect second-order motion terms; for sound levels within the normal range of hearing, this is a good approximation

The details of the hydrodynamic analysis and reasoning about physical approximations are too lengthy to include in this chapter [Lyon et al., 1988], but we can summarize the results by the short-wave dispersion relation (with complex k), which is

$$\omega^2 \rho = \pm k[S - j\omega(\beta + k^2\gamma)] \qquad (16.1)$$

where β is a low-order (viscous) loss coefficient (which may be negative in the actively undamped case), γ is a high-order (bending) loss coefficient, S is the membrane stiffness, and ρ is the mass density of the fluid. Parameters S and γ are functions of place, but at any given place are fixed for all time. The active negative damping term β also is a function of place, and changes slowly with time as the system adapts to changes in incoming sound level. The sign of the right-hand side of Equation 16.1 is taken as positive for positive ω, and negative for negative ω.

Because the physical parameters in Equation 16.1 are changing with x, a closed-form solution is not possible except under specific restrictions of form. Nevertheless, excellent approximate solutions for wave propagation in such nonuniform media are well known, and correspond to a wave propagating locally according to local wavenumber solutions. Any small section of the medium, of length Δx, over which the properties change slowly behaves just as would a small section in a uniform medium: It contributes a phase shift, $k_r \Delta x$, and a log gain, $-k_i \Delta x$. We also may need to adjust the amplitude $A(x)$ to conserve energy as energy-storage parameters such as the membrane stiffness change, even in a lossless medium.

In the cochlea, the amplitude of the pressure wave remains nearly constant as the wave propagates, but the amplitude of the velocity or displacement wave grows to conserve energy as the stiffness decreases.

Scaling

A wave medium is said to **scale** (or be **scale-invariant**) if the response properties at any point are just like those at any other point, with a change in time scale. The response properties of the cochleas of all known animals are approximately scale-invariant over most of the length of the basilar membrane. This scaling property is achieved by an exponential slowing of the wave-propagation velocity with the distance x. In a system that scales, the response for all places can be specified as a single transfer function $H(f)$,

$$f = \omega/\omega_N$$

where f is a nondimensional normalized frequency, and ω_N is any conveniently defined natural frequency that depends on the place—for example, the peak in the frequency response. Because of the assumed exponential form for the variation of parameters, we can write ω_N as

$$\omega_N = \omega_0 e^{-x/d_\omega}$$

where ω_0 is the natural frequency at $x = 0$ (at the base), and d_ω is the characteristic distance in which the velocity, and therefore ω_N, decreases by a factor of e.

Changing to a log-frequency scale in terms of $l_f = \log f$, we define the function $G(l_f) = H(f)$, which we can write as

$$G(l_f) = G\left(\log \frac{\omega}{\omega_N}\right) = G\left(\log \frac{\omega}{\omega_0} + \frac{x}{d_\omega}\right)$$

This equation shows that the transfer function G expressed as a function of log frequency l_f is identical to the transfer function for a particular frequency ω expressed as a function of place x, for an appropriate offset and place scaling. Thus, we can label the horizontal axes of transfer-function plots interchangeably with either place or log-frequency units, for a particular frequency or place respectively.

In the cochlea, the function G will be lowpass. Above a certain cutoff frequency, depending on the place, the magnitude of the response will quickly approach zero; equivalently, beyond a certain place, depending on frequency, the response will quickly approach zero.

The stiffness is the most important parameter of the cochlear partition that changes from base to apex, and it has the effect of changing the characteristic frequency scale with place (ω_N varies as the square root of stiffness if other parameters, such as duct size, are constant). Over much of the x dimension of real cochleas, the stiffness varies approximately exponentially [Dallos, 1978]. The scaling assumption simply allows us the convenience of summarizing the response of the entire system by a single function G, and does not prevent us from adopting more realistic parameter variations in the region where the variation is not exponential.

Approximate Wavenumber Behavior

It is instructive to look at approximate solutions to Equation 16.1 that make clear the dependence of the wavenumber on the parameters, because it is this dependence that relates the fluid dynamics to the circuit model we will describe later. In practice, more exact solutions for k may be achieved by Newton's method, starting from simple approximations such as those we discuss here.

Starting with real k, we obtain a first approximation to the dispersion relation by setting the imaginary part of Equation 16.1 to zero. This lossless approximation is

$$k_r \approx \frac{\omega^2 \rho}{S}$$

Using this approximate solution for k_r, we can obtain a first approximation for the imaginary part k_i by solving for the imaginary part of Equation 16.1, assuming that k_i is much less than k_r and ignoring terms with k_i^2 and k_i^3:

$$k_i \approx \frac{k_r \beta \omega}{S} + \frac{k_r^3 \gamma \omega}{S}$$

$$\approx \frac{\beta \omega^3 \rho}{S^2} + \frac{\gamma \omega^7 \rho^3}{S^4}$$

Because these relations are derived in the short-wavelength limit, they are not applicable at very low frequencies. However, they can give us an excellent representation for the behavior of the peak frequency and the characteristics of the high-frequency cutoff.

We can interpret these complex wavenumber approximations either as *frequency-dependent* at a constant place (constant S, β, and γ), or as *place-dependent* at a constant frequency (constant ω). Thus, a wave of frequency ω will propagate until the damping gets large; the loss per distance, k_i, grows ultimately as ω^7 or e^{7x/d_ω} (assuming the exponential dependence of S discussed earlier, and with γ proportional to ω_N and therefore to e^{-x/d_ω}). For a given frequency, the damping is near zero for small x and becomes dominant very quickly as x approaches a **cutoff place** x_C. Similarly, at a given place, low frequencies are propagated with little loss; as ω grows, however, the loss grows quickly, and waves above a **cutoff frequency** ω_C are heavily attenuated.

The cochlea is known to have sharp cutoff behavior, so it is reasonable to suppose that only the high-order γ loss term is significant in determining the cutoff points. We can estimate the cutoff frequency to be near the point where k_i becomes comparable to k_r. Based on the previous simple approximations,

$$\omega_C \approx (S^3/\gamma\rho^2)^{1/5}$$

If the system scales, cutoff frequencies and cutoff places are related exponentially:

$$\omega_C \approx \left(S_0^3/\gamma_0\rho^2\right)^{1/5} e^{-x/d_\omega}$$

$$x_C \approx -d_\omega \log \frac{\omega}{(S_0^3/\gamma_0 \rho^2)^{1/5}}$$

where the subscript 0 refers to values at the base $(x = 0)$. If the damping and stiffness coefficients do not scale exponentially, there is still a cutoff place as a function of frequency, but it is not a simple function of $\log \omega$.

The **best frequency**, or frequency of highest wave amplitude, will be somewhat less than the cutoff frequency, for any place. Because the cilia of the hair cells sense the velocity or displacement of the membrane, we should calculate the best frequency using the velocity rather than the displacement of the cochlear partition. Conversion from pressure to velocity involves a spatial differentiation, contributing another factor of k, or a tilt in the place response of about 12 decibels per octave. The velocity will peak within less than an octave of cutoff.

The effect of the variable damping on the cutoff points is not included in our approximation, due to the assumption that the higher-order loss mechanism mainly determines the sharp cutoff. According to this model, the best frequency should shift by nearly an octave (depending on parameters) as the damping is changed. The cutoff point, however, measured as the frequency where the response decreases with a particular high slope, changes relatively little. Experimentally, a shift in best frequency of up to 0.75 octave has been observed from healthy cochleas with active outer hair cells to traumatized cochleas where the outer hair cells could no longer provide active mechanical undamping [Cody, 1980]. In these experiments, the steep high-frequency side of the response was unchanged, as we would expect.

SILICON COCHLEA

All auditory processing starts with a cochlea. Silicon auditory processing must start with a *silicon cochlea*. The fundamental structure in a cochlea is the basilar membrane. The silicon basilar membrane is a transmission line with a velocity of propagation that can be tuned electrically. Output *taps*, where the signal can be observed, are located at intervals along the line. We can think about the taps as crude inner hair cells. Unfortunately, we cannot build a system with as many taps as living systems have hair cells. Human ears have about 3500; we will be lucky to have 1000. On the other hand, we can make many delay-line elements; the delay element we use in this delay line is the second-order section, described in Chapter 11. We expect this model delay line to be good enough to duplicate approximately the dynamics of the second-order system of fluid mass and membrane stiffness, including the active role of the outer hair cells.

Basilar-Membrane Delay Line

Our basilar-membrane model is fabricated with 480 sections in the boustrophedonic arrangement illustrated by the 100-section version in Figure 16.3. The only reason for using this serpentine structure instead of a straight line is that

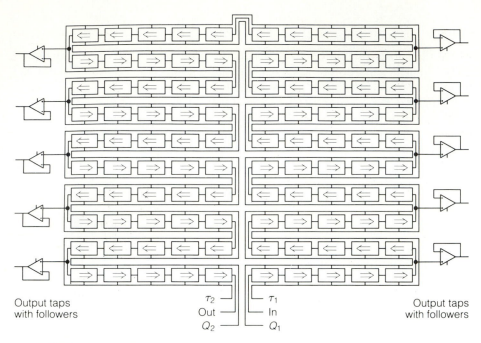

FIGURE 16.3   Floorplan of 100-stage cochlea chip, in serpentine arrangement. The wires that are shown connecting the τ and Q control terminals of the filter stages are built using a resistive polysilicon line, which acts as a voltage divider that adjusts the bias currents in the cascade as an exponential function of distance from the input. The second-order section used in this composition is shown in Figure 11.1 (p. 180).

there are many sections, each of which is longer than it is high. The chip has a reasonable aspect ratio with this floorplan. Circuit yields are good enough that we regularly are able to propagate a signal through the entire 480-stage delay line on chips from several fabrication runs.

The τ and Q bias inputs on the second-order sections are connected to polysilicon lines that run along one edge of the sections. We connect both ends of each of these resistive polysilicon lines to pads, so that we can set the voltages from offchip. Due to the subthreshold characteristics of the bias transistors in the amplifiers, the time constants of the sections are exponentially related to the voltages on the τ control line. If we put a different voltage on the two ends of the τ line, we get a gradient in voltage along the length of the polysilicon line. The subthreshold bias transistors in the transconductance amplifiers will turn this linear gradient in voltage into an exponential gradient in the delay per section. We can thereby easily make a transmission line where the velocity of propagation and cutoff frequency are exponential functions of the distance x along the line. We adjust all the sections to have the same Q value by putting a similar gradient on the Q control line, with a voltage offset that determines the ratio of feedback gain to forward gain in each section.

For a cochlea operating in the range of human hearing, time constants of about 10^{-5} to 10^{-2} second are needed. A convenient capacitor size is a fraction of a picofarad (10^{-12} farad), so the range of transconductance values needed is between 10^{-7} and 10^{-11} mho. If $kT/(q\kappa)$ is 40 millivolts, the range of bias currents will be between 10^{-8} and 10^{-12} amp. This range leaves several orders of magnitude of leeway from room-temperature thermal leakage currents at the low end, and from space-charge–limited behavior (transistors operating above threshold) at the high end, so the circuits are in many ways ideal. The total current supplied to a cascade of 480 stages is less than a microamp.

Second-Order Sections in Cascade

We can spatially discretize a nonuniform wave medium such as the cochlea by looking at the outputs of N short sections of length Δx; the section outputs are indexed by n, an integer place designator that corresponds to the x location $n\Delta x$. A cascade of second-order sections with transfer functions $H_1, H_2, \ldots, H_n, \ldots,$ H_N can be designed to approximate the response of the wave medium at the section outputs. In passing from output $n-1$ to output n, a propagating (complex) wave will be modified by a factor of $H_n(\omega)$, which should match the effect of the wave medium.

The equivalent transfer function $H_n(\omega)$, a function of place (output number n) and frequency, is thus directly related to the complex wavenumber $k(\omega, x)$, a function of place and frequency. The relation between the cascade of second-order sections and the wave medium is

$$H_n(\omega) = e^{jk\Delta x} \qquad \text{with } k \text{ evaluated at} \qquad x = n\Delta x \qquad (16.2)$$

or

$$k(\omega, x) = \frac{\log H_n(\omega)}{j\Delta x} \qquad \text{for} \qquad x = n\Delta x$$

Because H and k both can be complex, we can separate the phase and loss terms using $\log H = \log|H| + j\arg H$:

$$\log H = jk\Delta x = jk_r\Delta x - k_i\Delta x$$

$$\log \text{ gain} = \log|H| = -k_i\Delta x$$

$$\text{phase lag} = \arg H = k_r\Delta x$$

Therefore, if we want to model the action of the cochlea by a cascade of second-order sections, we should design each section to have a phase lag or delay that matches k_r and a gain or loss that matches k_i, all as a function of frequency:

$$\text{gain} = e^{-k_i\Delta x}$$

$$\text{group delay} = \frac{d\text{phase}}{d\omega} = \frac{dk_r}{d\omega}\Delta x = \frac{\Delta x}{U} \qquad (16.3)$$

where U is the group velocity; Equation 16.3 implies that the previous definition of group velocity, $d\omega/dk$, is correctly generalized to $d\omega/dk_r$. The overall transfer function of the cascade of second-order sections, from input to output m, which we call H^m, is

$$\mathrm{H}^m(\omega) = \prod_{n=0}^{m} H_n(\omega)$$

$$= \exp \sum_{n=0}^{m} \log H_n(\omega)$$

$$= \exp j \sum_{n=0}^{m} k(\omega, n\Delta x)\Delta x \tag{16.4}$$

In the cochlea, k is nearly real for frequencies significantly below cutoff; that is, the second-order sections are simply lossless delay stages at low frequencies. The gains may be slightly greater than unity at middle frequencies, when the input signal is small and the cochlea is actively undamped; at high frequencies, however, the gains always approach zero. Near cutoff, a small change in the value of k_i corresponds to a small change in the gain of any one section, but to a potentially large change in the overall gain of the cascade.

These formulae (from Equation 16.2 through Equation 16.4) provide a way to translate between a distributed-parameter wave view and a discrete delay-section view of the cochlea. The discrete-section model will be realistic to the extent that waves do not reflect back toward the base and that the sections are small enough that the value of k does not change much within a section. In our experimental circuits, k may change appreciably between the rather widely spaced output taps, so several delay sections are used per tap.

Figure 16.4(a) shows the response of a single second-order section from the transmission line. The curves were computed from Equation 16.4 for Q values of 0.7, 0.8, and 0.9; scaled versions of the $Q = 0.9$ transfer function, from earlier stages in a cascade, also are shown. For this application, we use Q values of less than 1.0, which means that the peak of the single-section response is very broad and has a maximum value just slightly greater than unity for Q greater than 0.707.

Because the system scales, each second-order section should have a similar response curve. The time-constant of each section is larger than that of its predecessor by a constant factor $e^{\Delta x/d_\omega}$, so each curve will be shifted along the log-frequency scale by a constant amount $\Delta x/d_\omega$. The overall response is the product of all the individual curves; the log response is the sum of all of the logs, as shown in Figure 16.4(b). In terms of the normalized log–log response G, the overall response is simply

$$\log \mathrm{H}^m(\omega) = \sum_{n=0}^{m} \log G \left(\log \frac{\omega}{\omega_0} + \frac{n\Delta x}{d_\omega} \right)$$

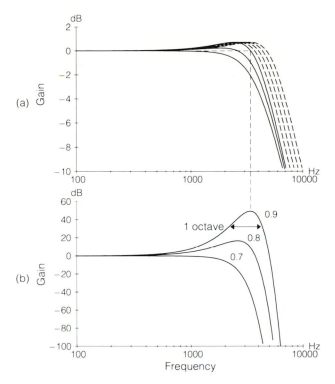

FIGURE 16.4 (a) Frequency response of a single second-order filter section, for Q values 0.7, 0.8, and 0.9, including scaled copies (dashed lines) of the $Q = 0.9$ response to represent earlier sections in a cascade. (b) Corresponding overall response of a cascade of 120 stages with a factor of 1.0139 scaling between adjacent stages. The dashed line between (a) and (b) indicates that the overall response peak occurs at the frequency for which the final section gain crosses unity. Note the different decibel scale factors on the ordinates.

Taking the section illustrated in Figure 16.4(a) as the last section before the output tap and working backward to sections of shorter time constants, we obtain the overall response in Figure 16.4(b). Each response curve has a maximum gain slightly larger than unity. There are many sections, and each one is shifted over from the other by an amount that is small compared with the width of the peak. Although there is not much gain in each section, the cumulative gain causes a large peak in the response. This overall-gain peak is termed a **pseudoresonance**, and is much broader (less sharply tuned) than is a single resonance of the same gain.

Figure 16.5 shows the s-plane plot of the poles of an exponentially scaling cascade of second-order sections with $Q = 0.707$. The time constant τ of the final stage of the cascade determines the smallest $\omega_N = 1/\tau$, indicated by the circle in the figure. For clarity, only six stages per octave (a factor of 1.122), covering only three octaves, are used for this illustration.

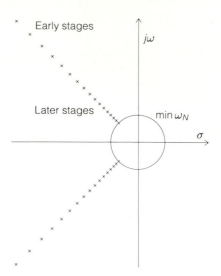

FIGURE 16.5 Plot in the s-plane of the poles of an exponentially scaled cascade of second-order sections with $Q = 0.707$ (maximally flat frequency response). The time constant τ of the final stage of the cascade determines the smallest ω_N, indicated by the circle. Six stages per octave (a factor of 1.122 scaling between stages) are used for this illustration, covering three octaves. Each pair of poles corresponds to a single second-order section, as shown in Figure 11.1 (p. 180).

Because each stage of the delay line has nearly unity gain at DC, we interpret the propagating signal as a pressure wave in the cochlea, which should propagate with a roughly constant amplitude in the passive case (the amplitude should be exactly constant in the short-wave region with zero damping). In the active case, a significant gain (for example, 10 to 100) can be achieved, measured in terms of the pressure wave.

We can design output-tap circuits to convert the propagating pressure wave into a signal analogous to a membrane deflection-velocity wave. Ideally, we would do this by a spatial differentiation to convert pressure to acceleration, followed by a time integration to convert to velocity. The combination would be exactly equivalent to a single time-domain filter, which can be approximated in the short-wave region by the approximate differentiator $\tau s/(\tau s + 1)$, with τ adjusted to correspond roughly to the τ of each section; this filter tilts the low side of the response to 6 decibels per octave, without having much effect on the shape or sharp cutoff of the pseudoresonance. The most effective such circuit we have built and tested is the hysteretic differentiator described in Chapter 10. The results reported in this chapter, however, are based on the second-order delay line alone.

Transistor Parameter Variation

Our electronic cochlea would be ideal if Figure 16.4 showed the real picture. As we have noted in Chapter 5, however, MOS transistors are not inherently well matched. For a given gate voltage, the current in the subthreshold region where our circuits operate can vary randomly over a range of a factor of about two. In the response curves of the real second-order sections, there is a dispersion in the center frequencies of the sections because of this random variation in currents.

That dispersion would not be too great a problem, but the Q values also vary, because the threshold of the Q control transistor varies randomly and is not well correlated with the τ adjustment on the same stage.

If the responses of too many sections fall off without peaking, the collective response will be depressed at high frequencies, and we will not be able to maintain a good bandwidth and gain in the transmission line. If we try to increase the value of Q too much, however, to make up for the depressed response, some of the sections will start to oscillate. The large-signal stability limit described in Chapter 11 places an additional constraint on the range of Q values than can be tolerated in the face of threshold variation. Thus, there is a range of variations beyond which this scheme will not work. Fortunately, ordinary CMOS processes are capable of yielding transistors that have currents sufficiently well controlled to obtain cochlear behavior with no oscillation.

Figure 16.6 illustrates a possible random distribution of pole positions, based on a uniform distribution of threshold-voltage offsets that would cause currents and transconductances to vary over a range of a factor of two. The nominal Q value and the τ scaling factor are set as in the experimental conditions discussed the next two sections. The bounded distributions allow us to compute that α (the ratio of feedback transconductance to total forward transconductance in the second-order section of Chapter 11) will change by a factor of two above and below nominal, and we can see that for this condition it is not difficult to avoid the large-signal instability. The effect of the large Q variation on the overall response of the system is more difficult to estimate.

Frequency Response

The most straightforward behavior of the silicon cochlea that can be compared with theory is the magnitude of the frequency response. The circuit is set up with a gradient in the τ such that each section is slower than its predecessor by a factor of 1.0139. With this value, the auditory range is covered in the 480 sections. The Q control voltage is set so that the peak response is about five times the DC response, as seen at several different output taps. Experimental data were taken with a sine wave of 14 millivolts peak-to-peak amplitude applied to the input. Results for two taps 120 sections apart are shown in Figure 16.7. The solid points are measured values, and the smooth curves are theoretical predictions. Each curve is constructed as a product of individual section response curves as given by Equation 11.4 (p. 181). The value of the DC gain of the amplifiers is determined from the ratio of the response peaks. The value of Q used in the theory is adjusted until the predicted peak heights agreed with observation. The resulting Q value is 0.79. The lower-frequency peak corresponds to a tap farther from the input by 120 sections than is the higher-frequency peak; the signal level at the second tap has thus suffered a degradation due to the DC gain of 120 followers in cascade. The open-circuit amplifier gain inferred from this observation is 1800, in good agreement with measurements on other amplifiers of similar design.

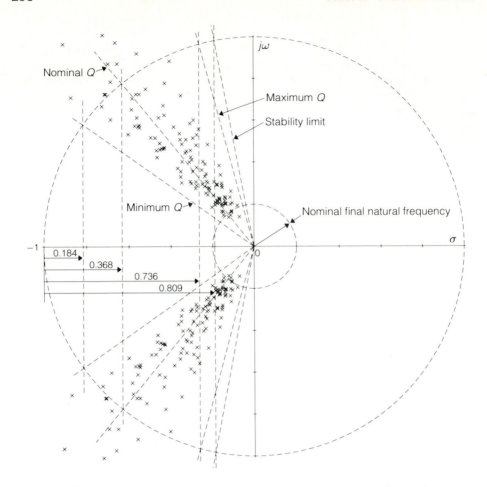

FIGURE 16.6 Plot in the s-plane of the poles of an exponential cascade of second-order filter sections with random threshold offsets ($Q = 0.79$ nominal, stage ratio = 1.0139, 120 stages covering about a factor of five in frequency). The threshold offset was modeled as a uniform distribution of bias current over a factor-of-two range, resulting in α parameter variation of up to a factor of two above and below nominal (factor-of-four range).

The remarkable agreement between theory and experiment is surprising in view of known random variations in transistor input offset voltages. We would expect a variation in Q and τ values for each section that is much larger than is the systematic progression between adjacent amplifiers. This variation need not, however, have a drastic effect on the result. The total response is the product of the responses of a large number of amplifiers. The product is an associative operation—it does not depend on the order of the terms. The fact that amplifiers in a particular physical location do not have precisely the τ value that we desire does not matter. Some amplifier somewhere will have that τ value, and it will make its contribution as required. It is more surprising that the random variation

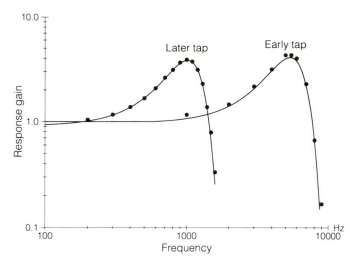

FIGURE 16.7 Log–log frequency response measured at two output taps of an experimental silicon cochlea 120 sections apart. The experimentally measured points (dots) agree quite well with the theoretical curves (using empirically fitted values of Q = 0.79, stage ratio = 1.0139, and DC gain = 1800). The DC-gain parameter (or open-loop gain of the transconductance amplifier) provides a correction that shifts the response at the later tap downward by $(1800/1801)^{120}$ = 0.936 relative to the earlier tap.

of Q values does not affect the result in a more violent way. As of now, we do not have a satisfactory theory explaining the composite response curve resulting from many curves of different individual Q values.

Transient Response

The response at one tap of the cochlea to a step input is shown in Figure 16.8. In part (a), the Q value of the delay line has been adjusted to be just slightly less than 0.707; the trace shows only a slight resonant overshoot. In part (b), the Q value has been increased, and more overshoot is evident. In part (c), the Q value is considerably higher, and the delay line rings for several cycles. If the Q value were automatically adjusted, as it is in living systems, part (a) would correspond to the response at high background sound levels, and part (c) would correspond to a very quiet environment. With the Q value adjustment corresponding to part (c), we can observe the response at the two taps along the delay line where the frequency response of Figure 16.7 was measured. The result is shown in Figure 16.9. These results illustrate the scale-invariance property that is unique and valuable about this structure: When we adjust the time scale on the oscilloscope to correspond to the τ value of the particular section being observed, we obtain a similar output waveform at every tap. Living systems use this principle so that the detection machinery does not depend on the position along the basilar membrane. We will use it for the same purpose.

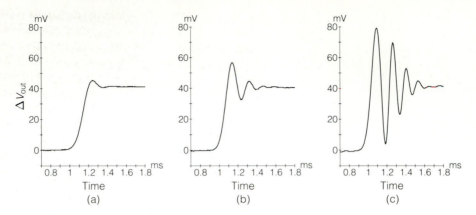

FIGURE 16.8   Step response at one tap of the cochlea. In (a), the Q value of the delay line has been adjusted to be less than maximally flat (about 0.69); the trace shows only a slight resonant overshoot. In (b), the Q value has been increased to about 0.74, and more overshoot is evident. In (c), the Q value is considerably higher (about 0.79), and the delay line "rings" for several cycles.

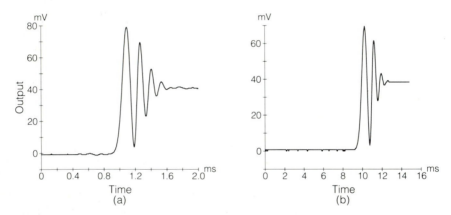

FIGURE 16.9   Step responses at two taps separated by 120 delay stages. Note that the second response (b) has about 10 times as much delay as the first one has (a), and that it has a slightly faster rise time relative to the delay. Aside from the relation of rise time to delay, the response at the two taps is similar, with the time scaled by about a factor of 10. This behavior gives rise to the scale-invariance property of the cochlea.

GAIN CONTROL

The function of the outer-hair-cell arrangement is to provide not just gain, but also control of the gain, which it does by a factor of about 100 in amplitude (10,000 in energy). When the signal is small, the outer hair cells are not inhibited and they feed back energy. This AGC system works for sound power levels within a few decades of the bottom end of our hearing range by making the

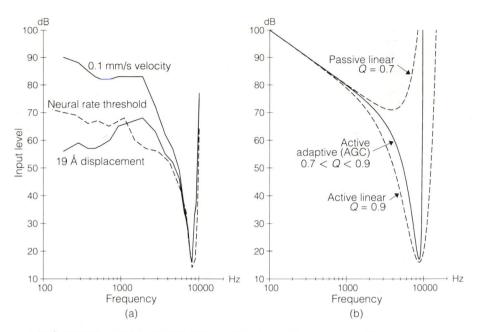

FIGURE 16.10 (a) Mechanical and neural iso-output tuning curves. Based on data from Robles and his associates [Robles et al., 1986]. The mechanical measurements (amount of input needed to get 1 millimeter per second basilar-membrane displacement velocity, or 19-angstrom basilar-membrane displacement amplitude) were made by measuring doppler-shifted gamma rays (Mössbauer effect) from a small radioactive source mounted on the cochlear partition. The neural tuning curve was measured by looking for a specified increase in firing rate of a single fiber in the cochlear nerve. (b) Iso-output tuning curves for the second-order model described in this chapter, under three operating conditions. The dashed curves are the response for fixed Q, independent of input level. The solid curve is the result for a particular nonlinear AGC scheme that reduces the Q of the cascaded filter stages as the output signal increases. The similarity in the response area shape and width between the active adaptive model and the biological system (a) is striking. For this simulation, all filter-stage Q values are equal, and are computed from a feedback gain α that is a maximum value (0.5) minus a constant, times the total output of 100 channels covering about an octave in each direction from the channel being measured. The relation of Q values to overall gains and overall transfer functions is discussed in the text.

structure slightly more resonant and thereby of much higher gain—by reducing the damping until it is negative in some regions.

Figure 16.10(a) shows data from a biological cochlea. The sound-pressure level required to produce a fixed membrane-displacement amplitude and velocity is plotted as a function of frequency. Also plotted is the input level required to produce a certain increase in the rate of firing of a single auditory nerve fiber. The data were obtained by Robles and his associates [Robles et al., 1985], using the Mössbauer effect in the chinchilla cochlea. Curves such as these are termed **iso-output** curves, because the input level is adjusted to produce the same output level at each frequency; the region above an iso-output curve is known as the **response area**. The curves show reasonable agreement between neural and mechanical data, implying that the response area is already determined at the mechanical level. Without the outer hair cells, the sensitivity is at least 30 decibels less, and the curve tips are much broader [Kim, 1984]. The sharpness of such **tuning curves** (response widths of only about one-fourth to one-tenth of the center frequency) often misleads model developers into thinking that the system is narrowly tuned, when in fact the curves are quite different from transfer functions. As frequency changes, the input level changes enormously, and the AGC system causes a change in the opposite direction to keep the output at a constant level. The response of the cochlea as a linear filter is difficult to infer from this kind of measurement, but it must be considerably broader than are the iso-output tuning-curve shapes [Lyon et al., 1986].

This use of controlled mechanical feedback provides an extremely effective gain-control system. This gain-control system takes effect before the signal is translated into nerve pulses, just as does the visual gain-control system in the retina. Nerve pulses are, by their very nature, a horrible medium into which to translate sound. They are noisy and erratic, and can work over only a limited dynamic range of firing rates. It is essential to have a first level of AGC *before* the signal is turned into nerve pulses, because this approach reduces the noise associated with the quantization of the signal.

We can model the effect of the outer hair cells as a negative damping. When the low-order loss term β in Equation 16.1 is negative, the system exhibits gain until, at high enough frequency, the higher-order γ loss mechanism dominates. If we were to model such a traveling-wave system with active gain as a time-invariant linear system, the system would have a fixed gain, independent of the sound input level. The live cochlea, however, is known to be highly adaptive and compressive, such that the mechanical gain is much less for loud inputs than for soft inputs. This nonlinear (but short-term nearly linear) behavior is necessary for two reasons. First, the mechanism that adds energy must be energy-supply limited, and therefore the gain cannot extend to arbitrarily high signal levels. Second, even at relatively low sound levels, the variation of the gain is needed to compress inputs into a usable dynamic range, without causing excessive distortion.

Many researchers who have attempted to model active wave amplification in the cochlea have met with difficulties, especially when the place dimension was discretized for numerical solution. De Boer has shown that slight irregularities in the cochlea can reflect enough energy to make the system break into unstable oscillations (as in tinnitus) [de Boer, 1983]; models that use discrete sections and allow waves to propagate in both directions sometimes suffer from the same problem. By taking advantage of the known normal mode of cochlea operation in which signals propagate in only one direction, our circuit model avoids the stability problem, as long as each section is independently stable.

We have not, at the present time, integrated the control system for automatically adjusting the Q values of the second-order sections onto the same silicon as the basilar-membrane model. We have, however, built a computer simulation of such a control system, which we describe later in this section. The results from this model shed considerable light on the operation of biological cochleas, and are guiding our design of a silicon cochlea with a completely integrated AGC system.

We have seen that the gain of a delay line composed of second-order sections is a sensitive function of the Q value of the individual sections. For Q less than 0.707, the gain of each stage will be less than unity at all frequencies; for slightly higher Q values, the stage is a simple but reasonable model of an actively undamped section of the cochlear transmission line, with gain exceeding unity over a limited bandwidth. By varying the filter's Q value adaptively in response to sound, we can cause the delay line to model a range of positive and negative damping, and can thereby cause large overall gain changes. In our model, the Q value for 120 sections before a given tap was adjusted downward from a maximum value of 1.0 as the average output-signal amplitude increased. The average output-signal amplitude was defined as the average of the amplitudes of output-signals from 50 sections on either side of the given tap; the model is thus a **coupled AGC system**, because a range of output channels can affect the gain of any particular channel. In a silicon implementation, this average would be computed by a one-dimensional resistive network, as described in Chapter 7.

Figure 16.10(b) shows iso-output curves for the cochlear model described in the previous paragraph, under two linear conditions (a passive low-gain condition, as in a cochlea with dead or damaged outer hair cells, and an active high-gain condition, as in a hypothetical cochlea with active outer hairs of constant gain and unlimited energy), and under the condition where the AGC system acts to adapt the gain between the two linear conditions in response to the output level averaged over nearby channels. The curves show that a simple coupled gain-control loop can cause a broadly tuned filter to appear to have a much narrower response than does a similar filter without AGC, when observed with an iso-output criterion; this result is in excellent agreement with the experimental data on the biological system in Figure 16.10(a).[1] The model also predicts that higher signal levels will cause an increase in effective bandwidth and a reduction in phase shift or delay near the best frequency (but a slightly increased phase lag below the best frequency), in agreement with physiological observations [Pickles, 1985; Sellick et al., 1982].

SUMMARY

The cochlea is a traveling-wave structure that creates the first-level representation in the auditory system. It converts time-domain information into spatially encoded information by spreading out signals in space according to their time

---

[1] Our scale-invariant model produces tuning curves that are similar to those observed in biological systems in the basal region, but are too sharp in the apical region [Dallos, 1988]. In the real cochlea the frequency-place mapping becomes nearly linear in the apical region, so waves are amplified over a more limited region, resulting in less AGC effect and less iso-output sharpness.

scale. The velocity of propagation along the structure decreases exponentially with distance, so the spatial pattern generated by a certain time sequence is independent of the rate at which the sequence is presented. Faster sequences create output patterns closer to the input of the structure; slower sequences generate output patterns nearer the output of the structure.

The silicon model of this traveling-wave structure exhibits behaviors that bear an uncanny resemblance to those of the living system. The effect of variation in transistor parameters is insignificant in the operation of the system, which is determined by the collective action of many sections. This model has allowed us to sharpen our understanding of nature's solution to the hearing problem. It also is an effective solution to a difficult engineering problem.

REFERENCES

Dallos, P. Biophysics of the cochlea. In Carterette, E.C. and Friedman, M.P. (eds), *Handbook of Perception*, vol 4. New York: Academic Press, 1978, p. 125.

Dallos, P. Personal communication, 1988.

de Boer, E. Wave reflection in passive and active cochlea models. In de Boer, E. and Viergever, M.A. (eds), *Mechanics of Hearing. Proceedings of the IUTAM/ICA Symposium,* The Hague: The Netherlands, Martinus Nijhoff Publishers, 1983, p. 135.

Kim, D.O. Functional roles of the inner– and outer–hair-cell subsystems in the cochlea and brainstem. In Berlin, C.I. (ed), *Hearing Science: Recent Advances.* San Diego, CA: College-Hill Press, 1984, p. 241.

Lyon, R.F. and Dyer, L. Experiments with a computational model of the cochlea. *Proceedings of the IEEE International Conference on Acoustical Speech and Signal Processing,* vol 3. Tokyo, Japan: IEEE, 1986, p. 1975.

Pickles, J.O. Recent advances in cochlear physiology. *Progress in Neurobiology,* 24:1, 1985.

Robles, L., Ruggero, M.A., and Rich, N.C. Mössbauer measurements of the mechanical response to single-tone and two-tone stimuli at the base of the chinchilla cochlea. In Allen, J.B., Hall, J.L., Hubbard, A., Neely, S.T., and Tubis, A. (eds), *Peripheral Auditory Mechanisms.* Berlin, New York: Springer-Verlag, 1986.

Sellick, P.M., Patuzzi, R., and Johnstone, B.M. Measurement of basilar membrane motion in the guinea pig using the Mössbauer technique. *Journal of the Acoustical Society of America,* 72:131, 1982.

von Békésy, G. *Sensory Inhibition.* Princeton, NJ: Princeton University Press, 1967.

Zurek, P.M. and Clark, W.W. Narrow-band acoustic signals emitted by chinchilla ears after noise exposure. *Journal of the Acoustical Society of America,* 70:446, 1981.

APPENDIXES

Is it not a joy when,
in reconsidering old things, we come to know the new?
—Confucius *Lun Yü* (1979)

APPENDIX

A

CMOS FABRICATION

The series of steps by which a geometric pattern or set of geometric patterns is transformed into an operating integrated system is called a **wafer-fabrication process**, or simply a *process*. An integrated system in MOS technology consists of a number of superimposed layers of conducting, insulating, and transistor-forming materials. By arranging predetermined geometric shapes in each of these layers, we can construct a system of the required function. The task of designers of integrated systems is to devise the geometric shapes and to determine the locations of these shapes in each of the various layers of the system. The task of the process itself is to create the layers and to transfer into each of them the geometric shapes determined by the system design.

Modern wafer fabrication probably is the most exacting production process ever developed. Since the 1950s, enormous human resources have been expended by the industry to perfect the myriad details involved. The impurities in materials and chemical reagents are measured in parts per billion. Dimensions are controlled to a few parts per million. Each step has been carefully devised to produce some circuit feature with the minimum possible deviation from the ideal behavior. The results have been little short of spectacular: Chips with many hundreds of thousands

Adapted with permission from Mead, C. and Conway, L., *Introduction to VLSI Systems.* © 1980, Reading, MA: Addison-Wesley.

of transistors are being produced for under \$10 each. In addition, wafer fabrication has reached a level of maturity such that the system designer need not be concerned with the fine details of its execution. The following sections present a broad overview sufficient to convey the ideas involved; in particular, we will examine those processes relevant to system design. Our formulation of the basic concepts anticipates the evolution of the technology toward ever finer dimensions.

In this appendix, we describe what the patterning sequence is and how it is applied in a simple, specific integrated-system process: CMOS. As in any other integrated technology, CMOS circuits are built up on the flat surface of a highly polished slab of single-crystal silicon; such a slab is called a **wafer**.

PATTERNING

The overall fabrication process consists of the **patterning** of a particular *sequence* of successive *layers*. These layers are built up in the dimension perpendicular to the surface. The complexity of the circuit along the surface can be very large, but that perpendicular to the surface is limited by the number of layers in the process. The patterning steps by which geometrical shapes are transferred into a layer of the final system are similar for each of the layers. We will be able to visualize the overall process more easily if we first describe the details of patterning one layer. We can then examine the particular sequence of layers used in the process to build up an integrated system, without repeating the details of patterning for each of the layers.

A common step in many processes is the creation of a silicon-dioxide insulating layer on the surface of a silicon wafer. Sections of the insulating layer are then removed selectively, exposing the underlying silicon. We will use this step for our patterning example. It begins with a bare, polished silicon wafer, shown in cross-section in Figure A.1(a). The wafer is exposed to oxygen in a high-temperature furnace to grow a uniform layer of silicon dioxide on its surface (Figure A.1b). After the wafer is cooled, it is coated with a thin film of organic "resist" material (Figure A.1c). The resist is thoroughly dried and baked to ensure its integrity. The wafer is now ready for the patterning to begin.

At the time of wafer fabrication, the pattern to be transferred to the wafer surface exists as a **mask**. A mask is merely a transparent support material coated with a thin layer of opaque material. Certain portions of the coating are removed, leaving opaque material on the mask in the precise pattern required on the silicon surface. The dark areas of opaque material on the surface of the mask are located where the designer wants to leave silicon dioxide on the surface of the silicon. Openings in the mask correspond to areas where the designer wants to remove silicon dioxide from the silicon surface. An image of the mask is projected onto the wafer surface using an intense source of ionizing radiation, such as ultraviolet light or low-energy X rays. (Figure A.1d.) The radiation is stopped in areas where the mask has opaque material on its surface. Where there is no opaque material on the mask surface, the ionizing radiation passes through into the resist, the

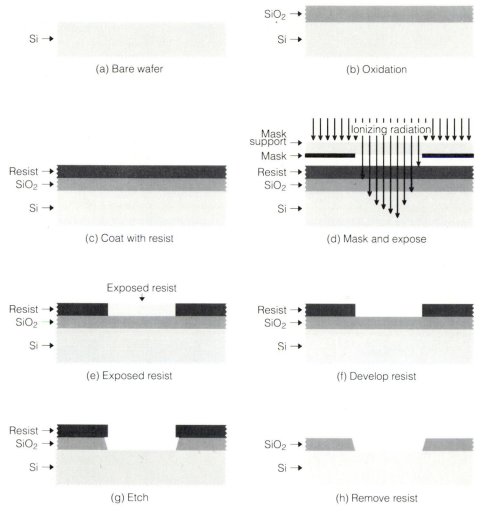

FIGURE A.1 Patterning.

silicon dioxide, and the silicon. The ionizing radiation has little effect on the silicon dioxide and on the silicon, but it breaks down the molecular structure of the resist into considerably smaller molecules.

We have chosen as an illustration a **positive-resist** process—in which case the resist material remaining after exposure and development corresponds to the dark areas in the original pattern. Negative resists can also be used, but positive resists typically are workable to finer feature sizes and have become dominant for that reason.

After exposure to the ionizing radiation, the wafer has the characteristics shown in Figure A.1(e). In areas exposed to the radiation, the resist molecules have been broken down to much lighter molecular weight than that of unexposed resist molecules. The solubility of organic molecules in various organic solvents is a very steep function of the molecular weight of the molecules. It is possible to dissolve exposed resist material in solvents that will not dissolve the unexposed resist material. We can thus "develop" the resist (Figure A.1f) by merely immersing the silicon wafer in a suitable solvent.

Up to this point, the original pattern has been transferred as a corresponding pattern into the resist material on the surface of the silicon dioxide. We can now transfer the same pattern to the silicon dioxide itself by exposing the wafer to an **etchant**—a reactive ionized gas that will etch silicon dioxide but will not attack either the organic resist material or the silicon wafer surface. The etching step usually is done with gaseous hydrofluoric acid, which etches silicon dioxide, but not organic materials or silicon. The result of the etching step is shown in Figure A.1(g).

The final step in patterning is removal of the remaining organic resist material. There are three techniques to remove resist materials: (1) using strong organic solvents that dissolve even unexposed resist material; (2) using strong acids, such as chromic acid, that actively attack organics; (3) exposing the wafer to atomic oxygen, which will oxidize away any organic materials present on its surface. Once the resist material is removed, the finished pattern on the wafer surface is as shown in Figure A.1(h). Notice that we have transferred the original geometric pattern directly into the silicon dioxide on the wafer surface. Although a foreign material was present on the wafer surface during the patterning process, it has now disappeared, and the only materials left are those that will be part of the finished wafer.

A similar sequence of steps is used to pattern selectively each of the layers of the integrated system. The steps differ primarily in the types of etchants used. Thus, as we study the processing of the various layers, you need not visualize all the details of the patterning sequence for each layer. Just recognize that the original pattern for a layer can be transferred into a pattern in the material of that layer.

THE SILICON-GATE CMOS PROCESS

We now describe the particular sequence of patterned layers used to build up CMOS integrated circuits and systems. Plates 1 through 3 illustrate a simple sequence of patterning and processing steps that are sufficient to fabricate a complete integrated system. The example follows the fabrication of one simple circuit within a system; all other circuits are simultaneously implemented by the same process. The example is the basic transconductance-amplifier circuit, described in Chapter 5. The top illustration in each part of the plates shows the top view of the layers of the circuit layout. The lower illustration in each of those pictures shows the cross-section through the cut indicated by the downward arrows. (The vertical scale in these cross-sections has been greatly exaggerated for illustrative purposes.)

The first step is to create a **well** of lightly doped n-type material in the p-type substrate. An opening in the overlying oxide, as defined by the yellow mask in the top portion of Plate 1, is created as we described. Ions of arsenic, antimony, or phosphorus are implanted into the surface, and reach the silicon only where there is no oxide. After the ion-implantation step, the remaining oxide is stripped, and the wafer is placed in a high-temperature furnace with an oxygen atmosphere. The result is shown in Plate 1(a). The n-type dopant atoms have diffused deep (2 to 4 microns in present processes) into the substrate, and a new thick (typically 0.5 micron) oxide has been grown over the entire surface.

The second pattern is shown by the green outline in the top portion of Plate 1(b). This pattern is used to expose all areas that eventually will be the *active* level. It includes the sources and drains of all transistors in the circuit, together with the transistor gate areas, and any diffusion-level circuit interconnection paths. This pattern is used for the second step in the process—the patterning of silicon dioxide on silicon, as described in the previous section. The wafer is then heated while exposed to oxygen, to grow a very thin layer of *gate oxide* over its entire surface. The resulting cross-section is shown in the lower portion of Plate 1(b).

The wafer is then entirely coated with a thin layer of polycrystalline silicon, or poly. Note that the polysilicon layer is insulated everywhere from the underlying materials by the layer of thin gate oxide and, in addition, by thicker oxide in some areas. The polysilicon will form the gates of all the transistors in the circuit and will also serve as a second layer for circuit interconnections. A third mask is used to pattern the polysilicon by steps similar to those previously described, with the result shown in red in Plate 1(c). The leftmost polysilicon area will function as the gate of the p-channel transistors of the amplifier we are constructing, whereas the area to the right will function as the gate of the n-channel transistors.

Once the polysilicon areas have been defined, n-type regions can be diffused into the p-type silicon substrate, forming the sources and drains of the n-channel transistors and the first level of interconnections. We do this step by first removing the thin gate oxide in all (green) active areas not covered by the (red) polysilicon. The wafer is then overcoated with resist material; the resist material is exposed through openings in a **select** mask and is developed in the manner described previously. This patterning step is not used to mask against an etchant, but leaves openings in the resist material over selected areas that are to be turned into n-channel transistors. The actual conversion of the underlying silicon is then done through implantation of ions of arsenic or antimony into the silicon surface. The resist material, where present, acts to prevent the ions from reaching the silicon surface. Therefore, ions are implanted in only the silicon area that is free of resist.

The areas of resulting n-type material are shown in green in the cross-section of Plate 2(d). They include the sources and drains of n-channel transistors, along with any $n+$ contacts to the n-type well. Notice that the red polysilicon area and the thin oxide under it act to prevent impurities from reaching the underlying silicon. Therefore, the impurities reach the silicon substrate in only those areas not covered by either polysilicon or photoresist, and not overlain by the thick original oxide. In this way, the active transistor area is formed in all selected places where the patterned polysilicon overlies the thin oxide area defined in the previous step. The active-level sources and drains of the transistors are filled in automatically between the polysilicon areas and extend up to the edges of the thick oxide areas. The major advantage of the silicon-gate process is that it does not require a critical alignment between a mask that defines the green source and drain areas and a separate mask that defines the red gate areas. Rather, the transistors are formed by the intersection of three masks, and the conducting n-type regions are formed in all selected areas where the green mask is not covered by the red mask.

The select photoresist is now stripped, and a new layer of resist is patterned with the *complement* of the select pattern. In this way, the only exposed areas are those that are to be implanted with p-type impurities. The sources and drains of p-channel transistors, along with any $p+$ contacts to the p-type substrate, are formed by implantation of aluminum, gallium, or boron. Once again, the polysilicon prevents the implanted ions from reaching the substrate, and thus defines the self-aligned p-channel transistors. A cross-section of the wafer after this step is shown in Plate 2(e).

To allow the implanted impurities to assume their proper place in the silicon lattice we hold the wafer at a high temperature, and allow the implanted impurities to *diffuse* into the underlying silicon. For this reason, the green (active) areas not covered by poly are often referred to as **diffusion**.

All the transistors of the basic amplifier circuit are now defined. The next step is to lay down connections to the input gate, between the drains of the p- and n-channel transistors, and to V_{DD} and ground. These interconnections will be formed with a metal layer that can make contact with both the diffused areas and the polycrystalline areas. To ensure that the metal does not make contact with underlying areas except where intended, we coat the entire circuit with another layer of insulating oxide. At the places where the overlying metal is to make contact with either the polysilicon or the diffused areas, we remove the overlying oxide selectively by patterning with a **contact** mask. The result of coating the wafer with the overlying oxide and then removing the oxide in places where contacts are desired is shown in Plate 2(f). In the top view, the black areas are those defined by the contact pattern, the sixth in the process's sequence of mask patterns. In the cross-section, notice that in the contact areas all oxide has been removed down to either the polycrystalline silicon or the diffused area.

Once the overlying oxide has been patterned in this way, the entire wafer is coated with metal (usually aluminum), and the metal is patterned with a seventh (blue) mask to form the conducting areas required by the circuit. The top view in Plate 3(g) shows four short metal segments running horizontally; the left connects to V_{DD}, and the right connects to ground. Notice the well contact at the left where a small select area surrounds a contact to an active region.

There is a similar substrate contact at the right, where no select or well region surrounds the active contact. The center two metal segments connect the drains of n-channel transistors to those of their p-channel counterparts. In addition, the lower center segment connects to the gate of the p-channel current mirror. In general, it is good practice to avoid placing polysilicon contacts over an active transistor area; the design rules we present later in this appendix do not allow such contacts.

The inherent properties of the silicon-gate process allow the blue metal layer to cross either the red polysilicon layer or the green active areas, without making contact unless one is specifically provided. The red polysilicon areas, however, cannot cross the green diffused areas without forming a transistor. The transistors formed by the intersection of these two masks can be either n-channel (if they are included in an area defined by the select mask), or p-channel (if they are outside a selected area). Hence, n-channel transistors are defined by the intersection of the select, green, and red masks; p-channel transistors are defined by the intersection of only the green and red masks.

After the metal level is patterned, the wafer surface is coated with yet another layer of oxide. This step provides electrical isolation between the two levels of metal interconnect. An eighth **via** mask is then used to pattern contact cuts in this glass layer at the locations where the second metal level is to contact the first, as shown in Plate 3(h).

The second level of metal is deposited and patterned with a ninth (gray) mask much as the first-level metal was. The V_{DD} line is running vertically at the left, and the ground line is running at the right, in Plate 3(i). At this point, the circuit is perfectly functional, and no more process steps are needed. It is common practice, however, to cover the completed chip with a last layer of oxide. This step protects the circuit from random impurities in the environment, and also from mechanical abuse. A final mask is used to open areas over the second metal at the locations of the (relatively large) **bonding pads**, where contacts are made to the macroscopic outside world.

Each wafer contains many individual chips. The chips are separated using a laser beam or a diamond saw. Each individual chip is then cemented in place in a package, and fine metal wire leads are bonded from the metal contact pads on the chip to pads in the package that connect with its external pins. A cover is then cemented over the recess in the package that contains the silicon chip, and the completed system is ready for testing and use.

YIELD STATISTICS

Of the large number of individual integrated-system chips fabricated on a single silicon wafer, only a fraction will be completely functional. Flaws in the masks, dust particles on the wafer surface, defects in the underlying silicon, and so on, all cause certain devices to be less than perfect. With traditional design techniques, any single flaw of sufficient size will kill an entire chip.

The simplest model for the **yield**—the fraction of the chips fabricated that do not contain fatal flaws—assumes (naively) that the flaws are randomly distributed over the wafer and that one or more flaws anywhere on a chip will cause that chip to be nonoperative. If there are N fatal flaws per unit area, and the area of an individual chip is A, the probability that a chip has n flaws is given by the Poisson distribution, $P_n(NA)$. The probability of a chip being good is

$$P_0(NA) = e^{-NA}$$

Although this equation does not accurately represent the detailed behavior of real fabrication processes, it is a good approximate model for estimating the yield of traditional designs. The exponential is such a steep function that a simple rule is possible: Chips with areas many times $1/N$ simply never will be fabricated without flaws. We must ensure that the chip area is less than a few times $1/N$ if one flaw will kill a system. The largest permissible chips in 1988 technology were approximately 1 square centimeter in area. Design forms developed in this book can permit systems to work even in the presence of flaws. When we use such design forms, the entire notion of yield is changed completely, and we can make much larger chips, including full-wafer systems, that are totally functional.

GEOMETRIC CONSTRAINTS

Perhaps the most powerful attribute of modern wafer-fabrication processes is that they are *pattern-independent*. That is, there is a clean separation between the processing done during wafer fabrication and the design work that creates the patterns to be implemented. This separation requires that the designer be given a precise definition of the capabilities of the processing line. The specification usually takes the form of a set of permissible geometries that the designer can use with the knowledge that the geometries are within the resolution of the process itself, and that they do not violate the device physics required for proper operation of transistors and interconnections formed by the process. When reduced to their simplest form, such geometrical constraints are called **geometric design rules**. The constraints are of the form of minimum allowable values for certain *widths*, *separations*, *extensions*, and *overlaps* of geometrical objects patterned in the various levels of the process.

As processes have improved over the years, the absolute values of the permissible sizes and spacings of various layers have become progressively smaller. There is no evidence that this trend is abating. In fact, there is every reason to believe that nearly another order of magnitude of shrinkage in linear dimensions is possible. For this reason, we will present a set of design rules in dimensionless form, as constraints on the allowable ratios of certain distances to a basic length unit. The basic unit of length measurement used is equal to the fundamental resolution of the process itself; it is the distance by which a geometrical feature on any one layer may stray from another geometrical feature on the same layer or on another layer, all processing factors considered and an appropriate safety factor added. It is set by phenomena such as overetching, misalignment between mask levels, distortion of the silicon wafer due to high-temperature processing, and overexposure or underexposure of resist. All dimensions are given in terms of this elementary distance unit, which we call the **length-unit** λ. In 1988, the length-unit for typical commercial processes is slightly less than 1 micron (written μm or simply μ); 1 micron is equal to 10^{-6} meter.

Geometric Design Rules

The rules we will discuss have been abstracted from a number of processes over a range of values of λ, corresponding to different points in time at different fabrication areas. They represent somewhat of a "least common denominator" likely to be representative of CMOS design rules for a reasonable time, as the value of λ decreases in the future. These rules were developed by the author and Richard Lyon in collaboration with other groups, in an effort coordinated by George Lewicki of the MOSIS organization [MOSIS, 1981].

Active layer A typical minimum for the line width of the diffused regions is $3\ \lambda$, as shown in Plate 4(a). The spacing required between two electrically separate active regions is a parameter that depends on not merely the geometric resolution of the process, but also the physics of the devices formed. If two diffused regions are spaced too closely, the depletion layers, associated with the junctions formed by these regions may overlap, resulting in a current flowing between the two regions when none was intended. In typical processes, a safe rule of thumb is to allow $3\ \lambda$ of separation between any two diffused regions that are unconnected, as show in Plate 4(b). The width of a depletion layer associated with any diffused region depends on the voltage on that region. If one of the regions is at ground potential, its depletion layer will of necessity be quite thin. In addition, some processes provide a heavier doping level at the surface of the wafer between the diffused areas in order to alleviate the problem of overlap of depletion layers.

Polysilicon layer The minimum for width of polysilicon lines is $2\ \lambda$. No depletion layers are associated with polysilicon lines, and therefore the separation of two such lines may be as little as $2\ \lambda$. These rules are illustrated in Plate 4 (c) and (d).

Polysilicon and active layers We have so far considered the diffused and polysilicon layers separately. Another type of design rule concerns how these two layers interact with each other. Plate 4(e) shows a diffused line running parallel to an independent polysilicon line, to which it is not connected at any point. The only requirement here is that the two unconnected lines not overlap. If they did, they would form an unwanted capacitor. Avoidance of this overlap requires a separation of only $1\ \lambda$ between the two regions, as shown in Plate 4(e). A slightly more complex situation is shown in Plate 4(f); here, a polysilicon gate area intentionally crosses a diffused area, thereby forming a transistor. So that the diffused region does not reach around the end of the gate and short-circuit the drain-to-source path of the transistor with a thin diffused area, the polysilicon gate must extend a distance of at least 2 λ beyond the nominal boundary of the diffused area. This gate-overlap rule is shown in Plate 4(f). It applies to both p- and n-channel transistors. There is no formal rule for the minimum channel length of a transistor, apart from the minimum width of the poly line that forms its gate. For analog circuits, however, we will normally use channel lengths considerably longer than the 2 λ minimum. The choice of channel length is a tradeoff between increased area and more ideal and repeatable transistor characteristics. A detailed discussion of the dependence of the transistor drain conductance on channel length is given in Appendix B.

Note that the minimum width for a diffused region applies to diffused regions formed between a normal boundary of the diffused region and an edge of a transistor, as well as to a diffused line formed by two normal boundaries.

Metal 1   Now we will consider the design rules for the metal layer. Notice that this layer in general runs over much more rugged terrain than does any other level; see the cross-section of Plate 3(g). For this reason, it is generally accepted practice to allow somewhat wider minimum lines and spaces for the metal layer than are allowed for the other layers. A good working rule is to provide widths and separations of 3 λ between independent metal lines, as shown in Plate 4 (g) and (h).

Metal 2   The comments concerning rugged terrain that we made with respect to the first metal layer apply with even more force to the design rules for the second metal layer, as we can see by referring to the cross-section of Plate 3(i). For this reason, it is generally accepted practice to allow a somewhat wider minimum space for the second metal layer than is allowed for the first. A good working rule is to provide widths of 3 λ and separations of 4 λ between independent metal-2 lines, as shown in Plate 4 (i) and (j).

Contacts   We can form a contact between the metal layer and either the diffused level or the polysilicon level by using the contact mask. A set of rules delimit the amount by which each layer must provide an area surrounding any contact to it, so that the contact opening will not find its way around the layer to something unintended below it. The physical factors that apply here are the relative registration of three levels. Our simple set of design rules, which requires that the level involved in a given contact must extend beyond the outer boundary of the contact cut by 2 λ at all points, is illustrated in Plate 5 (a) and (b). More compact rules are possible, but involve many special cases. The contacts themselves, like the minimum-width lines in the other levels, must be exactly 2 λ square. The use of fixed-size contact cuts greatly improves processing uniformity. Contact between a large metal region and a large diffused or poly region is made with many small contacts spaced 2 λ apart, as shown in Plate 5(c).

The metal layer must surround the contact layer in much the same way that the diffused and polysilicon layers did. Because the resist material used for patterning the metal generally accumulates in the low areas of the wafer, it tends to be thicker in the neighborhood of a contact than it is elsewhere. For this reason, metal tends to align itself to the contact, and it is generally sufficient for the metal to surround the contact by only 1 λ.

Contact cuts to diffusion should be at least 2 λ from the nearest gate region, as shown in Plate 5(d). Similarly, contact cuts to poly should be at least 2 λ from the nearest active region, as shown in Plate 5(d). There is an internal consistency in the rules shown, which is easy to lose if more complex special cases are spelled out. When two minimum-sized contacts, such as those shown in Plate 5 (a) and (b), are spaced as close as possible according to the poly–diffusion rule of Plate 4(e), the metal-to-metal spacing rule of Plate 5(a) will be satisfied automatically. Similarly, when a minimum-sized poly contact, such as that shown in Plate 5(b), is spaced as close to an active region as possible according to the poly–diffusion rule of Plate 4(e), the poly-contact-to-active-spacing rule of Plate 5(d) will be satisfied automatically.

Note that a cut down to the polysilicon level does not penetrate the polysilicon. Thus, we can, in principle, make a contact cut to poly over a gate region. Such contacts are not permitted in our design rules.

Via   We form a contact between the first and second metal layers by using the **via** mask. A set of rules dictate the amount by which each layer must surround the via. As before, the physical factors that apply here are the relative registration of three levels. We use a simple set of design rules, which requires that both levels involved surround the outer boundary of the contact cut by 1 λ at all points, as illustrated in Plate 5(e). The vias themselves, like ordinary contacts to other levels, must be exactly 2 λ long and 2 λ wide.

When contact is made from a large metal-2 region to a large metal-1 region, many small vias spaced 3 λ apart should be used, as shown in Plate 5(f). Via contacts must penetrate a thick layer of deposited oxide, and must stop when they reach the metal layer to which they make contact. Processing is much more reliable if the metal region to which a via is made is on a flat surface. That flat surface can be over a poly or active region, over a transistor, or merely on top of the thick oxide. In the fabrication example of Plates 1 through 3, the V_{DD} contact is over thick oxide, whereas the ground contact is over diffusion. To ensure flatness of the underlying metal, we should place vias at least 2 λ from the nearest poly or active edge, as shown in Plate 5(g).

Well   The well is a lightly doped, deep diffusion. A well region forms a junction with the underlying silicon-crystal substrate. On some occasions, the well is not used in a conventional manner; normally, however, it is used to contain the p-type transistors. Several rules associated with the well are shown in Plate 6. Wells that must be electrically isolated must be spaced 10 λ apart. A p-type active region inside the well must be at least 5 λ from the edge of the well. For an n-type region outside the well to be electrically isolated from the well, it must be spaced from the well by at least 5 λ.

Select   Active regions within a select region are n-type; those outside a select region are p-type. The basic rule is that the select boundary should be at least 2 λ from the active region. This rule ensures that no active area will be ambivalent about its type. Where an active region crosses a select boundary, a diode is (or may be) formed. We cannot assume that this diode has any particular characteristics. Such diodes are allowed only if they are shorted. Two examples of shorted diodes are shown in Plate 6.

Well contacts   Because the well is lightly doped, a contact to it will not automatically form a good electrical connection. For that reason, a patch of $n+$ diffused region is placed in the well, and a contact is made to the $n+$ region. If a select area surrounds the $n+$ patch by 2 λ, there is no constraint on where it can be placed; it is like any other n-type active area in the substrate. However, if we are to ensure that the patch contacts the well, it must overlap the well by at least 4 λ. We can form another type of well contact, also shown in Plate 6, by extending an existing active region, and surrounding the extension with select. If the active region is 5 λ inside the well, there is no hazard concerning part of the region not covered by select. We require only that the *contact-cut itself* be surrounded by 2 λ of select.

Substrate contacts   As is true of the well, we cannot ensure electrical connection to the substrate by simply placing a contact on the naked silicon surface. Instead, we place a $p+$ patch in the p-type substrate, and make a contact to the patch. Two kinds of substrate contact are shown in Plate 6. The most straightforward contact is formed by an active area spaced 2 λ from the select edge. The second form is made using a shorted diode. As is true of the well contact, the contact-cut itself, but not the entire active area, must be 2 λ outside the select.

Generic Rules

The design rules we have presented will not exactly match those of any specific process at any given value of λ. For that reason, the layout artwork representing a design usually is subjected to several *sizing operations*, in which the patterns representing individual layers are expanded or shrunk to fit the constraints of the target process as closely as possible. This operation allows many different vendors to fabricate a design with minimal area penalty. These sizing operations are not part of the design itself, but rather are part of the interface between the designer and the fabrication vendor. The best current example of such an interface is the MOSIS system [MOSIS, 1981].

We have used an n-well process to illustrate how a fabrication process is carried out, and to describe the constraints enforced by the design rules. A simple interchange of p- and n-type regions will result in a p-well process. In fact, designs done with the layers we have described can be fabricated equally well in either p- or n-well processes. From the designer's point of view, it is not necessary to know which process will be (or has been) used until the finished parts are returned from fabrication. The only difference the type of process makes is that the power supply for n-well parts will be positive, whereas that for p-well parts will be negative. The same convention holds for signal levels. The chips described in this book have been fabricated successfully in both p- and n-well technologies, with λ values ranging from 0.6 to 2.5 microns.

Our design rules are likely to remain valid as the length-unit λ scales down with the passage of time. Occasionally, for specific commercial fabrication processes, some one or more of these rules may be relaxed, or may be replaced by more complex rules, enabling slight reductions in the area of a system. Although these details may be important for competitive commercial products, they have the disadvantage of making the system design a captive of the specific design rules of the process. Extensive redesign and checking is required to scale down a system design as the length-unit scales down. For this reason, we recommend use of the dimensionless rules we have presented, especially for prototype items. Designs implemented according to these rules are easy to scale, and may have reasonable longevity.

REFERENCES

MOS Implementation System (MOSIS) User's Manual. Marina Del Rey, CA: USC Information Sciences Institute, 1981.

FINE POINTS OF TRANSISTOR PHYSICS

Mary Ann Maher   Carver Mead

In Chapter 3, we derived the behavior of an MOS transistor operating in the subthreshold region. There we gave the most abbreviated analysis that could explain how the drain current I was related to the gate, source, and drain voltages. We will now revisit the basic electrostatics of the device, first in the subthreshold region, where the mobile charge q_m per unit area in the channel is much smaller than the depletion charge in the substrate (Figure B.1). This treatment will allow us to understand the interaction of the surface potential of the channel with the substrate potential, an effect that we previously lumped into the constant κ that expressed the effectiveness of the gate in determining the surface potential. We will derive an expression for κ, and for the gate voltage required to produce a given drain current as the source voltage V_s is changed. We also will analyze how the drain current in saturation increases with increasing drain voltage, as a result of the channel-length shortening by the drain depletion layer.

We then will examine the general solution for current flow in the channel, including the effect of mobile charge on the electrostatics, and the effect of carrier velocity saturation at high electric fields along the channel.

Portions reprinted with permission from Maher, M. and Mead, C., A physical charge-controlled model for MOS transistors. Copyright © 1987, *Advanced Research in VLSI*. Proceedings of the 1987 Stanford Conference, edited by Losleben, P., Cambridge, MA: MIT Press.

The general problem is difficult because the surface potential depends on mobile-charge density through the electrostatics, the mobile-charge density depends on surface potential through the current-flow equations, and the boundary conditions on the mobile-charge density depend on surface potential through the Fermi distribution. This cycle of dependency is broken in the subthreshold range, because the mobile charge can be neglected in the electrostatics.

The experimental data presented in this chapter were taken on a set of transistors with several channel lengths, down to 0.7 micron. These devices were fabricated with an advanced process (by 1988 standards), and have a gate-oxide thickness of 125 angstroms.

SUBTHRESHOLD OPERATION

Throughout this book, we have adopted an approximation in which the surface potential is affected by the substrate ("bulk") potential; we have defined a constant κ such that, in the region of operation, the surface potential ψ is related to the gate voltage V_g by

$$\kappa = \frac{\partial \psi}{\partial V_g}$$

We will now treat the subthreshold transistor in more detail, derive an expression for κ, and predict how the gate–source voltage V_{gs} required to produce a given drain current depends on the source voltage V_s.

Electrostatics

In the subthreshold region, the mobile charge q_m per unit area is much smaller than is the depletion charge in the substrate. We therefore neglect the effect of mobile charge on the electrostatics of the device. In this way, we can calculate the energy barriers at source and drain from the terminal potentials relative to substrate, and we can use those barrier energies to determine the boundary conditions on the current-flow equations.

The energy diagram of a cross-section through the channel region of an n-channel MOS transistor[1] is shown in Figure B.1. We assume that the substrate is uniformly doped with N_A acceptors per unit volume; hence, the depletion layer contains a constant charge density per unit volume $\rho = qN_A$. In our coordinate system, x is measured perpendicular to the surface, with $x = 0$ at the substrate edge of the depletion layer. By simple application of Gauss' law, we know that the electric field at any x is equal to the total charge per unit area between the edge of the depletion layer ($x = 0$) and the point x, divided by ϵ_s, the permittivity of the silicon. We obtain the surface potential ψ by integrating this electric field

---

[1] An excellent background reference for the material in this chapter is presented by Grove [Grove, 1967].

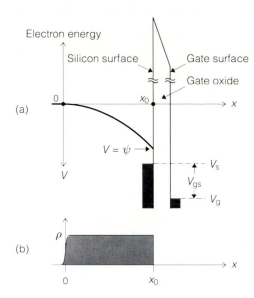

(a)

(b)

FIGURE B.1 Energy diagram of a cross-section through an *n*-channel MOS transistor. The cross-section runs normal to the surface through the potential maximum. The positive gate voltage repels holes from the semiconductor surface, and electric-field lines terminate on uncovered fixed-dopant ions creating a depletion layer. (a) The potential variation caused by the electric field. The zero of potential is the potential deep in the bulk, where the electric field is zero. (b) The charge distribution of uncovered dopant atoms.

from $x = 0$ to the surface ($x = x_0$):

$$\psi = -\frac{1}{\epsilon_s}\frac{\rho x_0^2}{2} \tag{B.1}$$

To take the charge in the substrate into account, we will henceforth use the potential deep in the substrate as the reference for the surface potential. Using this convention, the surface potential ψ is zero when the potential is flat all the way to the interface. For any value of surface potential, Equation B.1 gives the depletion-layer thickness. The total charge per unit area Q_{dep} in the depletion layer is this thickness times the bulk charge density ρ:

$$Q_{\text{dep}} = \rho x_0 = \pm\sqrt{-2\rho\epsilon_s\psi} \tag{B.2}$$

This expression allows us to define a **depletion-layer capacitance** C_{dep}:

$$C_{\text{dep}} = -\frac{\partial Q_{\text{dep}}}{\partial \psi} = \sqrt{-\frac{\rho\epsilon_s}{2\psi}} = \frac{\epsilon_s}{x_0} \tag{B.3}$$

The applied gate voltage appears partially across the gate oxide and partially across the silicon substrate. The voltage across the gate oxide is the oxide electric field times the oxide thickness t_{ox}. The electric field is just the total depletion-layer charge Q_{dep} divided by ϵ_{ox}:

$$V_{\text{g}} = \psi - \frac{t_{\text{ox}}}{\epsilon_{\text{ox}}}Q_{\text{dep}} = \psi + \frac{1}{C_{\text{ox}}}\sqrt{-2\rho\epsilon_s\psi} \tag{B.4}$$

where $C_{\text{ox}} = \epsilon_{\text{ox}}/t_{\text{ox}}$ is the oxide capacitance per unit area. Because the gate and substrate are made of differently doped materials, a built-in potential Φ_{ms} exists between them with zero applied gate voltage [Grove, 1967]. Equation B.4 also assumes that there is no charge at the surface. The silicon-oxide interface often has a fixed charge associated with it; in addition, process technologists implant a fixed concentration of charged impurities very near the interface to shift the gate voltage required for a given current. We take into account the fixed charge Q_{ss} and the built-in potential by adding the term $V_{fb} = \Phi_{ms} - Q_{ss}/C_{ox}$ to V_g. When $V_g = V_{fb}$, the surface potential is equal to zero and hence V_{fb} is called the **flat-band voltage**.

$$V_g = \psi + V_{fb} - \frac{1}{C_{ox}}Q_{dep} \tag{B.5}$$

For small changes in voltage around some operating point, we can derive the dependence of surface potential on gate voltage, and hence can derive an explicit expression for κ. Differentiating Equation B.5 with respect to ψ, we obtain

$$\frac{1}{\kappa} = \frac{\partial V_g}{\partial \psi} = 1 + \frac{1}{C_{ox}}\sqrt{-\frac{\rho\epsilon_s}{2\psi}}$$

We notice that, as the doping approaches zero, κ approaches unity; it is this limit that formed the basis for our conceptual discussion in Chapter 3. We also observe that κ is inversely related to the doping. For a highly doped substrate, more ions per unit depletion width are available to be uncovered, and the depletion width is shorter. As a result, the capacitance C_{dep} is greater and the current increases with gate voltage less rapidly than it does for a lightly doped substrate.

Current Flow

In a subthreshold MOS transistor, the current flow I from source to drain is due to the diffusion of carriers. From Equations 2.8 (p. 22) and 2.10 (p. 23),

$$I = -wqD\frac{\partial N}{\partial z}$$

where w is the transistor width, D is the diffusion constant, and N is the density of carriers in the channel. Because no carriers are lost on their journey from source to drain, N decreases linearly with distance z along the channel ($z = 0$ at the source):

$$I = -wqD\frac{N_d - N_s}{l} \tag{B.6}$$

where N_s and N_d are the density of carriers at the source and drain, respectively, and l is the channel length. The boundary conditions, N_s and N_d, are generated by the Boltzmann distribution, as described in Equations 3.4 (p. 35) and 3.5 (p. 35). We no longer make the approximation that the gate voltage is 100 percent effective in determining the surface potential. We assume that the surface potential does not vary along the channel, and use the surface potential at the source ψ_s in place of V_g in Equations 3.6 (p. 35) and 3.7 (p. 35).

$$N_s = N_1 e^{\frac{-q\psi_s}{kT}} e^{\frac{qV_s}{kT}} \tag{B.7}$$

$$N_d = N_1 e^{\frac{-q\psi_s}{kT}} e^{\frac{qV_d}{kT}} \tag{B.8}$$

where N_0 is the effective number of states per unit area in the channel and $N_1 = N_0 e^{-\phi_0/(kT)}$. The boundary conditions N_s and N_d actually apply at the boundaries where the channel meets the source and drain depletion layers. Because the bulk and gate potentials are constant along the channel, the fact that the mobile charge can be neglected compared with the gate and bulk charges implies that the surface potential is constant along the channel. This self-consistent set of conditions define the **subthreshold** regime of operation. Because there is no electric field *along* the channel, current cannot flow by drift; hence, diffusion must be the dominant current-flow mechanism. Applying the boundary conditions of Equations B.7 and B.8 to Equation B.6, we obtain

$$I = \frac{qw}{l} N_1 D e^{\frac{-q\psi_s}{kT}} \left(e^{\frac{qV_s}{kT}} - e^{\frac{qV_d}{kT}} \right) \tag{B.9}$$

If we absorb the preexponential factors into a constant I_0, and assume that for small excursions around the particular operating point ψ_0, $\psi_s = \psi_0 + \kappa V_g$, Equation B.9 becomes

$$I = I_0 e^{\frac{-q\kappa V_g}{kT}} \left(e^{\frac{qV_s}{kT}} - e^{\frac{qV_d}{kT}} \right)$$

We must remember that all voltages are referenced to the bulk voltage. Defining $V_{ds} = V_d - V_s$, we obtain a working form for the current:

$$I = I_0 e^{\frac{-q\kappa V_g}{kT}} e^{\frac{qV_s}{kT}} \left(1 - e^{\frac{qV_{ds}}{kT}} \right) \tag{B.10}$$

We notice that κ appears in the gate-voltage term, but not in the terms containing the source and drain potentials.

Drain Conductance

In the preceding discussion, we treated the channel length l as a constant. In reality, l is determined by the distance between the depletion regions surrounding the source and drain. The widths of these regions are functions of the source-to-substrate and drain-to-substrate biases. The width of the drain depletion layer increases with drain voltage, thereby decreasing the channel length. This decrease in channel length increases the gradient of carrier density, and therefore increases the channel current. This increase in channel current due to channel-length modulation is called the **Early effect**, after Jim Early, who first analyzed it in bipolar transistors [Early, 1952]. Because the dependence of I on l is explicit in Equation B.9, we can solve directly for the drain conductance g_d of the transistor in saturation:

$$\frac{\partial I}{\partial V_d} = g_d = \frac{\partial I}{\partial l}\frac{\partial l}{\partial V_d}$$

Because the current in Equation B.10 is inversely proportional to l,

$$g_d = -\frac{I}{l}\frac{\partial l}{\partial V_d} \tag{B.11}$$

Thus, the drain conductance g_d (which manifests itself as a nonzero slope on the drain characteristic-curves for large V_d) is proportional to $I \approx I_{sat}$ and is inversely proportional to l.

For hand calculations, we can approximate the derivative in Equation B.11 by

$$\frac{1}{l}\frac{\partial l}{\partial V_d} \approx -\frac{1}{V_0} \tag{B.12}$$

where V_0 is taken to be a constant for a given process and for a given transistor length. Because the conductance is proportional to the drain current, in this approximation the extrapolated drain curves all intersect the voltage axis at a single point, which is $-V_0$.

Taking the drain conductance into account, our equation for the current becomes

$$I = I_0\, e^{\frac{-q\kappa V_g}{kT}}\, e^{\frac{qV_s}{kT}} \left(1 - e^{\frac{qV_{ds}}{kT}}\right) + g_d V_{ds}$$

where we have used the approximation $g_d \Delta V_d \approx g_d \Delta V_{ds}$. In the V_0 approximation,

$$I = I_0\, e^{\frac{-q\kappa V_g}{kT}}\, e^{\frac{qV_s}{kT}} \left(1 - e^{\frac{qV_{ds}}{kT}} + \frac{V_{ds}}{V_0}\right) \tag{B.13}$$

For transistors in saturation, with a given voltage on their gates, Equation B.13 reduces to the following simple dependence on V_0, and therefore on l:

$$I = \text{constant} \left(1 + \frac{V_{ds}}{V_0}\right)$$

This functional form can represent the behavior of real transistors surprisingly well, as we can see in Figure B.2. The product of the drain current and the channel length for each transistor is a nearly straight line. Furthermore, within the voltage offsets among the transistors, all these lines extrapolate to a single value for $V_{ds} = 0$. From Equation B.12, the value of V_0 should be directly proportional to the channel length l. This dependence can be seen in Figure B.3.

Because the mobile charge is small in subthreshold devices, the voltage–current relationships are relatively simple. When high gate voltages induce large charge densities in the channel, the entire problem becomes more difficult. Before we undertake the general analysis of the transistor, we will consider one more effect that can be analyzed in the subthreshold region.

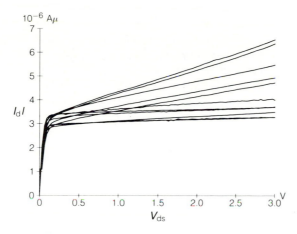

FIGURE B.2   The product of saturation current and channel length in microns is plotted versus drain–source voltage for transistors in subthreshold (V_g = 0.5 volt). Transistor lengths varied from 0.7 to 50 microns. All devices were measured on the same die, with gate-oxide thickness of 125 angstroms. Channel length was determined by comparing low-field conductance with a long-channel device.

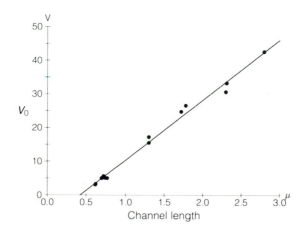

FIGURE B.3 V_0 versus channel length for the devices of Figure B.2. We determined V_0 by extrapolating the least-squares fit to the drain conductance to the x axis. Longer devices have larger V_0 and hence higher drain resistance. This result can be seen in Figure B.2, where the slopes of the current versus voltage plots are higher for shorter devices.

BODY EFFECT

We can see from the expressions for drain current given in the previous section that the gate voltage has less effect on the current flow than does the source voltage. As we increase the source voltage, we must increase the gate voltage even more to keep the current constant. We must deplete more charge in the substrate to lower the barrier energy (make the channel potential more positive). That additional charge increases the electric field in the gate oxide, and thus increases the voltage across the gate oxide. This increase in the gate–source voltage required to maintain the same current as we increase the source voltage is called the **body effect** (also known as the *bulk effect* or the *back-gate effect*). Equation B.10 is based on the approximation of constant κ that we derive by linearizing the surface potential about the operating point.

For any given current, there must be a certain charge in the channel. Whether the mobile charge is large or small compared with the bulk charge, it will be constant if the current is held constant. Hence, for computing the change in gate voltage required to keep the current constant as the source voltage is increased, the charge in the channel can, to first order, be ignored. The total effect is thus captured in Equation B.5, for operation either above or below threshold. The gate–source voltage required would be constant if the square-root term in Equation B.5 were zero. Hence, that term represents the body effect directly. The effect usually is expressed in terms of the increase in threshold voltage of the transistor with source voltage, but, as we have seen, it applies equally well to any level of current flowing in the transistor. From Equation B.5, the increase in gate voltage is proportional to the square root of the surface potential ψ, which, for a given current, is a constant $\Delta\psi$ above the source voltage:

$$V_g = V_s + \Delta\psi + V_{fb} + \frac{1}{C_{ox}}\sqrt{-2\rho\epsilon_s(V_s + \Delta\psi)}$$

$$= V_s + \Delta\psi + V_{fb} + \gamma\sqrt{V_s + \Delta\psi}$$

where $\gamma = \sqrt{-2\rho\epsilon_s}/C_{ox}$ often is called the back-gate coefficient, and γ is a

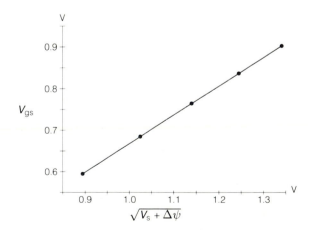

FIGURE B.4   Determination of substrate doping. Gate–source voltage is plotted versus $\sqrt{V_s + \Delta\psi}$, for a fixed current level. The slope of the line is proportional to the doping density. Using a value of 125 angstroms for the oxide thickness, we determined the density ρ to be 10^{17} per cubic centimeter.

function of the doping density, as a result of the quantity of charge that must be depleted in the substrate or "body" to lower the energy barrier. The most instructive way to evaluate the effect in a real transistor is to plot V_{gs} as a function of $\sqrt{V_s + \Delta\psi}$, for a fixed current level. The result is a straight line, as shown in Figure B.4. The slope of the line is γ.

THE GENERAL MOS MODEL

We will now undertake the derivation of the current flow in an MOS transistor for arbitrary voltages on its terminals. The model we will develop is valid above or below threshold, in saturation or in the "ohmic" (low V_{ds}) range. It takes into account the finite velocity attained by carriers as they are accelerated in very high electric fields (velocity saturation).

We shall begin by obtaining the channel current for a transistor in saturation. We define **saturation** as the region of operation in which, except for the Early effect, the channel current is not a function of drain voltage V_d. This condition is equivalent to the assumption that the mobile charge at the drain is moving at the saturated velocity v_0. Our strategy is to choose a value for the mobile charge q_m per unit area at the barrier maximum near the source. This value q_s is the integral, from the surface potential at the source end of the channel ψ_s up to infinite energy, of the Fermi distribution in the source times the density of states in the channel region. Given the source potential V_s, we can compute ψ_s for a given q_s by inverting this integration. Once we know ψ_s, we can compute the depletion layer width x_0 from strictly electrostatic considerations, because we know the bulk charge density ρ. Given x_0 and q_s, we can compute the gate potential V_g.

We can obtain the channel current I by integrating the current-flow equations from one end of the channel to the other, using q_s as a boundary condition. Thus, for each choice of mobile-charge density, we can compute separately the gate voltage and the corresponding channel current.

The more detailed treatment of the transistor when it is not in saturation is an extension of the saturation case where q_d, the mobile charge density at the drain end of the channel, is set not by velocity saturation, but rather by a boundary condition involving the drain voltage. Using this condition, we can build a complete model for the transistor, covering all regimes of operation. The characteristics are completely continuous above and below threshold, in saturation or otherwise.

We will first derive a complete closed-form solution for the transistor, assuming that the channel length and the mobility are constant for a given device. In a more complete treatment, these restrictions are not required [Maher et al., 1987]. This analysis takes into account all the effects of mobile-carrier–velocity saturation. The channel-length modulation (Early effect) is treated as a perturbation on the zero-order model. An excellent review of these and other effects is given by Tsividis [Tsividis, 1987].

Electrostatics

The actual electrostatics of the MOS device are extremely complicated, as they involve three independent potentials (source, drain, and gate) relative to the substrate. To simplify the problem, we observe that the current through the channel is always controlled by the point along the channel where the potential barrier is maximum. For sufficiently large l, this point is near the source except when the voltage drop along the channel is near zero. Conditions on either side of this maximum point become progressively less important in determining the current. Because the potential is a maximum, the variation of any quantity of interest in the direction parallel to the surface will be zero; therefore, we can determine the solution normal to the channel by using a one-dimensional analysis. The approximation used throughout this chapter is to extend the conditions found from this one-dimensional solution toward the drain until the drain depletion layer is encountered. This approach factors an otherwise intractable problem into simpler subproblems that can be solved separately.

The mobile charge is quantum-mechanically distributed over some depth, but we will assume that it is all located at the surface. Under this approximation, conditions in the bulk are not affected by the presence of mobile charge at the surface; thus, all the expressions derived in our subthreshold electrostatics analysis are valid, except those for the gate voltage. The voltage across the gate oxide is the oxide electric field times the oxide thickness t_{ox}. The electric field is proportional to the total charge to the left of the oxide, which is the depletion layer charge Q_{dep} plus the mobile charge per unit area q_m. We thus can extend Equation B.4 to take into account the mobile charge:

$$V_g = \psi + V_{fb} - \frac{1}{C_{ox}}(Q_{dep} + q_m)$$

(B.14)

The mobile-charge density q_m is a smooth function of the position z along the channel. The surface potential ψ is dependent on q_m; hence, both ψ and Q_{dep} will be functions of z as well. The gate, however, is an equipotential surface, so V_g is independent of z. Solving Equation B.14 for q_m, we obtain

$$-q_m = C_{ox}(V_g - \psi - V_{fb}) + Q_{dep}$$

(B.15)

In subthreshold, the gate voltage follows the surface potential, because the mobile charge can be neglected. Above threshold, however, the surface potential changes little, and most of the new electric-field lines from the gate terminate on mobile charges. These relationships are shown in Figure B.5.

We can relate ψ to q_m by defining an **effective channel capacitance** C per unit area. This quantity represents the additional mobile charge that must be injected into the channel per unit increase in surface potential. Differentiating Equation B.15 with respect to ψ, and applying Equation B.3, we obtain

$$C = \frac{\partial q_m}{\partial \psi} = (C_{ox} + C_{dep})$$

(B.16)

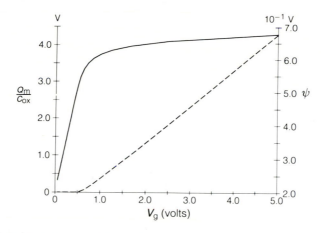

FIGURE B.5 Contributions of the surface-potential ψ (solid line) and of the mobile-charge Q_m/C_{ox} (dashed line) terms to the gate voltage as expressed in Equation B.14. In subthreshold, the gate voltage follows the surface potential, because the mobile charge is negligible. Above threshold, the major contribution to the change in gate voltage is the mobile charge.

Intuitively, the mobile charge is fixed by a boundary condition at the source. As it flows through the channel, there is a fixed relation between mobile charge and surface potential, given by Equation B.15. Thus, the presence of mobile charge creates an electric field E along the channel. The **thermal charge** $Q_T = CkT/q$ is the mobile charge per unit area required to change the surface potential by exactly kT/q.

Source Boundary Condition

The mobile charge per unit area q_m in the channel region is a function of the distance z along the channel. At the barrier maximum just into the channel from the source ($z = 0$), the boundary condition on the mobile-charge density q_s at the source end of the channel is given by the integral with respect to the energy $\mathcal{E}$ of the carrier density in the source region (a Fermi distribution), times the two-dimensional density of states $N(\mathcal{E})$ (number per unit area, per unit energy) in the channel:

$$q_s = q \int_{q\psi_s + \phi_0 - qV_s}^{\infty} \left(N(\mathcal{E}) \frac{1}{e^{\mathcal{E}/(kT)} + 1} \right) d\mathcal{E}$$

where ψ_s is the surface potential at the barrier maximum just into the channel from the source, and V_s is the source voltage.

For any realizable bias conditions, even for submicron devices, the source Fermi level is always many kT below the surface potential at the barrier maximum. The treatment we applied in the subthreshold case, where the Fermi function is replaced by a Boltzmann approximation, is thus valid. The resulting expression can be written as

$$q_s = qN_0 e^{(-q\psi_s - \phi_0 + qV_s)/(kT)} \tag{B.17}$$

where N_0, the effective density of states in the channel, is given by

$$N_0 = \int_{q\psi_s + \phi_0 - qV_s}^{\infty} N(\mathcal{E})e^{-\mathcal{E}/(kT)}\,d\mathcal{E}$$

For a real channel, the form of $N(\mathcal{E})$ is not known; thus, we cannot compute N_0 with confidence. The spacing of the energy levels in the channel will be a function of the electric field at the surface and hence $N(\mathcal{E})$ will be proportional to $1/\sqrt{\psi}$, a slow dependence which we neglect compared with the exponential due to the Boltzmann function. As long as we have the value of N_0 in the right general order of magnitude, however, the effect of an error in the preexponential factor is easily masked by small changes in surface potential.

Solving Equation B.17 for ψ_s, we obtain

$$-\frac{\phi_0}{q} + V_s - \psi_s = \frac{kT}{q} \ln\left(\frac{q_s}{qN_0}\right) \tag{B.18}$$

We thus can compute the surface potential for any mobile-charge density from Equation B.18. Given the surface potential, the gate voltage can be determined from Equation B.14, as described.

Channel Current

Given the boundary conditions on mobile-charge density and surface potential at the source, we can evaluate the channel current I. The current in the channel can be dominated by diffusion under some circumstances; in other regimes of operation, the same transistor may have drift velocities near saturation over the entire length of the channel. We will approximate the current flow by a drift and a diffusion term, and will include the effects of velocity saturation in the drift term:

$$\frac{I}{w} = q_m v_{\text{drift}} - D\frac{\partial q_m}{\partial z} \tag{B.19}$$

where w is the width of the channel. The detailed functional form of drift velocity in the channel is not known with certainty. We adopt a simple relation that has the proper behavior at both high and low fields [Hoeneisen et al., 1972b]:

$$v_{\text{drift}} = v_0\left(\frac{\mu E}{v_0 + \mu E}\right)$$

where E is the electric field along the channel, and v_0 is the carrier saturated velocity [Jacoboni et al., 1977].

We now introduce an approximation with which we can, for any particular operating point, evaluate Equation B.19 in closed form. As devices scale to smaller channel lengths and correspondingly thinner oxides, the effective channel capacitance C defined in Equation B.16 between the mobile charge and the bulk and gate (fixed potentials) becomes less dependent on the mobile-charge density q_m. In what follows, we assume C (and hence Q_T) is independent of z. Even at a channel length l of 3 microns, the error in current due to this assumption is only about 10 percent, and it decreases rapidly for shorter channel lengths. This approximation allows us to define a set of natural units, which we will use throughout the rest of this chapter:

$$
\begin{array}{ll}
\text{velocity} & v_0 \\[4pt]
\text{energy} & kT \\[4pt]
\text{voltage} & \dfrac{kT}{q} \\[8pt]
\text{charge} & Q_T = \dfrac{kT}{q}C \\[8pt]
\text{current} & v_0 Q_T \\[8pt]
\text{length} & l_0 = \dfrac{D}{v_0} = \dfrac{\mu kT}{q v_0}
\end{array}
$$

All these units are intuitive except for the length unit l_0, which we can think of, in loose terms, as the mean free path of the carrier. By expressing all quantities in the problem in terms of these natural units, we simplify all equations into a dimensionless form that allows us to discern easily the natural relationships and regimes of operation.

In the following analysis, we compute all currents for a channel of unit width. We use Q for the dimensionless form of the mobile-charge density q_m. Because we know that

$$
\frac{\partial q_m}{\partial z} = \frac{\partial q_m}{\partial \psi} \frac{\partial \psi}{\partial z} = CE
$$

we can write Equation B.19 (in dimensionless form)

$$
I = \frac{QQ'}{Q'+1} + Q'
$$

$$
I(Q'+1) = QQ' + Q'(Q'+1) \tag{B.20}
$$

where the prime indicates derivative with respect to z, the distance along the channel.

The first term on the right-hand side of Equation B.20 is the drift term, and the second is the diffusion term. The shortest channel length for which a device can be made to operate is still much larger than is the mean-free path of a

carrier, so velocity saturation is not achieved for the diffusion process. We therefore assume that the Q'^2 term is negligible compared with either the QQ' term
(when Q is large) or the Q' term (when Q is small). This approximation is excellent as long as l_0 is much less than the device dimensions. For a typical n-channel
process, l_0 is about 0.007 micron. We thus can write Equation B.20 as

$$I(Q' + 1) \cong QQ' + Q' = Q'(Q + 1)$$

or as

$$I = QQ' - Q'(1 - I) = \frac{\partial}{\partial z}\left(\frac{Q^2}{2} + Q(1 - I)\right) \tag{B.21}$$

We now integrate both sides of Equation B.21 along the channel from source
$(z = 0)$ to drain $(z = l)$, noting that I is not a function of z:

$$Il = \frac{Q_s^2 - Q_d^2}{2} + (Q_s - Q_d)(1 - I) \tag{B.22}$$

Solving Equation B.22 explicitly for I gives

$$I = \frac{Q_s - Q_d}{Q_s - Q_d + l}\left(\frac{Q_s + Q_d}{2} + 1\right) \tag{B.23}$$

We can gain a number of important insights into the operation of MOS
devices from these equations. Tracing through the derivation, we see that the
quadratic term in Equation B.22 is a result of the drift term in Equation B.19,
and the linear term is a result of the diffusion term in Equation B.19. The
two terms make approximately equal contributions to the saturation current for
$q_s = Q_T$, in natural units $Q_s = 1$. The gate voltage at which Q_s is equal to 1
is defined as the **threshold voltage** V_{th}. For larger Q_s, the surface potential is
dominated by mobile charge; for smaller Q_s, the surface potential is determined
by the charge in the depletion layer. As we have observed before, *below threshold,
current flows by diffusion; above threshold, current flows by drift.*

Long-Channel Limit

For l large compared with Q_s and Q_d, the $Q_s - Q_d + l$ in the denominator
of Equation B.23 is approximately equal to l, and the current becomes

$$Il \approx \frac{Q_s^2 - Q_d^2}{2} + Q_s - Q_d \tag{B.24}$$

This approximation corresponds to the usual treatment, which ignores velocity-
saturation effects. For such a long-channel device in saturation, Q_d is much less
than Q_s, and Equation B.24 becomes

$$I_{sat}l \approx \frac{Q_s^2}{2} + Q_s \tag{B.25}$$

For operation in the subthreshold region, both I and Q are much less than 1;

$Q_s^2/2$ is less than Q_s, and Equation B.25 reduces to the dimensionless form of Equation B.6 in saturation:

$$I_{sat}l \approx Q_s$$

Well above threshold, Q_s is much greater than 1; and the electric-field lines from additional charges on the gate virtually all end on mobile charges in the channel. The mobile-charge density above threshold is thus $q_s \approx (V_{gs} - V_{th})C_{ox}$, where V_{th} is the *threshold voltage* of the transistor. This relationship is shown in Figure B.5. In natural units,

$$Q_s \approx (V_{gs} - V_{th})\frac{C_{ox}}{C} = \kappa(V_{gs} - V_{th})$$

In this approximation, which corresponds to the standard treatment of the device characteristics, the current flow (Equation B.25) becomes

$$I_{sat}l \approx \frac{\kappa^2}{2}(V_{gs} - V_{th})^2$$

In these expressions, the threshold voltage V_{th} depends on V_s through the body effect, as we discussed previously.

Short-Channel Transistor in Saturation

For extremely short devices operated in saturation, well above threshold, the $Q_s - Q_d$ in the denominator of Equation B.23 is much greater than l, so we can neglect l. Also, both Q_s and I are much greater than 1. For a transistor in saturation, the charge density q_d at the drain is moving at saturated velocity v_0. In natural units, we can write this condition as $Q_d \approx I$. Therefore, in this short-channel limit, Equation B.23 becomes

$$I \approx \frac{Q_s + I}{2} \Rightarrow I \propto V_{gs} - V_{th} \tag{B.26}$$

We can develop an intuition for this result by the following line of reasoning. For a very short-channel device, the entire population of electrons that surmount the barrier is moving at saturated velocity. In natural units, we can write this condition as $Q_s = I$, in agreement with the limit given in Equation B.26.

It is easy to push a small transistor into the short-channel limit. For a 100-angstrom oxide thickness, a gate voltage of 3 volts produces a source charge density Q_s of about 120 in natural units. The length unit l_0 is about 0.007 micron. Thus, the dimensionless length of a device with 0.8-micron channel length is about equal to the dimensionless charge at that gate voltage. Shorter devices will rapidly approach the limiting behavior of Equation B.26.

For channel lengths where the short-channel effects are important but where the limiting behavior has not been reached, we can proceed as follows. In saturation, $Q_d \approx I$, and Equation B.22 becomes a simple quadratic form in Q_s:

$$2I_{sat}l + 1 = (Q_s + 1 - I_{sat})^2 \tag{B.27}$$

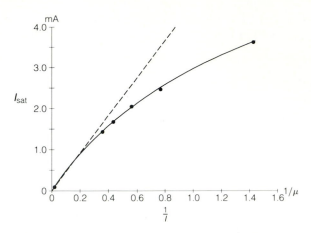

FIGURE B.6   Saturation current above threshold versus $1/l$. The solid line is Equation B.28; dots indicate data from experimental devices. The dashed line shows the long-channel approximation, in which saturation current is inversely proportional to channel length. In a transistor made with 1988 technology (1.5-micron feature size), the curve deviates substantially from the long-channel behavior.

The saturation currents of a number of transistors of different lengths are plotted as a function of $1/l$ in Figure B.6. The dashed line is the long-channel dependence given by Equation B.24. It is clear that devices with channel lengths of the order of 1 micron show large deviations from the long-channel limit. We can solve Equation B.27 explicitly for I_{sat}:

$$I_{sat} = Q_s + (l+1)\left(1 - \sqrt{1 + 2Q_s\frac{l}{(l+1)^2}}\right)$$

$$\approx Q_s + (l+1)\left(1 - \sqrt{1 + \frac{2Q_s}{l}}\right) \tag{B.28}$$

The solid line in Figure B.6 is Equation B.28, evaluated with the parameters mentioned above.

To evaluate the transistor terminal characteristics, we first choose a value for Q_s. We compute the saturation current directly from Equation B.27. Knowing V_s, we compute ψ_s at the source from Equation B.18. Given ψ_s, we compute x_0 from Equation B.1, and determine the depletion-layer charge Q_{dep} from Equation B.2. We now have Q_s, Q_{dep}, and V_s; thus, we can compute V_g from Equation B.14. We therefore can derive the channel current and gate voltage for any operating condition in saturation.

Short-Channel Transistor Below Saturation

For sufficiently low drain voltages, the mobile-charge density q_d at the drain is no longer moving at saturated velocity. We must determine the drain boundary condition for Equation B.23 to evaluate Q_d as a function of V_d. At every point along the channel, we will define a quasi–Fermi level or *imref* [Shockley, 1950] ξ such that

$$-\psi - \frac{\phi_0}{q} + \xi = \frac{kT}{q} \ln\left(\frac{q_m}{qN_0}\right) \tag{B.29}$$

This expression is, of course, just a generalization of Equation B.18.

Writing Equation B.29 for both source and drain with natural units, assuming $\xi_s = V_s$ at the source, and subtracting the two expressions yields a relation between the surface potentials at source and drain (ψ_s and ψ_d), the mobile-carrier densities at source and drain (Q_s and Q_d), and the imrefs at source and drain (V_s and ξ_d)

$$\psi_s - \psi_d + V_s - \xi_d = \ln\left(\frac{Q_d}{Q_s}\right) \tag{B.30}$$

We further assume, for the purpose of estimating the effect of small drain voltages on Q_d, that carriers at the drain end of the channel are Boltzmann distributed in energy with the same temperature as carriers in the drain. This assumption is fulfilled exactly in the limit of zero drain–source voltage. It obviously is not accurate when carriers are moving with saturated velocity. Refinements are possible, but we will not attempt them here.

We will derive the drain boundary condition by the following somewhat hand-waving argument. Let the density of states in the drain be N_d and that at the drain end of the channel be N_c. The probability P_{cd} of a carrier in the channel making a transition to a state in the drain is just the probability P_c of the state in the channel being occupied multiplied by the probability $1 - P_d$ that the corresponding state in the drain is unoccupied. A similar argument produces the probability that a carrier in the drain makes a transition back into the channel.

$$P_{cd} = N_c P_c N_d (1 - P_d)$$

and

$$P_{dc} = N_d P_d N_c (1 - P_c)$$

The net drain current is proportional to the difference of these two probabilities.

$$\frac{I}{K} = P_{net} = P_{cd} - P_{dc} = N_c N_d (P_c - P_d) \tag{B.31}$$

The actual value of the current is known only to within the large, horrible, complicated, and totally unknown constant K.

Substituting P_c and P_d in terms of the imrefs as given in Equation B.29, Equation B.31 becomes

$$I = K Q_d \left(1 - e^{-\xi_d + V_d}\right) \tag{B.32}$$

We notice that we can evaluate the constant K by considering operation at large drain voltages (V_d much greater than ξ_d). This condition corresponds to saturation, in which case carriers at the drain end of the channel are moving at saturated velocity. In natural units, this condition is written $Q_d = I$, and therefore, by some miracle, K is equal to one. We therefore can write Equation B.32 as

$$\ln\left(1 - \frac{I}{Q_d}\right) = V_d - \xi_d \tag{B.33}$$

Substituting Equation B.33 into Equation B.30, we arrive at the final form of the relation among carrier density, current, and drain voltage:

$$V_d - V_s = \psi_d - \psi_s - \ln\frac{Q_s}{Q_d} + \ln\left(1 - \frac{I}{Q_d}\right) \tag{B.34}$$

The second term is just the difference in the imrefs at the two ends of the channel. The third term is due to the *drain drop*—that is, to the difference between ξ_d and V_d. We can find the actual current for any given operating point by simultaneously solving Equations B.34 and B.23, using ψ_s from Equation B.17 and ψ_d from Equation B.14.

Drain Conductance

As in our discussion of subthreshold operation, we once again have treated the channel length l as a constant. From Equation B.27, it is obvious that the Early effect is more complicated in the general case than it was in subthreshold. Aside from the additional complexity, our previous approach to analyzing the drain conductance is still applicable. A more general form of Equation B.12 is

$$V_0 = \frac{I}{\frac{\partial I}{\partial V_d}} = \frac{I}{\frac{\partial I}{\partial l}\frac{\partial l}{\partial V_d}} \tag{B.35}$$

Differentiating Equation B.27 with respect to l, we obtain

$$\frac{\partial I}{\partial l}(l + Q_s + 1 - I) = -I$$

or

$$\frac{I}{\frac{\partial I}{\partial l}} = -(l + Q_s + 1 - I) \tag{B.36}$$

Substituting Equation B.36 into Equation B.35, we obtain the final form for the Early effect at any gate voltage:

$$V_0 = \frac{l + Q_s + 1 - I}{-\frac{\partial l}{\partial V_d}} \tag{B.37}$$

Measured values of V_0 versus length are plotted in Figure B.7 for several different values of V_g, each corresponding to a value for Q_s. The effect of above-threshold operation is to shift the entire curve to higher values, maintaining approximately the same slope. This behavior is suggested by Equation B.37.

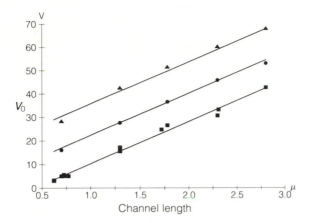

FIGURE B.7   The Early voltage V_0 versus channel length. Curves are plotted for three different gate voltages. Solid lines are the values predicted by Equation B.37. Dots indicate experimental data. The figure shows that, as in the subthreshold case, V_0 is proportional to l and the y-intercept value is proportional to Q_s.

It is a direct result of the saturation of carrier velocity at high electric fields, which makes the current less dependent on channel length. It is significant for devices that are several microns in length, and is a dominant characteristic of submicron devices.

SUMMARY

We have reviewed the behavior of transistors operating both above and below threshold, paying particular attention to the dependence of the transistors' characteristics on channel length. To this end, we have defined a set of natural units for the physical quantities involved in transistor operation. These units have allowed us to express the equations describing transistor operation in dimensionless form, and thus to simplify the analysis. We have seen that the functional form of the equations describing above-threshold operation are far from the long-channel limit, even with 1-micron channel lengths. Subthreshold devices, however, continue to conform to the simple model, even at very small dimensions. These conclusions have important consequences for the design of digital, as well as of analog, systems.

REFERENCES

Early, J.M. Effects of space-charge layer widening in junction transistors. *Proceedings of the IRE*, 40:1401, 1952.

Grove, A.S. *Physics and Technology of Semiconductor Devices*. New York: Wiley, 1967.

Hoeneisen, B. and Mead, C.A. Current–voltage characteristics of small size MOS transistors. *IEEE Transactions of Electron Devices*, 19:382, 1972b.

Jacoboni, C., Canali, C., Ottaviani, G., and Quaranta, A.A. A review of some charge transport properties of silicon. *Solid State Electronics*, 20:77, 1977.

Maher, M.A. and Mead, C. A physical charge-controlled model for MOS transistors. In Losleben, P. (ed), *Advanced Research in VLSI*. Cambridge, MA: MIT Press, 1987, p. 211.

Shockley, W. *Electrons and Holes in Semiconductors, With Applications to Transistor Electronics*. New York: Van Nostrand, 1950.

Tsividis, Y.P. *Operation and Modeling of the MOS Transistor*. New York: McGraw-Hill, 1987.

C

RESISTIVE NETWORKS

Resistive networks play a central role in level normalization in a great many neural systems; an example of such a network was presented in Chapter 15. Analyses of such networks are scattered throughout the literature, often couched in a terminology that is specific to another discipline. For this reason, it is desirable to gather the relevant material in a single place, using a consistent notation.

ONE-DIMENSIONAL CONTINUOUS NETWORKS

The simplest resistive network is shown in Figure 7.3 (p. 108). It has a longitudinal resistance R per unit length, and a conductance to ground G per unit length. A potential V_0 is applied to the left end of the process $(x = 0)$. The network is assumed to be semi-infinite, and R and G are assumed to be independent of x. We can determine how the input affects the voltage $V(x)$ on a node of the network at some value of x by writing the relations between the voltage and the current $I(x)$ flowing through the resistance R at that value of x, and of the same variables slightly farther along the line at $x + dx$:

$$V(x) = V(x + dx) + I(x + dx)R\,dx \qquad (C.1)$$

$$I(x) = I(x + dx) + V(x)G\,dx \qquad (C.2)$$

In the limit where dx becomes very small, I and V become continuous functions of x. Equation C.1 then becomes

$$\frac{dV}{dx} = -IR \tag{C.3}$$

and Equation C.2 becomes

$$\frac{dI}{dx} = -VG \tag{C.4}$$

Differentiating Equation C.3 with respect to x, and substituting Equation C.4 in the right-hand side, we obtain a second-order differential equation for V:

$$\frac{d^2V}{dx^2} = -R\frac{dI}{dx} = RGV \tag{C.5}$$

R and G are constant, so the solution to Equation C.5 has the form

$$V = V_0 e^{-\alpha x} = V_0 e^{-\frac{x}{L}} \tag{C.6}$$

We have ignored the $e^{\alpha x}$ solution because it diverges for large x. That solution will be appropriate, of course, for a network running in the $-x$ direction. The constant α is the *space constant* and L is the *characteristic length* or *diffusion length* of the network:

$$\alpha = \frac{1}{L} = \sqrt{RG} \tag{C.7}$$

As we noted in Chapter 6, a signal can be represented either by a voltage or by a current. If the signal is a current, it can be injected directly into a node of the network. We can determine the magnitude of the injected current required at $x = 0$ to produce the voltage V_0 by substituting Equation C.6 into Equation C.3:

$$I(0) = V_0 \frac{\alpha}{R} = V_0 \sqrt{\frac{G}{R}} = V_0 G_0 \tag{C.8}$$

The value $G_0 = \sqrt{G/R}$ is the **effective conductance** of the semi-infinite network. From the point of view of a signal source, the network acts just like a single conductance G_0.

If a signal is injected into a node in the middle of a very long process, the influence of that current spreads out in both directions, not just in the $+x$ direction. For a one-dimensional model, the solution for the $-x$ direction is just the mirror image of the solution for the $+x$ direction. For that reason, the effective conductance at a node of a network that extends in both directions is $2G_0$, because a current $V_0 G_0$ must be supplied for each direction.

DISCRETE NETWORKS

The results of the previous section are valid for only continuous or very nearly continuous networks—those for which RG is much less than 1. For most real applications, this restriction is not satisfied, and we must treat the general

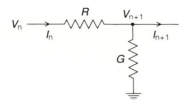

FIGURE C.1 Schematic showing relations between the voltages and currents in one section of a semi-infinite resistive network.

case where R and G can take on any values. We will begin by deriving a finite-difference equation for the voltage V_n on the nth node of the discrete line of Figure 7.3 (p. 108). The situation at one section of the line is shown in Figure C.1. We can derive the exact behavior of the discrete network by writing the circuit relations for two adjacent sections.

First, we express the current through the resistance R, connected between node n and node $n + 1$, in terms of the voltages on those two nodes:

$$I_n R = V_n - V_{n+1} \tag{C.9}$$

The same relation holds for the second section:

$$I_{n+1} R = V_{n+1} - V_{n+2} \tag{C.10}$$

The current through the conductance G is just the difference between I_n and I_{n+1}:

$$G V_{n+1} = I_n - I_{n+1} \tag{C.11}$$

Equation C.11 assumes that no current is injected directly into the node from an external source; in other words, we are looking for the natural spatial response of the network when current is injected into a single node. The effects of this excitation die out as we move away from the point $n = 0$ where the current is injected.

Substituting Equations C.9 and C.10 into Equation C.11, we obtain

$$GRV_{n+1} = V_n - V_{n+1} - V_{n+1} + V_{n+2}$$

Simplifying, we obtain the second-order finite-difference equation that the voltages of the nodes must satisfy:

$$V_{n+2} - (2 + RG)V_{n+1} + V_n = 0 \tag{C.12}$$

We expect a solution that dies out exponentially as we move away from the source. We construct a trial solution of the form

$$V_n = \gamma^{|n|} V_0 \tag{C.13}$$

Substituting this form for V_n in Equation C.12, and assuming $n > 0$, we obtain

$$V_0 \gamma^{n+2} - (2 + RG)V_0 \gamma^{n+1} + V_0 \gamma^n = 0$$

Dividing by $V_0 \gamma^n$, we obtain

$$\gamma^2 - (2 + RG)\gamma + 1 = 0 \tag{C.14}$$

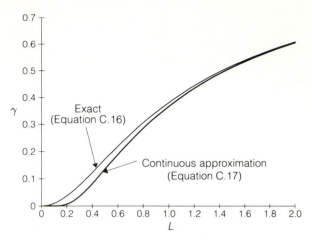

FIGURE C.2   Comparison of the continuous and discrete solutions for the exponential decay in a resistive network. The effective value of γ is plotted as a function of $L = 1/\sqrt{RG}$ The continuous approximation is excellent for $L > 1$.

We conclude that Equation C.13 is indeed a solution to Equation C.12, and that γ is specified by the quadratic form, Equation C.14. Applying the quadratic formula, the solution for γ is

$$\gamma = 1 + \frac{RG}{2} \pm \sqrt{RG + \frac{R^2 G^2}{4}} \tag{C.15}$$

We know that the voltage must approach zero for large n, and therefore that γ must be less than unity. We thus choose the negative sign for the square root in Equation C.15:

$$\gamma = 1 + \frac{RG}{2} - \sqrt{RG}\sqrt{1 + RG/4}$$

$$= 1 + \frac{1}{2L^2} - \frac{1}{L}\sqrt{1 + \frac{1}{4L^2}} \tag{C.16}$$

where, as in the continuous case, we have defined $L = 1/\sqrt{RG}$. The quantities are not directly comparable, because the discrete elements have discrete values, whereas in the continuous network we specified the conductance and resistance per unit length. We obtain the correspondence between the two cases by measuring distance in the discrete network in terms of sections; in other words, one section is the length unit in discrete networks.

We can examine how the value of γ given by Equation C.16 compares with the continuous solution. If the two solutions were identical, we could compute the value of γ by equating Equation C.6 with Equation C.13:

$$\frac{V}{V_0} = \gamma^x = e^{x \ln \gamma} \approx e^{-\frac{x}{L}}$$

from which we could infer

$$\gamma \approx e^{-\frac{1}{L}} = e^{-\sqrt{RG}} \tag{C.17}$$

We can compare this expression for the continuum limit of the discrete network with the exact result, given by Equation C.16, as shown in Figure C.2. At large L, the two expressions are in excellent agreement. For L less than about 1, however, we must use the expression for the discrete network. It is somewhat surprising that the expression derived for a continuous approximation is good to such a low value of L.

In the first section of this appendix, we characterized the continuous network by two quantities: the diffusion length L, and the effective conductance G_0. In Equation C.17 we have established the correspondence between the diffusion lengths in the continuous and discrete cases; we will now investigate the effective conductance of the discrete network. Dividing Equation C.9 by V_n yields

$$\frac{I_n}{V_n} R = 1 - \frac{V_{n+1}}{V_n} = 1 - \gamma \tag{C.18}$$

Applying Equation C.18 to the first section $(n = 0)$ of a semi-infinite network, and dividing by R, we obtain the conductance at the input to the network:

$$G_{\text{in}} = \frac{I_0}{V_0} = \frac{1 - \gamma}{R} \tag{C.19}$$

Substituting the value of γ from Equation C.15 into Equation C.19 yields

$$G_{\text{in}} = \sqrt{\frac{G}{R}} \sqrt{1 + \frac{RG}{4}} - \frac{G}{2} \tag{C.20}$$

We might be tempted to use the value of G_{in} given by Equation C.20 as the effective conductance of the network, by analogy with the continuous case (Equation C.8). We must exercise discretion, however, in dealing with the discrete network. The conductance of a node in the middle of a long network should be $2G_0$, as it was in the continuous case. If we join the ends of two semi-infinite discrete networks, one running to the left and the other to the right, we are faced with the situation shown in Figure C.3. The networks for

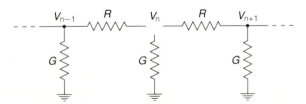

FIGURE C.3   Boundary condition at the point where two semi-infinite resistive networks are joined. An additional conductance to ground is required to form a homogeneous structure. This requirement is satisfied automatically if the open end of each network is terminated with a conductance $G/2$.

which we derived Equation C.19 cannot be joined to form a continuous network unless we add a conductance at the node that is formed when they are joined. If we want each discrete semi-infinite network to have a conductance G_0 at its open end, we must *terminate* the open end of the line with a conductance $G/2$. Once this termination is in place, the second term in Equation C.20 disappears, and we have the final form for the effective conductance of the discrete network:

$$G_0 = \sqrt{\frac{G}{R}} \sqrt{1 + \frac{RG}{4}} \tag{C.21}$$

For large $L = 1/\sqrt{RG}$, Equation C.21 reduces to the form given in Equation C.8, as expected. For discrete lines with small values of L, the line still has a well-defined effective conductance, but its value can be considerably different from that expected for a continuous line.

If the signals to be processed by the network are represented by voltages, a convenient way to launch these inputs into the network is to connect the bottoms of the conductances to the voltage sources, as shown in Figure 7.5 (p. 110). For linear resistors and conductances, the principle of superposition will hold for this arrangement as it did for current inputs, and we need to compute only the node voltage V due to a single input v.

We assume that the node driven by the input is in the center of a network that is infinite in both directions. The semi-infinite networks on each side of the center section each have an effective conductance G_{in}, given by Equation C.20. The relation between these two voltages can be derived from the simple equivalent circuit shown in Figure C.4.

The current I is related to the source voltage v by

$$v = I \left(\frac{1}{G} + \frac{1}{2G_{in}} \right) \tag{C.22}$$

The network node voltage V is

$$V = \frac{I}{2G_{in}} \tag{C.23}$$

FIGURE C.4 Equivalent circuit used for determining the voltage V at a network node generated by a source v at the corresponding position in the network.

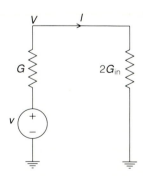

We obtain the ratio of source voltage to network voltage by dividing Equation C.22 by Equation C.23:

$$\frac{v}{V} = \frac{2G_{\text{in}}}{G} + 1 \tag{C.24}$$

We can obtain a more convenient form of Equation C.24 by using the definition of G_{in} from Equation C.20 and that of L from Equation C.16:

$$\frac{V}{v} = \frac{1}{\sqrt{4L^2 + 1}}$$

Discontinuities in Dendritic Processes

We will use the results we obtained in the previous section to analyze discontinuities in resistive networks. A **discontinuity** is a fork in a tree, or is a synapse that cannot be modeled as a simple voltage or current input. We will use the notion of an *equivalent circuit* when we need to join two or more segments of a linear network. Because the conductance of a discrete network can vary considerably depending on how it is terminated, we will assume that the ends of all networks are properly terminated. With this understanding, the results of this analysis apply to both discrete and continuous networks.

We have already mentioned the degenerate case of a junction between two networks, in which two identical semi-infinite networks are joined to form a single, infinite network. Let us revisit that case, to formalize the result and to clarify the treatment of more complex arrangements.

An equivalent circuit for a semi-infinite linear network is shown in Figure C.5. Inputs to the network generate the output voltage V_0. For the purpose of computing this voltage, the network can be replaced by its equivalent con-

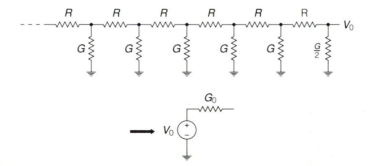

FIGURE C.5 Equivalent circuit of a semi-infinite network. Inputs at various points in a linear semi-infinite network (top) produce an output voltage V_0. For any computation in which the network is a component, it can be replaced by the equivalent circuit (bottom).

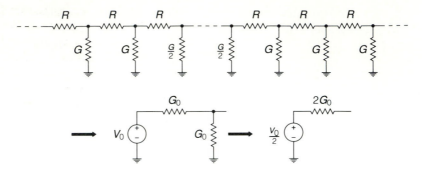

FIGURE C.6   Junction of two semi-infinite networks. The effect of continuing a semi-infinite network (top) to infinity can be computed from the equivalent circuits (bottom) of the two semi-infinite networks. In this example, the network on the right contains no sources.

ductance, G_0. We used a variant of this procedure to derive Equation C.24. The real trick in using equivalent circuits is to observe that the roles of the source and of the network can be interchanged. Suppose we have several signals injected into the far-left reaches of the network, safely hidden from our scrutiny by the border of Figure C.5. We do not need to know anything about them, save that they produce a voltage V_0 at the open-circuit end of the network. For any purpose, then, we can use that end of the network as a voltage source V_0, with a series conductance equal to G_0. No DC measurement we can make will allow us to distinguish between the two circuits. This trick allows us to *compose* semi-infinite network segments as though they were simple resistors and voltage sources.

The simplest composition is a continuation of the same network to infinity. The situation is shown in Figure C.6. The output of the open-circuit network is V_0. The effect of extending the network to infinity is to add a conductance G_0 to ground. The result is a voltage equal to $\frac{1}{2}V_0$ at the node where the networks are joined. In other words, the voltage at the open-circuit end of a cut network is just twice the voltage that would exist at the same point in an infinite network. This statement applies to only those networks in which all sources are to one side of the cut; it is equivalent to our comment regarding Equation C.24, that the effective conductance of an infinite network is one-half that of a semi-infinite network.

Of course, no network is infinite in extent, even in one direction. We can use the approach outlined in this section with finite networks if we note that L is, in rough terms, the distance a signal must traverse before it forgets its origins. Hence, we can, for our present purposes, treat any segment more than 1 or $2\,L$ units long as semi-infinite. We will now use the equivalent-circuit approach to analyze two important structures: shunting-inhibitory inputs and branches in the dendritic tree.

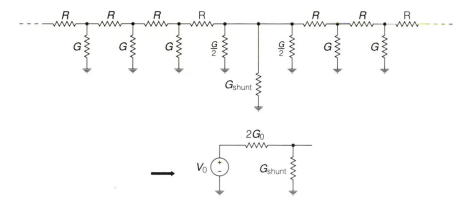

FIGURE C.7 Shunting-inhibition circuit. The effect of a shunting synapse can be computed using the equivalent circuit (bottom) of an infinite network (top). For large values of G_{shunt}, the synapse performs a division.

Shunting Inhibition

The simplest realization of shunting inhibition is implemented directly by the network of Figure 7.5 (p. 110); we merely make one conductance very large compared with the others. In this situation, a signal traveling in either direction in the network will be attenuated. We can estimate the attenuation a signal will suffer as it passes such a shunt in the following way. Assume that the signal is due to a source or to a set of sources many sections away from the shunt. The signal will be decaying gradually, according to Equation C.13. From the shunt's point of view, the signal is just a voltage source with a series conductance equal to the characteristic conductance $2G_0$ of the network. The equivalent circuit is shown in Figure C.7. We can obtain the output voltage by applying Kirchhoff's law to the shunted node:

$$V_{out} = \frac{V_0 G_0}{G_{shunt} + 2G_0}$$

where V_0 is the voltage that would have been present without the shunt. As G_{shunt} becomes large compared with G_0, the operation performed by such a synapse resembles a division by G_{shunt}.

Although simple network models often include the assumption that a synaptic input can be modeled as a current or voltage source, real synapses operate by opening specific channels in the membrane. These open channels increase the conductance of that patch of membrane to the reversal potential of the ion for which the channel is selective. This increase in conductance produces two effects: It adds a current to that location if the reversal potential of the ion is different from the resting potential of the neuron, and it acts as a shunt for additional synaptic input. For this reason, the current injected into a dendrite increases

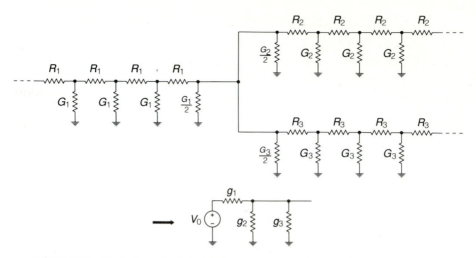

FIGURE C.8 Equivalent circuit (bottom) representation of a branched dendrite (top). A signal originating in branch 1 is attenuated by the branch according to Equation C.25.

less than linearly with increasing synaptic input. This self-shunting behavior of synapses was first analyzed by Rall [Rall, 1964].

Branches

A branching resistive network is shown in Figure C.8. The equivalent circuit, also shown, allows us to derive how much of a signal propagating in one branch makes it into another branch with a different effective conductance. From the equivalent circuit, we can write an expression for V_0, the voltage at the junction of the three branches:

$$V_0 = V_1 \frac{g_1}{g_1 + g_2 + g_3} \tag{C.25}$$

where the gs are the effective conductances of the three branches, and V_1 is the output voltage of the first (source) branch if the other branches are removed. A particularly symmetrical condition occurs when $g_1 = g_2 + g_3$. In this *matched condition,* no measurement in branch 1 can tell us that the network has branched. Any result for a semi-infinite network applies directly to a branched network with matched branches. This statement is true of only those signals traveling from the root of the tree toward the leaves. A signal originating in a terminal branch of a balanced matched tree ($2g_2 = 2g_3 = g_1$) will be attenuated by a factor of four at the branch—a factor of two more than that occasioned by a continuation of the originating branch to infinity. If equal signals originate in two branches of a matched tree, the resulting output will be the same as it would have been had the signal originated in the trunk segment.

The effects of branches on the electrical properties of the dendritic tree were first analyzed in detail by Rall [Rall, 1959].

TWO-DIMENSIONAL CONTINUOUS NETWORKS

The simplest two-dimensional network is a uniform, infinite sheet of resistive material. The sheet has a **sheet resistance** ρ, and a conductance to ground σ per unit area. The resistance R of any rectangle of material is $R = \rho(l/w)$, where l is the length of the rectangle in the direction of current flow, and w is the width. A square of material therefore will have resistance ρ, independent of the size of the square. The sheet resistance ρ thus has the dimensions of resistance, but often is given in *ohms per square*. The parameters ρ and σ are the continuous, two-dimensional counterparts of R and G in the one-dimensional case.

A top view of the resistive sheet, centered on the point at which an input is injected, is shown in Figure C.9. The entire solution will be symmetrical about the point $r = 0$ at which the input is injected. For any radius r, we can write the radial resistance dR and conductance dG of an annulus of thickness dr, using the previous definitions of ρ and σ:

$$dR = \rho \frac{dr}{2\pi r} \qquad (C.26)$$

$$dG = \sigma 2\pi r \, dr \qquad (C.27)$$

In crossing through the annulus, a current dI will be shunted to ground through the conductance dG:

$$dI = -V(r) \, dG \qquad (C.28)$$

The voltage will be decremented by dV due to current flow through the resistance dR:

$$dV = -I(r) \, dR \qquad (C.29)$$

Substituting Equation C.27 into Equation C.28, we obtain a differential equation for I:

$$\frac{dI}{dr} = -V\sigma 2\pi r \qquad (C.30)$$

Likewise, we obtain a differential equation for V by substituting Equation C.26

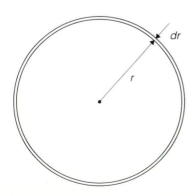

FIGURE C.9 Top view of a two-dimensional resistive sheet. A current injected in the center flows through a lateral resistance due to the sheet resistance of the layer, and is shunted by the area conductance to ground. At any radius r, the shunting conductance is proportional to $2\pi r \, dr$, whereas the lateral spreading resistance is proportional to $dr/2\pi r$.

into Equation C.29:

$$\frac{dV}{dr} = -I\frac{\rho}{2\pi r} \tag{C.31}$$

Taking the derivative of Equation C.31 with respect to r, and substituting into Equation C.30, we obtain a differential equation for the voltage:

$$\frac{d^2V}{dr^2} + \frac{1}{r}\frac{dV}{dr} - \alpha^2 V = 0 \tag{C.32}$$

where $\alpha = 1/L = \sqrt{\rho\sigma}$, as before. Equations of this form have been studied for many years, and their solutions are known as *Bessel functions*. The particular solution of Equation C.32 is the *modified Bessel function, K_0*:[1]

$$V = V_0\,K_0(\alpha r) \tag{C.33}$$

where V_0 is a constant.[2] The K_0 function diverges extremely rapidly as r approaches zero, and therefore the voltage at the origin is infinite. The solution begins to resemble an exponential decay for large values of r. There are numeri- •
cal algorithms that allow a computer program to evaluate K_0. When we have no computer at our elbows, we can use closed-form approximations to K_0 for large and small arguments:

$$K_0(\alpha r) \approx -\ln(\alpha r) \qquad \text{where} \qquad \alpha r \ll 1 \tag{C.34}$$

$$K_0(\alpha r) \approx \sqrt{\frac{\pi}{2\alpha r}}\,e^{-\alpha r} \qquad \text{where} \qquad \alpha r \gg 1 \tag{C.35}$$

At large distances, the decay law for a single input has not changed drastically from the one-dimensional case (Equation C.6). The solution is still a generally exponential decay, with a space constant that is analogous to that of the one-dimensional case given in Equation C.7. The $1/\sqrt{r}$ dependence is the sole contribution of the two-dimensional nature of the network to the asymptotic solution at large r. The expression given in Equation 7.8 (p. 114) is nearly identical to that in Equation C.35 when the unit distance in the circular approximation to the hexagonal network is the distance between the flat sides of the concentric hexagons [Feinstein, 1988]. At small r, the story is different.

As in the one-dimensional case, we need to evaluate the current required to produce the voltage V_0. For this purpose, we can use the solution for small values of r. Substituting Equation C.34 into Equation C.33 and differentiating with respect to r, we obtain

$$\frac{dV}{dr} = -\frac{V_0}{r} \qquad \text{where} \qquad \alpha r \ll 1 \tag{C.36}$$

---

[1] We have discarded the other solution $I_0(\alpha r)$ because we are interested in only those solutions that remain finite as r becomes large.

[2] V_0 is the value of $V(r)$ at $\alpha r \approx 0.458$.

Substituting Equation C.36 into Equation C.31, we obtain the r dependence of the current I flowing in the sheet:

$$I = \frac{2\pi V_0}{\rho} \qquad \text{where} \qquad \alpha r \ll 1$$

As we expected, for sufficiently small r, where the asymptotic approximation is valid, the area is too small for any appreciable current to be lost to ground, and therefore the total current is independent of r. We still have a problem, however: As r goes to zero, the logarithm in Equation C.34 diverges and the voltage becomes infinite. This behavior is an artifact of the continuous model we have made of the discrete physical system; we cannot resolve it without deriving the solution for the discrete system. A detailed treatment of the discrete hexagonal network, including a solution for the input conductance in terms of elliptic integrals, is given in Feinstein [Feinstein, 1988]. This report also gives an approximate closed-form solution for the discrete network, valid for L less than 100. For practical application, the algorithm described in Chapter 7 is an effective technique for evaluating the discrete-network node voltages, especially those close to the origin, which cannot be obtained from Equation C.35.

REFERENCES

Feinstein, D. The hexagonal resistive network and the circular approximation. *Caltech Computer Science Technical Report,* Caltech-CS-TR-88-7, California Institute of Technology, Pasadena, CA, 1988.

Rall, W. Branching dendritic trees and motoneuron membrane resistivity. *Experimental Neurology.* 1:491, 1959.

Rall, W. Theoretical significance of dendritic trees for neuronal input–output relations. In Reiss, R.F. (ed) *Neural Theory and Modeling; Proceedings of the 1962 Ojai Symposium.* Stanford, CA: Stanford University Press, 1964,

COMPLEXITY IN NEURAL SYSTEMS

Yaser Abu-Mostafa

Why do neurons have so many inputs? Although we do not have a complete understanding of the operation of individual neurons and of large neural systems, we know enough to see why the large number of neuron inputs matches the basic function of the neurons and the system. Two of the factors contributing to this match are what we call the **analog factor** and the **entropy factor**. We start by giving a brief description of these factors; then we discuss each in detail.

1. Analog factor: The analog mode of computation makes the computation power of an individual neuron proportional to the *square* of the number of inputs K, whereas the neuron's size is only linear in K. This result contrasts with traditional logic gates, such as AND gates, in which both computation power and size are linear in K, and hence would be equally well implemented by a tree of two-input gates of the same type. To simulate the function of a neuron with K inputs, we need the order of K^2 two-input neurons. Therefore, the saving in overall system size when we use the K-input neurons is proportional to K, and is several orders of magnitude for the known values of K in the brain.

2. Entropy factor: The typical input for the neural system comes from a natural environment that has a certain degree of disorder, or entropy. **Entropy** is a quantitative measure of the disorder or randomness of an

environment. An important part of the function of the neural system is to be able to learn from "training" samples drawn from the environment. Under what conditions is learning possible? If we assume that the learning mechanism is local, as in the case of Hebbian learning, where the strength of a synapse is incremented or decremented according to the states of the two neurons it connects, we can show that a relation holds between the entropy of the environment and the number of neuron inputs. The relation forces the number of neuron inputs to be at least equal to the entropy of the environment.

ANALOG FACTOR

A neuron, like any other logic device, makes a decision based on the values of its inputs. However, the decision-making mechanism in the case of neurons is analog; that is, it involves the processing of continuous-valued signals rather than of discrete-valued signals. For example, the function of certain neurons can be modeled as a **threshold rule**: The neuron will fire (will have output $+1$) if the weighted sum of its inputs exceeds an internal threshold; otherwise, it will not fire (will have output -1). Thus,

$$
u_i = \begin{cases} +1, & \text{if } \sum_{j=1}^{K} w_{ij} u_j \geq t_i \\[2ex] -1, & \text{if } \sum_{j=1}^{K} w_{ij} u_j < t_i \end{cases} \tag{D.1}
$$

where u_i is the output of neuron i, $\{u_j\}$ are the inputs to this neuron (and also are the outputs of other neurons), $\{w_{ij}\}$ are the weights of the synaptic connections, and t_i is the internal threshold. Although, in this equation, the inputs $u_1, u_2, \ldots, u_K$ and the output u_i are all discrete (binary), output depends on the input through the analog parameters $\{w_{ij}\}$ and t_i. The function of most neurons is more sophisticated than is this simple threshold rule; some neurons accept analog values for their inputs and generate analog outputs.

Why does the analog processing mode make the large number of inputs to the neuron vital? The techniques of circuit complexity provide a direct answer. Consider the neuron described by Equation D.1 for u_i. Suppose we replace this K-input neuron by a network of two-input neurons that does the same job. The idea of this hypothetical replacement is to see whether there is an inherent advantage to having neurons with a large number of inputs K, or whether we can do equally well with more neurons, each of which has fewer inputs. For example, if we considered K-input AND gates instead of K-input neurons, the replacement network would be a tree of two-input AND gates (see Figure D.1). Let us compare the sizes of the single K-input gate and of the tree. The size of the K-input gate is approximately proportional to K (it may vary from one physical implementation to another). The size of the tree is proportional to the number of two-input gates in the tree, which is approximately K. Hence, there is

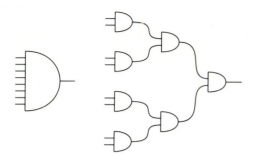

FIGURE D.1   A tree of two-input AND gates (right) replacing a single eight-input AND gate (left) and performing the same function.

no essential gain or loss in the overall system size if we use only two-input gates. Does the situation change when we consider neurons instead of AND gates?

It does. Here also, the size of the K-input neuron is approximately proportional to K. However, the neuron can be replaced by only a network of two-input neurons the size of which is proportional to *at least* K^2. Let us first see why the size of the K-input neuron is proportional to K. The synapses merge toward the neuron (see Figure 7.1, p. 102) in a treelike fashion (not necessarily a binary tree). As they merge, their signals $(w_{ij}u_j)$ are added, forming partial sums that accumulate to create the total signal $\sum_{j=1}^{K} w_{ij}u_j$. The neuron then compares the signal to the internal threshold t_i and determines the value of u_i. The overall size of the neuron including this merging tree is dominated by the size of the tree, which is proportional to K. Hence, the size of the K-input neuron is proportional to K, as we asserted. So why is it not possible to replace the K-input neuron by a tree of two-input neurons in exactly the same way as we did for the AND gate?

Because the neuron simulates a general threshold function of K variables, the network of two-input neurons should be able to simulate any threshold function of K variables. Any such network, however, must have at least the order of K^2 two-input neurons, a consequence of the circuit complexity of threshold functions. Suppose we have a network with M two-input neurons that can simulate any threshold function of K inputs. There are only 16 ways to program each neuron, because there are only 16 switching functions of two variables. Hence, there are at most 16^M different ways to program the network to simulate a given overall function. This number must be at least large enough to accommodate the number of different K-input threshold functions, which is at least $2^{K^2/2}$ [Muroga et al., 1966]. Hence,

$$16^M \geq 2^{K^2/2}$$

which forces M to be at least the order of K^2.

The argument does not guarantee that there is a network with K^2 two-input neurons that can replace the K-input neuron. It shows only that there is no smaller network that will do it, which is exactly what we were trying to prove. The situation becomes even worse when logic more sophisticated than threshold is involved. The fancier the logic, the more it pays to have plenty of inputs to the neuron. The ability of the neurons to handle analog signals makes it worthwhile to save the analog nature of the data and then to make a global decision. With a network of two-input neurons, the intermediate discrete decisions waste most of the information carried by the intermediate analog signals, and a bigger network is needed to make up for this lost analog information by providing an abundance of intermediate discrete decisions. For example, the intermediate analog signals may be soft decisions (analog values between 0 and 1, instead of just 0 or 1) carrying not only the decision (0 or 1, depending on which is closer), but also information about how reliable the decision is (how close). We need several bits to encode an approximate value of this reliability if we use discrete signals.

ENTROPY FACTOR

The ability of neural systems to learn spontaneously a desired function from training samples is these systems' most important feature. Clearly, a given neural system cannot learn any old function; there must be restrictions on which systems can learn which functions. We present a theorem describing such a restriction. The theorem imposes a lower bound on the number of neuron inputs, in terms of the entropy of the environment. For the theorem to hold, the learning mechanism is assumed to be local; when a training sample is loaded into the system, each neuron has access to only those bits that are carried by it and by the neurons to which it is directly connected. This strong assumption excludes the sophisticated learning mechanisms used in neural-network models, but it may be more plausible from a biological point of view.

The environment in our model produces patterns represented by N bits $\mathbf{x} = x_1 \cdots x_N$. Only h different patterns can be generated by a given environment, where $h < 2^N$ (the entropy is essentially $\log_2 h$). We do not assume any knowledge about which patterns the environment is likely to generate—we know only that there are h such patterns. In the learning process, a huge number of sample patterns are generated at random from the environment and are sent to the system, 1 bit per neuron. The system uses this information to set its internal parameters and gradually to tune itself to this particular environment. Because of the system architecture, each neuron knows only its own bit and (at best) the bits of the neurons to which it is directly connected by a synapse. Hence, the learning rules are local: A neuron does not have the benefit of the entire global pattern that is being learned.

After the learning process has taken place, each neuron is ready to perform a function defined by what it has learned. The collective interaction of the functions of the neurons is what defines the overall function of the network. The theorem reported here is that (roughly speaking), if the number of neuron inputs is less than the entropy, the system cannot learn about the environment. The idea used to prove the theorem is to show that, if the number of neuron inputs is small, then the final function of each neuron is independent of the environment. Hence, we can conclude that, in this situation, the overall system has accumulated no information about the environment. Let us formalize these ideas.

A neural system is an undirected graph (the vertices are the neurons and the edges are the synapses). We label the neurons $1, \ldots, N$ and define $K_n \subseteq \{1, \ldots, N\}$ to be the set of neurons connected by a synapse to neuron n, together with neuron n itself. An environment is a subset $e \subseteq \{0,1\}^N$ (each $\mathbf{x} \in e$ is a sample from the environment). During learning, $x_1, \ldots, x_N$ (the bits of $\mathbf{x}$) are loaded into the neurons $1, \ldots, N$, respectively. Now we consider an arbitrary neuron n and relabel everything to make K_n become $\{1, \ldots, K\}$. Thus, the neuron sees the first K coordinates of each $\mathbf{x}$.

Our result is asymptotic in N, so we specify K as a function of N; $K = \alpha N$, where $\alpha = \alpha(N)$ satisfies $\lim_{N \to \infty} \alpha(N) = \alpha_o$, for $0 < \alpha_o < 1$. The result also is statistical, so we consider the *ensemble* of environments $\mathcal{E}$

$$\mathcal{E} = \mathcal{E}(N) = \{e \subseteq \{0,1\}^N : |e| = h\}$$

where $h = 2^{\beta N}$, and $\beta = \beta(N)$ satisfies $\lim_{N \to \infty} \beta(N) = \beta_o$, for $0 < \beta_o < 1$. The probability distribution on $\mathcal{E}$ is uniform; any environment $e \in \mathcal{E}$ is as likely to occur as is any other.

The neuron sees only the first K coordinates of each $\mathbf{x}$ generated by the environment e. For each e, we define the function $n : \{0,1\}^K \to \{0,1,2,\ldots\}$, where

$$n(a_1 \cdots a_K) = |\{\mathbf{x} \in e : x_k = a_k \text{ for } k = 1, \ldots, K\}|$$

and the normalized version

$$\nu(a_1 \cdots a_K) = \frac{n(a_1 \cdots a_K)}{h}$$

The function ν describes the relative frequency of occurrence for each of the 2^K binary vectors $x_1 \cdots x_K$ as $\mathbf{x} = x_1 \cdots x_N$ runs through all h vectors in e. In other words, ν specifies the projection of e as seen by the neuron. Clearly, $\nu(\mathbf{a}) \geq 0$ for all $\mathbf{a} \in \{0,1\}^K$ and $\sum_{\mathbf{a} \in \{0,1\}^K} \nu(\mathbf{a}) = 1$.

Corresponding to two environments e_1 and e_2, we will have two functions ν_1 and ν_2. If ν_1 is not distinguishable from ν_2, the neuron cannot tell the difference between e_1 and e_2. The distinguishability between ν_1 and ν_2 can be measured by

$$d(\nu_1, \nu_2) = \tfrac{1}{2} \sum_{\mathbf{a} \in \{0,1\}^K} |\nu_1(\mathbf{a}) - \nu_2(\mathbf{a})|$$

The range of $d(\nu_1, \nu_2)$ is $0 \leq d(\nu_1, \nu_2) \leq 1$, where 0 corresponds to complete indistinguishability and 1 corresponds to maximum distinguishability. Let e_1 and e_2 be independently selected environments from $\mathcal{E}$ according to the uniform probability distribution. Now $d(\nu_1, \nu_2)$ is a random variable, and we are interested in the expected value $E(d(\nu_1, \nu_2))$. The case where $E(d(\nu_1, \nu_2)) = 0$ corresponds to the neuron getting no information about the environment; the case where $E(d(\nu_1, \nu_2)) = 1$ corresponds to the neuron getting maximum information. The following theorem predicts, in the limit, one of these extremes, depending on how the number of neuron inputs (represented by α_o) compares to the entropy (represented by β_o).

Theorem

1. If $\alpha_o > \beta_o$, then $\lim_{N \to \infty} E\left(d(\nu_1, \nu_2)\right) = 1$
2. If $\alpha_o < \beta_o$, then $\lim_{N \to \infty} E\left(d(\nu_1, \nu_2)\right) = 0$

A formal proof of the theorem is given in previous publications [Abu-Mostafa, 1988a; Abu-Mostafa, 1988b]. Here, we provide a sketch of that proof. Suppose $h = 2^{K+10}$ (corresponding to part 2 of the theorem). For most environments $e \in \mathcal{E}$, the first K bits of $\mathbf{x} \in e$ go through all 2^K possible values approximately 2^{10} times each as $\mathbf{x}$ goes through all h possible values once. Therefore, the patterns seen by the neuron are drawn from the fixed ensemble of all binary vectors of length K with essentially uniform probability distribution; that is, ν is the same for most environments. This observation means that, statistically, the neuron will end up performing the same function regardless of the environment in question.

What about the opposite case, where $h = 2^{K-10}$ (corresponding to part 1 of the theorem)? Now, with only 2^{K-10} patterns available from the environment, the first K bits of $\mathbf{x}$ can assume at most 2^{K-10} values out of the possible 2^K values a binary vector of length K can assume in principle. Furthermore, which values can be assumed depends on the particular environment in question; that is, ν depends on the environment. Therefore, although the neuron still does not have the global picture, the information it has provides some information about the environment.

In summary, we have contrasted two situations. In the first situation, the neuron sees too few bits and cannot observe any pattern in these bits that identifies the environment. In the second situation, the neuron sees enough bits to form up such a pattern. The critical value of the number of bits that differentiates between the two situations is equal to the entropy of the environment.

REFERENCES

Abu-Mostafa, Y. Connectivity versus entropy. In Anderson, D. (ed), *Neural Information Processing Systems*. New York: American Institute of Physics, 1988a, p. 1.

Abu-Mostafa, Y. Lower bound for connectivity in local-learning neural networks. *Journal of Complexity*, 4:246, 1988b.

Muroga, S. and Toda, I. Lower bound of the number of threshold functions. *IEEE Transactions on Electronic Computers*, EC-15:805, 1966.

CREDITS

FIGURES AND TABLES

4.1, p. 44, 4.1, p. 48, and 4.4, p. 51: Adapted with permission from Katz, B. *Nerve, Muscle, and Synapse.* Copyright © 1966, New York: McGraw-Hill.

4.5, p. 52: Adapted with permission from Katz, B. *Nerve, Muscle, and Synapse.* Copyright © 1966, New York: McGraw-Hill. After Hodgkin, A.L., Ionic movements and electrical activity in giant nerve fibres. 1958, *Proceedings of the Royal Society of London,* Series B, Vol. 148. After Hodgkin, A.L. and Huxley, A.F., Current carried by sodium and potassium ions through the membrane of the giant axon of Loligo. 1952, *Journal of Physiology,* Vol. 116.

4.6, p. 53: Adapted with permission from Hodgkin, A.L. and Huxley, A.F. Current carried by sodium and potassium ions through the membrane of the giant axon of Loligo. 1952, *Journal of Physiology,* Vol. 116.

4.7, p. 55: Reproduced from *The Journal of General Physiology,* 1986, Vol. 88, by copyright permission of the Rockefeller University Press.

4.10, p. 60: Reprinted with permission from Liley, A.W. The effects of presynaptic polarization on the spontaneous activity at the mammalian neuromuscular junction. 1956, *Journal of Physiology,* Vol. 134.

4.11, p. 61: Adapted with permission from Shepherd, G.M. *The Synaptic Organization of the Brain,* 2nd ed. Copyright © 1979. New York: Oxford University Press.

15.1, p. 258: Adapted with permission from Dowling, J. *The Retina: An Approachable Part of the Brain.* Copyright © 1987. Cambridge, MA: Belknap Press of Harvard University Press. After Dowling, J., Synaptic organization of the frog retina: an electron microscopic analysis comparing the retinas of frogs and primates. 1968, *Proceedings of the Royal Society of London*, Series B, Vol. 170.

15.8, p. 268 and 15.9, p. 270: Reproduced from *The Journal of General Physiology*, 1974, Vol. 63, by copyright permission of the Rockefeller University Press.

15.10, p. 271: Adapted with permission from Enroth-Cugell, C. and Robson, J.G. The contrast sensitivity of retinal ganglion cells of the cat. 1966, *Journal of Physiology*, Vol. 187.

16.10, p. 299: Adapted with permission from Robles, L., Ruggero, M.A., and Rich, N.C. Mössbauer measurements of the mechanical response to single-tone and two-tone stimuli at the base of the chinchilla cochlea. In Allen, J.B., Hall, J.L., Hubbard, A., Neely, S.T., and Tubis, A. (eds), *Peripheral Auditory Mechanisms*. Copyright © 1986. Berlin, New York: Springer-Verlag.

EPIGRAPHS AND QUOTES

Part I, p. 1: Reprinted with permission from Pantin, C.F.A., *Organic Design*, an address delivered on August 9, 1951; British Association: Edinburgh Meeting; as quoted in *The New Landscape in Art and Science*, by Gyorgy Kepes, Paul Theobald and Co., Chicago, 1956. Copyright © 1956 Gyorgy Kepes, Cambridge, MA.

Part II, p. 65: From Teilhard de Chardin, Pierre. *The Phenomenon of Man*, copyright © 1955 by Editions du Seuil. English translation copyright © 1959 by William Collins Sons and Co., and Harper and Row Publishers, Inc.

Part III, p. 125: Reprinted with permission from Mach, Ernst, *Popular Scientific Lectures*, 5th edition, translated by Thomas J. McCormack. Open Court Publishing Company, LaSalle, Illinois, 1943.

Part IV, p. 205: Reprinted with permission from Pantin, C.F.A., *Organic Design*, an address delivered on August 9, 1951; British Association: Edinburgh Meeting; as quoted in *The New Landscape in Art and Science*, by Gyorgy Kepes, Paul Theobald and Co., Chicago, 1956. Copyright © 1956 Gyorgy Kepes, Cambridge, MA.

Appendixes, p. 303: From *Confucius: The Analects*, translated by D.C. Lau. Penguin Classics, 1979, copyright © 1979 by D.C. Lau.

Chapter 4, p. 54: Reprinted with permission from Hodgkin, A.L. and Huxley, A.F. Current carried by sodium and potassium ions through the membrane of the giant axon of Loligo. 1952, *Journal of Physiology*, Vol. 116.

Chapter 11, p. 192: Reprinted with permission from Shepherd, G.M. *The Synaptic Organization of the Brain*, 2nd ed. Copyright © 1979. New York: Oxford University Press.

INDEX

absolute illumination, independence of, 218
absolute illumination level, 257
absolute value, 88
absolute value of complex number, 133
abstraction, 12, 81, 89, 151
acceptors, 33
acoustic cues, 210
acoustic event, 213
acoustic headshadow, 210, 215
action potential, 44, 50, 54, 111, 193, 259
active, 309
active devices, 20
active generation of sensory input, 127
active layer, 313
adaptation, 269, 300, 301
addition, 85, 87
addition of complex numbers, 132
aggregation of signals, 101, 257
all-or-nothing response, 45, 54, 195, 200
aluminum, 310
amacrine cells, 258
ambiguity, 231, 233, 237, 275
ampere, 15
amplifier, 195
amplitude-dependent bandwidth, 160
analog, 354
analog computation, 59

analog factor, 353
analog switches, 266
anatomy of retina, 258
AND gates, 353, 354
angstrom, 34, 147, 284, 333
antagonistic surround, 262
antimony, 309
aperture problem, 230, 232
apex, 281
apparent velocity, 210
approximation to derivative, 166, 167
arbitrary input waveform, 140
architecture, 356
arguments of function, 83
arsenic, 309
associative operation, 296
atomic number, 31
atoms, 31
attractor point, 249
auditory centers of brain, 279
auditory localization, 208
auditory nerve, 283, 299
auditory psychophysiology, 210
auditory system, 227
auditory-cue generator, 215
auditory-localization cues, 226
automatic gain control, 97, 128, 267, 284, 298, 300, 301

axial resistance, 155, 194, 201
axon, 44, 193, 259
axon hillock, 193, 194
axonal arborization, 194

back-gate effect, 326
background illumination, 260
bad data, 104, 106
balance of forces, 252
bandpass-filter, 281
bandwidth, 154, 158, 160, 275, 301
barber-pole illusion, 233
barrier, 34
barrier energy, 320
base, 260
basilar membrane, 280, 289
Bessel function, 350
best frequency, 289, 301
bias circuit, 262
bias circuit for resistive connection, 118
bias control, 264
bias current, 239, 273
bilayer, 45
binary signals, 354
binaural separation, 211
binaural time-disparity cue, 215
binaural-headshadow model, 215, 218,
        219, 221
bipolar cell, 258, 260, 262, 268
bipolar transistor, 219, 260
body effect, 325
body movements, 269
Boltzmann approximation, 330
Boltzmann distribution, 24, 57
bonding pads, 311
boundary condition, source, 329
boundary conditions, 322
Brownian motion, 20, 24
bubble on gate, 36
bulk effect, 326

capacitance, 16, 179, 201
capacitance, depletion-layer, 321
capacitance of nerve membrane, 147
capacitive voltage divider, 196, 200, 220
capacitor, 16, 151, 163, 175, 195, 291
cascade of second-order sections, 291
causality, 142
cell membrane, 45
center surround, 271, 272, 275
center-surround organization, 105
center-surround response, 262
channel, 33, 193, 322

channel capacitance, 328
channel current, 35, 327, 330, 334
channel length, minimum, 314
channel potential, 319
channels, 55, 197, 258
channels, ion specificity of, 57
characteristic distance, 287
characteristic length, 108, 121, 340
charge carriers, 33
charge in channel, 326
charge on capacitor, 16
charge on electron, 15. *See also* electrical
        charge.
chips, 311
cilia, 283, 285
circuit arrangements of synapses, 62
circuit complexity, 354
circular approximation, 113, 350
classical neuron doctrine, 44
clock rates, 265
closed state of channel, 57, 199
closed-form approximation, 350, 351
CMOS, 36
CMRR, 95
cochlea, 279, 289, 299
cochlear ducts, 281
cochlear partition, 280
cochlear place, 285
collective computation, 105, 237, 254,
        257, 302, 356
collector, 261
common mode, 241
common-mode rejection ratio, 95
complement of pattern, 310
complementary MOS, 36
complementary set–reset logic, 264
complex arguments, 131
complex conjugate, 133, 135, 181
complex conjugate roots, 145
complex exponential, 131, 132, 134, 138,
        285
complex number, 131, 152
complex plane, 131, 179
complex roots, 181
complex variable, 134
complex waveform, 135
complex wavenumber, 286, 291
complexity, 5
complexity in neural systems, 353
composite response curve, 297
composition, 151
composition of network segments, 346
composition of operators, 136

compressive nonlinearity, 97, 98, 300
computable approximation, 167
computation in nervous system, 58
concentration gradient, 48
conceptual framework, 12
conductance, 17, 67, 262, 272, 339, 349
cones, 261
confidence, 236
conformal map, 209
conformation change of channel, 56
connectivity, 5, 7, 116, 121
conservation of charge, 87, 196
conservation of energy, 286
constraint line, 230, 232, 234, 242, 247
constraint solver, 233, 237
constraints on system, 7, 276
contact, 314
contact mask, 310
context, 277
continuous intensity values, 232
continuous networks, 340
continuum approximation, 272
contrast ratio, 218, 236, 245, 260, 267
control quantity, 50
convergence, 102
convolution, 143
copies of signals, 84
copy of currents, 239
Cornsweet illusion, 275
correction force, 234, 242
correlation, 202
cortex, 277
cosine, 131, 133
coulomb, 15
coupled AGC system, 301
coupling between stages, 203
coupling capacitor, 220
covalent bonds, 32
cross-coupled inverters, 264
crystal, 32, 306
CSRL, 264
current, 35, 164
current density, 22
current flow, transistor, 322
current gain, 261
current mirror, 39, 69, 84, 88, 239
current source, 40, 241
current through capacitor, 163
current-sense amplifier, 266
current-type signals, 87
current–voltage characteristics of
    transistor, 37
cutoff frequency, 158, 281, 287, 288

cutoff place, 288

damped response, 283
damped sinusoid, 285
damped sinusoidal response, 135, 183
damping, 183, 184, 190
decay constant, 273, 274
decaying solutions, 191
decision, 101
defects, 311
delay, 154, 158, 193, 291
delay line, 150, 152, 201, 214, 216, 218,
    219, 221, 289, 294, 297
  follower–integrator, 152
  RC, 155
delay–add section, 216, 220
δ function, 166
dendrites, 43, 155, 259
dendritic tree, 111, 120, 193
denominator of transfer function, 145
density gradient, 22
depletion charge, 319
depletion layer, 320
  charge, 328
  width, 313, 322, 327
depolarization, 199
depolarize, 50, 53, 111
depolarized membrane, 197
depth, 128
depth information, 208, 209
derivative, 136
design rules, 312
develop resist, 308
diamond lattice, 32
dielectric constant, 13
diff1 circuit, 167, 270
diff2 circuit, 169
difference of Gaussians, 271
difference voltage, 67
differential amplifier, 67
differential equation, 340, 349
differential equation to algebraic
    equation, 135
differential input, 67
differential mode, 241
differential pair, 67, 90
differential signals, 86
differentiation, 127, 128, 163
differentiator, 238, 294
differentiator, realizable, 164
diffusion, 35, 49, 156, 331, 332
diffusion areas, 310
diffusion constant, 23, 156, 322

diffusion equation, 155
diffusion length, 108, 155, 340, 343
diffusion of carriers, 322
diffusion, of dopant, 309
diffusion of particles, 22
diffusion velocity, 22
dimensionless form of equations, 331
dimensions of representation, 103
diode-connected transistor, 39, 176, 219
direction of information flow, 60
discontinuity, 203, 271, 345
discrete decision, 356
discrete network, 340
discrete steps of conductance, 54
disorder, 353
dispersion relation, 285, 286
dispersive medium, 285
dissipative medium, 155
distinguishability, 357
distortion, 300
distortion of silicon wafer, 313
divergence, 102
donors, 32
dopamine, 272
dopant, 33, 309
doping, 32, 322
drain, 33, 177
drain conductance, 72, 75, 80, 314, 323, 336
drain drop, 336
drain voltage range, 39
drift, 49, 323, 331, 332
drift of particles, 21
drift velocity, 21, 330
drive, 130
driven solution, 137
driving function, 137
driving term, 130
ducts, 280
dynamic range, 97, 129, 268

ear canal, 216, 220
eardrum, 280
Early effect, 75, 323, 327, 336
Early voltage, 79
eclectronics, 11
edge, 230, 233, 247, 254
edge response, 270, 273
effective conductance, 340, 343, 344, 346
effective conductance of network, 109
effective resistance, 117, 118
effectiveness of gate at controlling the
        barrier energy, 38
efferent fibers, 283

eigenfunction, 134, 138
Einstein relation, 24
electric dipole, 47
electric field, 320, 321, 333
electric field, along channel, 323, 329, 330
electrical charges, 13
electrical current, 14, 15
electrical fluid, 14
electrical nodes, 17
electrical potential, 14
electrically compact, 111
electron volt, 15
electronic, 279
electronic cochlea, 279, 294
electrostatic energy, 47
electrostatics, 320, 328
electrotonic, 193
electrotonic spread, 108, 156, 262
element, 31
emergent property, 5
emitter, 260
encoding location of visual event, 213
encoding of data, 194
energy barrier, 12, 34, 48, 58, 260, 320,
        328
energy diagram, 320
energy landscape, 254
energy-supply limit, 300
engineer, 279
entropy, 353, 356
entropy factor, 353, 356
equilibrium, 252
equipotential regions, 17
equivalent circuit, 344, 345, 347
equivalent circuit of membrane, 49
error, 237, 251
error vector, 236
essential behavior, 12
essential dimensionality, 103
etch, 308
etchant, 308
events, 127, 194
evolution, 7, 208
exceptional event, 105
excitatory, 111
excitatory and inhibitory channels, 62
excitatory signal, 50
exponential, 97, 131
exponential atmosphere, 25, 27
exponential current–voltage relation, 58,
        272
exponential decay, 148, 157, 167, 262,
        272, 340, 350

exponential dependence of membrane conductance, 54
exponential function of voltage, 57
exponential gradient in velocity of propagation, 290
exponential growth, 184
exponential nonlinearity, 39
exponential response, 183
exponential slowing of wave, 287
extracellular fluid, 147

fabrication, 305
fan-in, 102
fan-out, 102
farad, 16
features, 103
feedback, 173, 179, 181, 182, 187, 189, 197, 237
Fermi distribution, 327, 329
Fermi level, 34, 329
Field, Lily, 28
finite impulse response, 143
finite pulse duration, 201
finite-difference equation, 341
first-order equation, 130
first-order sections, 152
floating sources, 86
fluid model, 14. *See also* hydraulic analogy.
follower, 84, 118, 147, 162, 169
follower-aggregation, 105, 121
follower–integrator, 147, 179, 180, 219, 269
force between electrical charges, 13
force toward local constraint, 233
formalism, 137
four-quadrant multiplier, 90
fractional power, 99
frequency, 152
frequency cutoff, 288
frequency of occurrence, 357
frequency response, 160, 165, 170, 184, 221, 295
full-wafer systems, 312
full-wave rectifier, 89
fuzzy data, 254

gain, 20, 269, 293
gain control, 275, 300
gain of delay line, 301
gap junctions, 107, 261
gate, 33, 177, 309
gate oxide, 309, 320

gate voltage sign convention, 36
gates, 101
gating charge, 57, 58
Gauss' law, 320
generic design rules, 316
geometric design rules, 312
Gilbert multiplier, 92
glass layer, 311
global average intensity, 270
global velocity, 233, 235, 237, 241
global wires, 253
global wiring, 267
golden ratio, 189
gradient descent, 251, 253
gradient in pinna–tragus delay, 220
graph, undirected, 357
gravitational force, 13
gravitational potential, 14
gray-scale image, 232
ground, 15
group velocity, 285, 292

hair cells, 50, 280, 283
half-wave rectifier, 89, 283
headshadow-model, 220
hearing, 279, 302
heat capacity, 156
Heaviside, Oliver, 136, 138
Heaviside operator calculus, 136
Hebbian learning, 354
Hermann–Hering illusion, 275
hexagonal array, 218, 262, 267
hexagonal network, 113, 350
higher-order differential equations, 135
high-pass filter, 163
Hodgkin and Huxley, 51, 54, 193
Hodgkin, Huxley, and Katz, 45
homogeneous, 130
homogeneous response, 145
homogeneous solution, 158
horizontal cells, 107, 258, 260, 261, 268
horizontal cues, 221
horizontal localization, 210, 226
horizontal resistor circuit, 116
horizontal resistor (HRes), 116
hydraulic analogy, 130
hydrocarbon chain, 46, 56
hydrodynamic analysis, 286
hydrodynamic wave, 281
hydrofluoric acid, 308
hydrophobic and hydrophilic forces, 47
hyperpolarize, 50, 111
hysteretic differentiator, 173, 219, 294

identity function, 83
image enhancement, 275
image gradient, 230
imaginary part, 131
impulse response, 138, 143, 144, 145, 183
inactivation, 199
incompressible fluid, 286
inert gases, 32
infinite network, 345
information generated by body
        movement, 219
inhibition, 192, 271
inhibitory, 111
inhibitory signal, 50
initial values, 145
initiation of action potential, 197
inner ear, 279
inner hair cells, 281, 283, 285, 289
inner-plexiform layer, 258
instability, 187
integer overflow, 161
integration, 127, 128, 136
intensity gradient, 209, 232, 236
intensity ramp, 275
interaural time disparities, 211, 220, 226
interconnection, 227
intrinsic semiconductor, 32
ion implantation, 309
ionic channels, 54
ionic radius, 47
ionized acceptor, 33
ionized donor, 33
ionizing radiation, 307
ion-specific conductance, 54
irrelevant information, 275
I_{sat}, 37
iso-output curves, 299, 301

joule, 15

κ, 319, 322, 323
Kirchhoff adder, 87
Kirchhoff's current law, 87
Kirchhoff's law, 218, 253, 347
kT/q, 36, 177
$kT/(q\kappa)$, 177, 186

ladder network, 108
Laplace transform, 136
Laplace transform of transfer function,
        144
Laplacian filter, 257, 271
large-signal behavior, 175, 186

large-signal instability, 295
large-signal response, 158, 172
lateral inhibition, 257, 269, 281
laws of physics, 4
layers, 306
layout, 151
learning, 354, 356, 357
least squares, 251
least-squares fit, 234
length of complex number, 133
length unit, 342
length-unit λ, 313
Lilienfeld, Julius Edgar, 33, 40
limitations of neural technology, 194
limit-cycle oscillation, 186, 191, 194
limited damage, 160
linear approximation, 18, 145
linear decay, 191
linear differential equation, 138
linear superposition, 19, 110, 142, 148,
        215, 218, 344
linear system, 128, 134, 159, 161
local average, 107, 269, 275
local derivatives, 232
local image information, 269
local learning rule, 356
location of sound, 210
log plot, 139
logarithm, 97, 351
logarithm of intensity, 209
logarithmic compression, 268
logarithmic dependence, 177
logarithmic photoreceptor, 219, 229
logarithmic response, 260
logic elements, 101
logic gates, 353
long-channel limit, 332
long-distance signal transmission, 194
loop gain, 197
loss mechanism, 285
low-pass filter, 281

Mach bands, 275
magnitude, 154, 157
magnitude of complex number, 132, 185
magnitude of transfer function, 139
map, 277
mapping, 208, 226
mask, 306
matched condition, 348
mathematical operations, 85
matrix notation, 251
maximum clock frequency, 265

maximum gain, 293
maximum rate, 159
mean, 107
mean free path of carrier, 331
mean free time, 21
mechanical oscillation, 283
median, 107
membrane, 147
membrane capacitance, 262
metabolic pumps, 15, 48
metal, 314
metal layer, 310
metal mask, 310
metal 2, 314
mho, 17
micron, 313
middle-ear ossicles, 280
misalignment between mask levels, 313
MKSA system of units, 15
mobile charge, 323, 326, 328, 333
mobility, 21
model, 18
model of the world, 208
modified Bessel function, 350
module, 151
modulus of complex number, 133
molecules, 32
monolayer, 47
MOS, 6
MOS transistor, 33
MOSIS, 313, 316
Mössbauer effect, 299
motion, 128, 229, 231
motion events, 258
motion information, 208
motion of observer, 213
motion parallax, 128, 209, 213
motion simulation, 242
moving light source, 226
moving objects, 229
moving-window average, 148, 167
multiplication of complex number, 132, 133, 153
multiplicative definition of motion, 247
multiplier, 90, 238
myelin, 45, 201

name convention, 17
natural mode, 145
natural response, 130, 170, 181
natural units, 331
natural voltage units, 161
n-channel, 36, 309

negative damping, 286, 299, 300, 301
negative feedback, 85, 169, 170, 241, 266
negative resist, 307
Nernst potential, 25
nerve channels, 193
nerve membrane, 45, 193
nerve pulse, 44, 111, 193, 300
neural network, 106
neural processes, 147
neural representations, 208
neuron, 43, 193
neurotransmitter, 61
nodes of Ranvier, 45, 194, 201
noise, 233
noise immunity, 177
nondispersive medium, 285
nonlinear, 123, 145, 173, 192, 300
nonlinear element, 174
nonlinearity, 18, 178, 189
nonoverlapping clocks, 265
normal equations, 252
normalization, 268, 339
normalized frequency, 184
$n+$ contacts, 309
n-type, 33
number of open channels, 57

offset voltage, 168, 170, 171, 173, 296
ohm, 16
ohmic nature of individual channel, 58
ohms per square, 349
one-dimensional model, 340
open state of channel, 57
open-circuit output, 75
operating point of system, 269
operator s, 136
optical illusions, 275
optical motion, 229
organ of Corti, 280
organizing principles, 5, 7
orthogonal constraints, 233
orthogonality, 234
oscillation, 172, 183, 186, 191, 239, 241, 283, 295, 300
oscillatory response, 173, 179
outer hair cells, 281, 283, 289
outer-plexiform layer, 257
output conductance, 73, 78
output-voltage limitation, 72
overconstrained problem, 234
overetching, 313
overflow, 173
oxidation, 306

oxide capacitance, 151, 321
oxide electric field, 328
oxide thickness, 34, 321, 333
oxygen, 309

package, 311
parallax, 209
parallel computation, 218
parameter change, 131
parasitic capacitance, 172, 262
pass transistors, 264
pattern, 308
pattern-independent nature of wafer
        fabrication, 312
patterning, 306
p-channel, 36, 309
peak frequency, 288
peak response, 295
peripheral vision, 128, 208
periphery, 128
permeability of nerve membranes, 55
permittivity, 13, 47
permittivity, silicon, 320
perpendicular force, 235
phase, 132, 139, 154
phase angle, 132
phase lag, 139, 291
phase velocity, 285
phosphorus, 309
photocurrent, 260, 261
photodetector, 260
photodetector gain, 219
photon, 261
photoreceptor, 50, 237, 257, 258, 260, 262
photoreceptor, logarithmic, 218
phototransistor, 219, 260
piecewise-linear analysis, 203
pinna, 210, 211, 218
pinna–tragus delay, 221, 226
pinna–tragus model, 216, 218, 220
pinna–tragus vertical cue, 216
pixel, 218, 267
polar form of complex number, 132, 153,
        181
polar head-groups, 46
polarizability, 47
polarization, 46
polarization, of neuron, 50
polarize, 46, 50
pole, 179, 244
poles of transfer function, 145
poly, 309
polysilicon, 33, 309, 313

polysilicon line, 220, 290. *See also* poly.
polysilicon, 33
population of channels, 58
positive damping, 301
positive feedback, 179, 184, 193, 197, 241,
        265, 283
positive real part, 145
positive resist, 307
potassium and sodium concentrations, 48
potassium current, 52
potential difference, 85
potential energy, 13
power dissipation, 39
power requirements, 208
power supply, 15, 48, 197
power-supply rails, 49
$p+$ contacts, 310
precision, 6
preprocessing, 275
pressure wave, 281, 286, 294
probability distribution, 357
process, 43, 258, 305
prolonged depolarization, 198
propagating wave, 281
propagation velocity, 281, 284
pseudoresonance, 293, 294
p-type, 33
pulse duration, 198, 200, 203
Pythagorean theorem, 185

Q, 183, 185, 186, 290, 292, 295, 296, 301
quadratic form, 342
quasi Fermi level, 335
quiescent value, 148

radial resistance, 349
rail, 168
random distribution of defects, 312
random sample patterns, 356
random variable, 357
random variation in current, 294
random walk, 20
randomness, 353
real part, 131, 135
real time, 269
receptive field, 209, 270, 272
recognition, 103
redundancy, 6
reference, 70, 86, 178, 269
reference level, 220
reference potential, 15
refractory period, 200
region of intersection, 234

region of smoothness, 105
removal of resist, 308
repeater, 194, 201
repolarization, 200
reported motion, 245, 247
reported velocity, 244
representation, 134, 135, 193
resetting neuron, 198
resist material, 306
resistance, 16, 272, 339, 349
resistant transformation, 107
resistive connection, 116, 261, 262
resistive network, 107, 162, 259, 261, 262,
    277, 301, 339
resistive sheet, 349
resistor, 16, 149, 164, 239
resistor bias circuit, 261
resonance, 186, 293
resonant overshoot, 297
resonant peak, 172
response amplitude, 274
response to arbitrary inputs, 140
resting potential, 50, 199
restoration of signal, 201
retina, 113, 127, 208, 209, 218, 219, 257
retinal ganglion cells, 209, 258
retinotopic array, 214
retinotopic map, 209, 213, 277
retinotopic projection, 207
reversal potential, 49, 197, 199
ringing in the ears, 283
rise time, 154, 158, 160
robustness, 6, 106
rolloff frequency, 244
roots, 157

s operator, 136
saturated velocity, 327, 330, 333
saturation, 324, 327
saturation current, 37, 334
scalae, 280
scale invariance, 287, 292, 297
scan register, 263
scanner, 263
schematic, 17
schematic symbols for transistors, 36
sea level, 15
second level metal, 311
second-order equations, 130
second-order section, 179, 289, 292
SeeHear, 207
segmentation, 122
select, 316

select mask, 309
self-adjusting circuits, 281
self-aligned transistors, 310
self-assembly, 47
self-compensation, 72
self-reinforcing reaction, 45, 51, 54
self-shunting of synapses, 348
semiconductors, 31
semi-infinite network, 339, 343
sensory input, 163
separation of variables, 156
serial access, 266
shared wire, 272, 277
sheet resistance, 349
shift register, 264
short channel length, 331
short-channel transistor, 333
short-wavelength limit, 288
shunting inhibition, 59, 62, 112, 347
siemens, 17
signal, 85, 134
signal types, 83
signal-to-noise ratio, 236
signed distance, 235
silicon axon, 203
silicon cochlea, 289
silicon dioxide, 306, 309
silicon retina, 257
simplicity of design, 218
simultaneous constraints, 233
sine, 131, 133
sine wave, 157, 163, 282, 295
sine-wave response, 138
sinusoidal signal, 152
sizing operations, 316
slew-rate limit, 160, 161, 172, 186, 187,
    191
small-signal approximation, 18
small-signal bandwidth, 161
small-signal behavior, 148
smooth function, fitting of, 105
smoothing, 106, 121
smoothing, temporal, 147
s-notation, 137, 180
sodium current, 52
soft decision, 356
sound analysis, 279
sound localization, 210
sound synthesis, 214
sound-pressure level, 299
source, 33, 177
source boundary condition, 329

space constant, 108, 121, 155, 157, 158, 262, 269, 272, 340
space domain, 162
space–time average, 268
spatial average, 268
spatial derivative, 209, 239, 271, 294
spatial frequency, 285
spatial intensity gradient, 242
spatial localization, 208
spatially weighted average, 262
spectral notch, 226
s-plane, 134
s-plane transfer function, 138
spontaneous acoustic emission, 284
square root, 98
squid axon, 45, 49
stability, 137, 145, 169, 180, 183, 184, 186, 191, 239, 241, 295, 300
stability limit, 187
static probe, 266
statistical computation, 104, 357
stereocilia, 283
stereopsis, 209
stiffness of cochlear partition, 287
submicron devices, 337
substrate, 309
substrate contact, 316
substrate potential, 319
subthreshold, 39, 208, 219, 239, 261, 290, 294, 319, 320, 323
subtraction, 85, 87
supercomputers, 4
surface potential, 320, 322, 332
survival, 128
sustained output, 270
symmetry, 113
symmetry of source and drain, 36
synapse, 43, 59, 103, 347, 354
synaptic outputs, 111
synthetic neuroscience, 8

tanh, 69, 107, 118, 119, 123, 159, 161, 170, 186, 268
tectorial membrane, 282
television display, 266
temperature, 23
temporal aliasing, 230
temporal changes, 163
temporal derivative, 207, 209, 218
temporal integration, 43
temporal patterns, 213
temporal response of retina, 269
termination, 344, 345

termination of nerve pulse, 198
test flash, 270
theorem, 357
thermal charge, 329
thermal motion, 20
thermal resistance, 156
thermal velocity, 23
thermal voltage, 36
threshold, 102, 195, 291, 327, 328
threshold function, 355
threshold, neuron, 44, 51, 354
threshold of hearing, 284
threshold voltage, 39, 332, 333
tile, 267
time coincidence of nerve pulses, 201
time constant, 130, 148, 156, 161, 167, 170, 180, 220, 269, 290, 293
time delay, 212
time derivative, 128, 209, 213, 214, 216, 239
time disparity, 226
time domain, 162, 301
time into the past, 142
time scale of events, 269
time-before-measurement, 142
time-dependent signals, 127
time-invariant linear system, 130, 203, 300
time-varying signal, 214
tinnitus, 283, 300
tragus, 210, 211
training, 356
transconductance, 60, 67, 169, 179, 181, 187, 291, 295
transconductance amplifier, 67, 147, 220, 238
transfer function, 85, 137, 138, 149, 170, 179, 287, 291, 300
transient, 203
transient inputs, response to, 136
transient response, 171, 183, 297
transistor mismatch, 71
transistor physics, 319
transistor variation, 294
transistors, 27
transition energy of channel, 57
transmission line, 289, 301
traveling wave, 158, 284, 301
traveling-wave structure, 281
tree of two-input gates, 353
tree of two-input neurons, 355
triad synapse, 258, 260, 262, 268
triads of molecules, 56

tuning curves, 300
two-dimensional network, 112, 349
two-rail signal, 264
two-state model, 57
tympanic membrane, 280

ultraviolet light, 306
undoped poly, 116
unidirectionality of transfer, 265
unit of voltage, 38
unity gain, 151
unity-gain follower, 84
unmyelinated processes, 262
unrealizable differentiator, 164

velocity, 158, 232
velocity ambiguity, 232
velocity of image, 229
velocity of propagation, 281, 289, 302
velocity of sound, 286
velocity plane, 230
velocity saturation, 319, 327, 330
velocity space, 230, 235, 239, 248
velocity, two-dimensional, 230
vertical cue, 226
vertical localization, 211
veto synapses, 112
via, 315
via mask, 311
viscosity of fluid, 283, 285
vision, 229
visual system, 227
VLSI, 6
V_{min} problem, 75, 79
voltage, 85, 164
voltage clamp, 52, 70
voltage controlled channels, 55
voltage difference, 220

voltage differences, 86
voltage drop, 18
voltage gain, 76, 81, 168, 171, 172, 175,
          195, 293, 295
voltage offset, 295
voltage source, 17, 262
voltage-dependent conductance, 53, 57
voltage-divider fraction, 196
voltage-type signals, 86

wafer, 306, 311
wafer fabrication, 305
wafer scale, 6, 312
waste of information, 356
water level, 15
wave propagation, 284
wave reflection, 292
waveform, 150, 187, 190
waveguide, 284
wavenumber, 285
waves in nonuniform media, 284
weight, 13, 167
weighted average, 106, 110, 148, 167, 262
weighting of inputs, 103
well, 309, 315
well contact, 316
wide-range amplifier, 79, 262
wide-range multiplier, 94, 241
windows, 280
wire, 7, 233, 276
wiring complexity, 116

X rays, 306
X-type ganglion cell, 271

yield statistics, 311

zero-contrast case, 247